5TH EDITION

HINOJOSA AND KRAMER'S

Evaluation
in Occupational Therapy

OBTAINING and INTERPRETING DATA

EDITED BY

Paula Kramer, PhD, OTR, FAOTA, and
Namrata Grampurohit, PhD, OTR/L

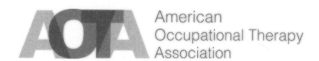

American
Occupational Therapy
Association

AOTA Vision 2025
Occupational therapy maximizes health, well-being, and quality of life for all people, populations, and communities through effective solutions that facilitate participation in everyday living.

Mission Statement
The American Occupational Therapy Association advances occupational therapy practice, education, and research through standard-setting and advocacy on behalf of its members, the profession, and the public.

AOTA Staff
Sherry Keramidas, *Executive Director*
Matthew Clark, *Chief Officer, Innovation & Engagement*

Elizabeth Dooley, *Vice President, Strategic Marketing & Communications*
Laura Collins, *Director of Communications*
Caroline Polk, *Digital Manager and AJOT Managing Editor*
Ashley Hofmann, *Development/Acquisitions Editor*
Barbara Dickson, *Production Editor*

Rebecca Rutberg, *Director, Marketing*
Amanda Goldman, *Marketing Manager*
Jennifer Folden, *Marketing Specialist*

American Occupational Therapy Association, Inc.
6116 Executive Boulevard, Suite 200
North Bethesda, MD 20852-4929
Phone: 301-652-AOTA (2682)
Fax: 301-652-7711
www.aota.org
To order: 1-877-404-AOTA or store.aota.org

Disclaimers
This publication is designed to provide accurate and authoritative information in regard to the subject matter covered. It is sold or distributed with the understanding that the publisher is not engaged in rendering legal, accounting, or other professional service. If legal advice or other expert assistance is required, the services of a competent professional person should be sought.
—*From the Declaration of Principles jointly adopted by the American Bar Association and a Committee of Publishers and Associations*

It is the objective of the American Occupational Therapy Association to be a forum for free expression and interchange of ideas. The opinions expressed by the contributors to this work are their own and not necessarily those of the American Occupational Therapy Association.

ISBN: 978-1-56900-595-8
Ebook ISBN: 978-1-56900-596-5
Library of Congress Control Number: 2020941649

Cover design by Debra Naylor, Naylor Design, Inc., Washington, DC
Composition by Manila Typesetting Company, Manila, Philippines
Printed by P.A. Hutchison, Mayfield, PA

Dedication

 This book is dedicated to Jim Hinojosa, PhD, OT, FAOTA. Jim was a dear friend, a fine therapist, an outstanding educator, a scholar, and a major contributor to the profession. He first identified the need for this book and worked diligently through the first four editions to make it a significant work. We hope that this fifth edition lives up to his standards.

Acknowledgments

It was difficult to begin this book as it was the first book I worked on without my dear friend, Dr. Jim Hinojosa. I was fortunate enough to have met a brilliant young woman, Dr. Namrata Grampurohit, while teaching at University of the Sciences. She used the fourth edition of this text in her class and shared with me a few ideas that might be added to an update in the next edition. Although I didn't know it at the time, she was clearly the right person to become a co-editor of this book. She has added substantially to the book. Namrata is so bright and creative and has brought new ideas to the project. I am grateful that I met her and for her wonderful collaboration on this edition.

Putting together a book is not an easy task and there are many people to thank for bringing this edition to fruition. Ashley Hofmann and her team at AOTA have been wonderful to work with and supportive throughout. As we faced the coronavirus pandemic amidst copyedits to the book, the AOTA team stood strong and continued to provide outstanding service to us and this book. Our contributing authors are the best and brightest, and have provided up-to-date information that will be useful to new and experienced practitioners alike. We are grateful to them for their time and effort and to their spouses, significant others, families, and friends who have supported them to furnish such fine work.

Finally, we are very thankful to our families, David and Andrew Hunt, and Kapil, Neil and Keya Chiravarambath. Without their encouragement and support, we would not have been able to undertake this project. Our professional colleagues have always given us encouragement, support, and thoughtful feedback, and we are forever grateful to them for enhancing our development.

Contents

List of Figures, Tables, Exhibits, Case Examples, and Appendixes

Case Examples

Appendixes

About the Editors

Paula Kramer, PhD, OTR, FAOTA, is a Professor Emerita of the University of the Sciences in Philadelphia. She has been an occupational therapist for 47 years, practicing predominantly in pediatrics, and has been an educator for almost 40 years. Dr. Kramer's primary areas of interest are in theory development and the importance of using theory in practice. She is a Fellow of the American Occupational Therapy Association (AOTA); a recipient of the A. Jean Ayres Award from the American Occupational Therapy Foundation; and received the AOTA Award of Merit, the highest award of the Association. She has co-authored more than 10 books and over 90 book chapters.

Namrata Grampurohit, PhD, OTR/L, teaches at Jefferson University (Thomas Jefferson University + Philadelphia University) in Philadelphia as an Assistant Professor in the Department of Occupational Therapy, Jefferson College of Rehabilitation Sciences. She completed her bachelor's and master's degrees in occupational therapy from the University of Mumbai, India, and her PhD in rehabilitation sciences from University of Washington. She has been an occupational practitioner for 20 years; her past clinical work involved practice in critical care, acute care, and inpatient rehabilitation at Evergreen Health in Washington.

Dr. Grampurohit's research is focused on measurement of function in individuals with neurological conditions, which is supported by her lab within the Center for Outcomes and Measurement. She is also interested in evidence-informed interventions that support clients and their families, which was highlighted in her 2020 Intervention Research Grant Award through the American Occupational Therapy Foundation. As a 2020 graduate of the AOTA Academic Leadership Institute, Dr. Grampurohit leads the field of measurement and outcomes in rehabilitation, and believes in bringing occupational therapy into the forefront of research and practice.

Contributors

Julie D. Bass, PhD, OTR/L, FAOTA
Professor, Department of Occupational Therapy
Henrietta Schmoll School of Health
St. Catherine University
St. Paul, MN

Yu-Lun Chen, MS, OT/L
Adjunct Faculty
Department of Occupational Therapy
Steinhardt School of Culture, Education, and Human
  Development
New York University
New York

Denise Chisholm, PhD, OTR/L, FAOTA
Professor and Vice Chair
Department of Occupational Therapy
School of Health and Rehabilitation Science
University of Pittsburgh
Pittsburgh, PA

Namrata Grampurohit, PhD, OTR/L
Assistant Professor
Department of Occupational Therapy
Jefferson College of Rehabilitation Sciences
Jefferson University
Philadelphia

Lou Ann Griswold, PhD, OTR/L, FAOTA
Associate Professor and Chair
Occupational Therapy Department
University of New Hampshire
Durham

Razan Hamed, PhD, OTR/L
Associate Professor, Programs in Occupational Therapy
Department of Rehabilitation and Regenerative Medicine
Vagelos College of Physicians and Surgeons
Columbia University
New York

Paula Kramer, PhD, OTR, FAOTA
Professor Emerita
Department of Occupational Therapy
Samson College of Health Sciences
University of the Sciences
Philadelphia

Lauren Little, PhD, OTR/L
Associate Professor, Occupational Therapy
Rush University
Chicago

Aimee J. Luebben, EdD, OTR, FAOTA
Professor Emerita
Department of Occupational Therapy
University of Southern Indiana
Evansville

Keli Mu, PhD, OTR
Associate Dean for International Relations
Chair and Professor of Occupational Therapy
School of Pharmacy and Health Professions
Creighton University
Omaha, NE

MJ Mulcahey, PhD, OTR/L, CLCP, FASIA
Professor, Occupational Therapy, Rehabilitation Medicine
Jefferson College of Rehabilitation Sciences
Sidney Kimmel Medical College
Thomas Jefferson University
Philadelphia

Laurette Olson, PhD, OTR/L, FAOTA
Professor and Program Director
Graduate Occupational Therapy Program
Iona College
School of Arts and Science
New Rochelle, NY

Cristina C. Parsons, MOT, OTR/L
PhD Student
Occupation and Rehabilitation Science Program
Colorado State University
Fort Collins

Kristie K. Patten, PhD, OTR/L, FAOTA
Associate Professor and Department Chair
NYU Steinhardt School of Culture, Education and Human
  Development
Department of Occupational Therapy
New York

Andrew C. Persch, PhD, OTR/L, BCP
Assistant Professor
Department of Occupational Therapy
Colorado State University
Fort Collins

Jennifer S. Pitonyak, PhD, OTR/L, SCFES
Associate Professor and Associate Director
School of Occupational Therapy
University of Puget Sound
Tacoma, WA

Charlotte Brasic Royeen, PhD, OTR, FAOTA, FASAHP, FNAP
A. Watson Armour III Presidential Professor
Dean, College of Health Sciences
Rush University Medical Center
Chicago

Lydia Royeen, PhD, OTR/L
Senior Occupational Therapist
Rush University Medical Center
Chicago

Rebecca L. Simon, EdD, OTR, FAOTA
Associate Professor and Academic Fieldwork Coordinator
Occupational Therapy Doctorate Program
Johnson & Wales University
Providence, RI

Wendy E. Walsh, PhD, OTR/L
Chair, Department of Occupational Therapy
Samson College of Health Sciences
University of the Sciences
Philadelphia

Rondalyn V. Whitney, PhD, OTR/L, FAOTA
Associate Professor
Division of Occupational Therapy
School of Medicine
West Virginia University
Morgantown

Wayne L. Winistorfer, MPA, OTR, FAOTA
Regional Director
Rehabilitation Services Ascension
NE Wisconsin
Adjunct Instructor
Occupational Therapy Assistant Program
Fox Valley Technical College
Appleton, WI

Foreword

It is a bittersweet honor to write the foreword to the fifth edition of *Evaluation in Occupational Therapy: Obtaining and Interpreting Data.* Now with updated the title *Hinojosa and Kramer's Evaluation in Occupational Therapy: Obtaining and Interpreting Data* in honor of the late Dr. Jim Hinojosa's memory and his outstanding contributions to this textbook. Beyond this classic textbook, Dr. Hinojosa is remembered as a scholar, scientist, researcher, master educator, and a true leader in the field of occupational therapy. He is missed, but his legacy will last forever.

The sweet part is that this textbook has influenced occupational therapy practitioners for years. Because of this textbook, we are better clinicians, educators, and researchers. It does not matter what practice area that we are involved in; this book will have a tremendous impact and shift our paradigms. Additionally, this is a text that can be used to start shaping the thinking of entry-level occupational therapy students as well as postprofessional students.

For this fifth edition Paula Kramer, PhD, OTR, FAOTA, is joined by Namrata Grampurohit, PhD, OTR/L, and they have assembled an author list that challenges the superlatives. The authors are composed of master educators and researchers. I invite you to sit back and enjoy this read, which will change the way you think!

—*Glen Gillen, EdD, OTR, FAOTA*

Preface

Paula Kramer, PhD, OTR, FAOTA, and Namrata Grampurohit, PhD, OTR/L

The focus of this book is on the evaluation and assessment of people seeking occupational therapy services. It is intended for students and all occupational therapists to help them gain a comprehensive understanding of the evaluation process. In some chapters, authors mention specific assessments and processes to illustrate concepts, but no chapter presents or reviews the use of specific assessments or evaluations within specific disability areas. Choosing appropriate assessments from all those available requires sound clinical judgment, which is an important professional responsibility.

As in the previous editions of this text, evaluation is described as a vehicle for determining the need for intervention and developing or changing intervention plans. The book also covers some new areas, such as outcomes assessment because this is a growing and important area in the occupational therapy profession. Also new to this edition is the discussion of evaluation in emerging areas of practice. Primary care, telehealth (which has become increasingly important during the COVID-19 pandemic), and the evaluation of groups and populations are used as examples of how evaluation may be different in emerging areas.

This book does not deal with the complex topic of the non-client–related evaluations in which occupational therapists engage, such as systems, facilities, or programmatic evaluations. These types of evaluations are critically important, and systematic, well-planned evaluation is essential for reviewing the goals of each occupational therapy program, whether clinical or educational.

A critical element of this book is its emphasis on the *process* of evaluation. Understanding the entire evaluation process helps occupational therapists determine the need for intervention, establish an appropriate treatment plan, and discern the outcomes of intervention. Moreover, the ongoing process of evaluation provides therapists with an understanding of when and how to modify the intervention plan by using clinical reasoning and monitoring of intervention effectiveness.

Collaboration with clients is essential to ensuring that the occupational therapy intervention has the desired effect of enabling them to engage in meaningful occupation. Once therapists thoroughly understand the various concepts foundational to evaluation, they are in a better position to choose the most appropriate assessments for the situation at hand. Chapter 1, "Evaluation: Where Do We Begin?" provides an overview of evaluation and serves as an introduction to this book.

Chapter 2, "Philosophical and Theoretical Influences on Evaluation," continues the discussion of the general theoretical issues in evaluation introduced in Chapter 1. It describes the philosophical basis of evaluation and its relationship to occupational therapy theory and, in particular, to frames of reference. It also provides an overview of the evaluation process from these perspectives.

Chapters 3–6 center on the use of assessments throughout the occupational therapy evaluation process. Chapter 3, "Assessment Identification and Selection," describes a process for identifying and selecting assessments to use in practice; Chapter 4, "Practical Aspects of the Evaluation Process," discusses evaluation issues in today's complex practice environments; and Chapter 5, "Evaluation in the Intervention Planning Process," discusses the critical importance of evaluation in the intervention planning process. Chapter 6, "Administration of Evaluation and Assessments," articulates the importance of understanding concepts related to administration in the process of evaluation. Chapter 7, "Contextual Evaluation to Support Participation," explores the influence of context on the client and the evaluation process and discusses its influence on participation in society.

Subsequent chapters discuss the use of nonstandardized assessments (Chapter 8, "Nonstandardized Assessments"), the psychometrics of standardized assessments, including reliability, validity, and responsiveness (Chapter 9, "Psychometric Properties Related to Standardized Assessments: Understanding the Evidence for Reliability, Validity, and Responsiveness"), and the scoring and interpretation of assessment results (Chapter 10, "Scoring and Interpreting Results").

Chapter 11, "Interpretation and Documentation of the Evaluation Process," discusses the critical aspect of documentation, which is necessary for all evaluation, including the more contemporary aspects of electronic documentation. Chapter 12, "Outcomes Assessment," is a new addition to this book. Outcomes assessment is an area that is growing in importance for occupational therapists to demonstrate the changes that have occurred through intervention, supporting the profession's unique value. The next chapter "Addressing Diversity in Occupational Therapy Assessment," Chapter 13, focuses on current issues that therapists need to be aware of as they evaluate diverse populations.

Chapter 14, "Evaluation in Emerging Practice Areas," is also a new addition to the book, scoping the issue of evaluation in emerging areas of practice. As occupational therapists move into new areas of practice, different issues are brought forth in the evaluation process. This chapter explores three different emerging practice areas as examples. It does not focus on specific assessments but rather on the role of therapists in evaluation within these emerging areas of practice.

Chapter 15, "Ethics of Evaluation," focuses on the ethical dilemmas that arise during the evaluation process. The final chapter of the book, Chapter 16, "Occupational Therapy Evaluation and Evidence-Based Practice," presents matters of evaluation as they relate to evidence-based practice, research, and program development.

Finally, this fifth edition has a revised title—*Hinojosa and Kramer's Evaluation in Occupational Therapy: Obtaining and Interpreting Data.* This is to honor Dr. Jim Hinojosa, who developed the original idea for this text, and to acknowledge its longevity as an important contribution to our understanding of evaluation in occupational therapy. We hope that this text continues to provide a clear and comprehensive overview of the evaluation process for new and seasoned occupational therapists in all areas of practice.

Evaluation: Where Do We Begin?

Paula Kramer, PhD, OTR, FAOTA, and Namrata Grampurohit, PhD, OTR/L

CHAPTER HIGHLIGHTS

- Importance of evaluation in occupational therapy
- Definition of terms used in this text
- Foundational documents in occupational therapy
- Effective evaluation and occupational therapist's responsibilities
- Influence of evaluation on intervention planning
- External influences on the evaluation process

KEY TERMS AND CONCEPTS

- Accountable evaluation
- Accreditation Council for Occupational Therapy Education® Standards
- Analysis of occupational performance
- Assessment
- Autonomy
- Beneficence
- Clinical reasoning
- Data-driven decision making
- Evaluation
- Evaluation report
- Evidence-based evaluation
- Fidelity
- Formative process
- *International Classification of Functioning, Disability and Health*
- Justice
- Nonmaleficence
- Occupational profile
- *Occupational Therapy Code of Ethics*
- *Occupational Therapy Practice Framework: Domain and Process*
- Outcome
- Outcome-focused evaluation
- Outcome measures
- Practice standards
- Reassessment
- Reevaluation
- *Scope of Practice*
- Screening
- *Standards of Practice for Occupational Therapy*
- Summative process
- Team approach
- Veracity

INTRODUCTION

Evaluation is a fundamental step in the occupational therapy process, and it is dynamic and iterative by design. ***Clinical reasoning*** is at the core of an evaluation and guides the decisions made by occupational therapists on the basis of the information collected (Cronin & Graebe, 2018). This information is gathered continuously from multiple sources that drive the formation of a data-driven intervention plan. Well-defined intervention plans can ultimately lead to beneficial client outcomes. Client outcomes across a setting or an intervention program can be aggregated to evaluate program-level outcomes.

In this chapter, we define the terms related to evaluation, explain evaluation in the context of practice-related guidelines and publications, and outline the responsibilities of occupational therapists and occupational therapy assistants in this process. We also discuss intervention planning with clinical reasoning that follows an evaluation, along with the external factors that must be considered in this process.

Finally, we describe important concepts in occupational therapy evaluation, such as accountable evaluation, evidence-based evaluation, and outcome-focused evaluation, that lead to data-driven decision making.

This book focuses primarily on occupational therapy evaluation of a person, and the evaluation of groups is discussed to a lesser degree. Program evaluation terminology and methods differ from traditional approaches to personal evaluation, and readers are referred to other excellent resources on program evaluation (Longest, 2014; Newcomer et al., 2015). The purpose of this chapter is to introduce the foundational content of the process of evaluating an individual, and the other chapters delve into details on the various components of an evaluation.

The core professional principles key to occupational therapy evaluation are presented with reference to published practice frameworks from the American Occupational Therapy Association (AOTA). Although these foundational evaluation concepts are similar across nations, readers outside of the United States are encouraged to seek similar guidance documents from their national professional association for a more relevant application—for example, the Australian *Occupational Therapy Scope of Practice Framework* (Occupational Therapy Australia, 2017), the *Canadian Practice Process Framework* (Townsend & Polatajko, 2007), and the United Kingdom's *Professional Standards for Occupational Therapy Practice* (College of Occupational Therapists, 2017). The basic evaluation knowledge presented in this chapter prepares occupational therapists for practice-based evaluation that can be extended to any setting.

IMPORTANCE OF EVALUATION IN OCCUPATIONAL THERAPY

Occupational therapists recognize the importance of a thorough evaluation to answer the following questions:

- What are the priorities for my client that occupational therapy can address?
- What information can I collect during a session to inform the next steps of intervention planning or discharge? How can I best justify this decision?
- What essential components of occupational performance can I assess to develop an effective intervention plan?
- How can I document, using appropriate terminology, the needs of the client, the justification for intervention, and the outcomes of intervention that are meaningful to the client?
- How can I best inform a client's intervention plan in new and emerging practice settings?

Current best practices in occupational therapy evaluation can equip therapists with efficient tools to answer each of these questions. Advances in practice guidelines, assessment tools, and technology can aid in identifying the optimal way to gather information for a meaningful and high-quality evaluation. Traditionally, the occupational therapy literature has placed greater emphasis on treatment strategies than on evaluation, and this emphasis has been reflected in the lack of confidence in planning and conducting an evaluation that is expressed by therapists in practice (Asaba et al., 2017; Clemson & Fitzgerald, 1998; Wales et al., 2012). The profession has in recent years realized the value of client-centered evaluation, as indicated by the Centers for Medicare and Medicaid Services' advocacy for the inclusion of the occupational profile as a mandatory part of occupational therapy evaluation for Medicare clients (AOTA, 2018).

An integral part of evidence-based practice is the use of robust measures with strong evidence of reliability and validity to support their use with clients. Measures such as the occupational profile provide consistent, descriptive, and client-centered data and are critical for a comprehensive evaluation, but they potentially lack the standardization needed to track outcomes. Reimbursement guidelines demand standardized assessment data, and occupational therapists must carefully select appropriate outcome measures that meet their needs.

One area commonly assessed by occupational therapists is occupational performance. Although this area is difficult to measure, great advances in occupational performance measurement across varied ages, diagnoses, and cultures should be noted, such as the development of the Assessment of Motor and Process Skills (Fisher & Bray Jones, 2014) and the School Assessment of Motor and Process Skills (Fisher et al., 2007).

Beyond occupational performance, many evaluation components are measurable and need to be incorporated in an evaluation to underscore the occupational therapy scope of practice and to optimally address client needs. For example, the School Function Assessment (Davies et al., 2004) for children and the Social Profile (Donohue, 2013) for children and adults address frequently targeted results in occupational therapy with readily available outcome measurement scales, but adoption of these outcome measures across practice settings has been minimal. Internal and external barriers to administering standardized assessments specific to occupational therapy are reported to be lack of consistent use; negative perceptions of colleagues; and a lack of time, space, and team communication (Asaba et al., 2017). Occupational therapists encounter numerous challenges in selection, purchase, administration, and implementation of outcome measures for comprehensive client evaluation.

Textbooks in occupational therapy provide detailed listings of assessment tools with overview, administration, and interpretation guidelines. However, they leave out important aspects of selection of measures, the meaning of their psychometric properties, and their appropriate use for a comprehensive evaluation. This book provides a holistic approach to evaluation, including frameworks, the evaluation process, and use of clinical reasoning to guide intervention planning. It also brings into the spotlight evaluation in emerging practice settings, computerized assessments, and rarely discussed but essential aspects of cultural diversity and ethics in evaluation.

DEFINING TERMS

Defining the terms related to evaluation is necessary to avoid confusion resulting from their interchangeable and variable use in practice and the literature. In this book, the terms *screening, evaluation, assessment, reassessment,* and *outcome* have distinct meanings based on their purpose, content, and timing and are discussed in detail in this section. They are also defined in Exhibit 1.1.

Screening

Screening refers to the process used with a potential client involving review of available data, observation of the client, administration of screening tools, or all of these, to identify the client's strengths and weaknesses and document the need for a formal evaluation. The duration of screening is generally shorter than a full evaluation, and it should never replace a full evaluation. Screening does not include identifying specific occupational performance deficits or intervention planning. In AOTA's (2015b) *Standards of Practice for Occupational Therapy,* screening is defined as "obtaining and reviewing data relevant to a potential client to determine the need for further evaluation and intervention" (p. 2).

Evaluation

Evaluation refers to the comprehensive process that involves obtaining and interpreting the data needed to

EXHIBIT 1.1.	Key Terms Related to Evaluation

Screening: Reviewing available data, observing a potential client, or administering screening instruments to identify strengths and limitations and make a determination regarding a formal evaluation.

Evaluation: The overall process of obtaining and interpreting the data to understand the person, system, or situation for intervention planning, progress, or discharge.

Reevaluation: The comprehensive review of a client, system, or situation at some point after the initial evaluation; it involves interpreting the data to inform intervention planning, progress, or discharge.

Assessment: Tool, instrument, or systematic interaction to measure or determine a client's occupational profile, occupational performance, or deficits in function.

Reassessment: Reviewing client performance at any time other than at initial evaluation; it involves the use of observations, an assessment tool or instrument, or systematic interaction. Reassessment usually occurs continuously throughout the intervention process.

Outcome: Final result of occupational therapy evaluation and intervention.

understand the person, system, or situation. As defined in the *Standards of Practice for Occupational Therapy*, evaluation is "the process of obtaining and interpreting data necessary for intervention. This includes planning for and documenting the evaluation process and results" (AOTA, 2015b, p. 2).

An essential element of evaluation is the occupational therapist's clinical reasoning; therapists draw on their judgment to determine the potential value of a planned outcome on the basis of the data from multiple assessments. Evaluation requires the synthesis of collected data, both standardized and nonstandardized; analysis and interpretation of the data; reflective reasoning; and consideration of client factors, performance skills, performance patterns, context, environment, and activity demands (AOTA, 2015b). An *evaluation report* includes the process and tools used to collect data and synthesize the findings, and it states the results and makes data-driven recommendations for occupational therapy intervention. If the need for intervention is not established during the evaluation process, the report includes a summary of the client's current function and recommendations for other possible types of intervention.

Reevaluation

Reevaluation refers to the comprehensive process that involves review of the client, system, or situation at some point after the initial evaluation. According to the *Standards of Practice for Occupational Therapy*, *reevaluation* is "the process of critical analysis of client response to intervention. This analysis enables the therapist to make necessary changes to the intervention plan" (AOTA, 2015b, p. 2). A reevaluation involves collecting data and interpreting the findings to modify the intervention plan, make a discharge recommendation, or both. Changes to an intervention plan also need to be data driven; however, the data

may be observable because standardized assessments may or may not be administered depending on the reason for reevaluation and potential reimbursement issues. Clinical reasoning should always be supported by evidence to guide the appropriate professional decisions.

Assessment

Assessment refers to a specific tool, instrument, or systematic protocol used as part of an evaluation to gather data and describe a client's occupational profile, client factors, performance skills, performance patterns, environment, or activity demands. Assessments are component parts of an evaluation or reevaluation process used to obtain data. An assessment construct, also known as a trait, is the central concept that is the focus of an assessment tool. Assessment tools allow measurement of a specific trait, and clinicians at times use tools for purposes different than those intended by the developers. Unintended consequences of improper use of assessments can invalidate the results obtained by clinicians. Clinicians should closely follow recommendations for the administration, use, and interpretation of assessments.

Reassessment

Reassessment refers to the review of client performance at any time other than the initial evaluation. Reassessment is an ongoing process of appraisal of client performance to more easily inform immediate intervention changes or establish the need for a reevaluation. In this regard, reassessment is an ongoing process of reviewing, assessing, and reassessing to determine progress during the intervention period. Reassessment can be done by using nonstandardized or standardized assessments used in previous sessions or by introducing new, more appropriate assessments on the basis of client need.

Outcome

The *outcome* is the final consequence of occupational therapy evaluation and treatment. The *Standards of Practice* define *outcome* as the "end result of the occupational therapy process; what clients can achieve through occupational therapy intervention" (AOTA, 2015b, p. 2). The choice of assessment tools to assist with the development of measurable goals can help in defining successful outcomes.

The measures used for the purpose of defining outcomes are commonly referred to as *outcome measures*. Outcome measures are standardized or nonstandardized assessments that provide specific data. Some assessments can be repeated to determine outcomes, whereas the reliability and validity of others are negatively affected by repetition.

Formative, Evaluative, and Summative Processes

Formative and *summative processes* are other terms related to evaluation that have emerged in the field of education (Swearingen, 2002; Figure 1.1). **Formative process** refers to the gathering of data for monitoring; it is used by therapists when they are beginning to form ideas about aspects

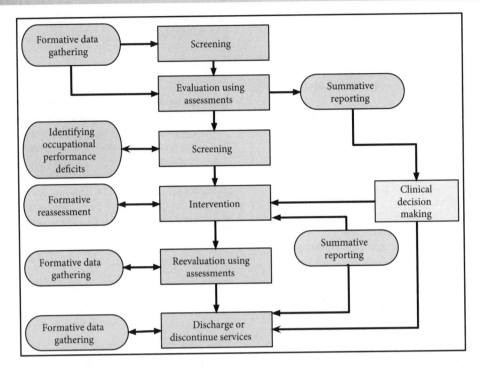

Source. N. Grampurohit. Used with permission.

of the client's performance that need attention or for ongoing monitoring of performance. An *evaluative process,* for identifying problems in occupational performance deficits, seeks to ascertain the ideas developed during the formative process and establish the strengths and weaknesses observed in the client's performance. A *summative process,* however, refers to the data-driven decisions that therapists make to map out the client's next steps; in this process, therapists summarize or synthesize the information to inform intervention planning or discharge.

Although the educational literature may refer to these three processes as different types of assessment with distinct testing tools, for the purpose of this book we refer to them as processes that a therapist uses during evaluation. The three processes appear linear, with sequential formative–evaluative–summative components, but in reality they are iterative and can inform clinical decisions during evaluation and reevaluation.

FOUNDATIONAL DOCUMENTS FOR EVALUATION IN OCCUPATIONAL THERAPY

Occupation-centered and client-focused practices have enhanced occupational therapy evaluation in recent years, and the profession embraces several principles inherent to the science of occupational therapy. Key professional documents published and updated periodically provide guidance for practice and highlight the importance of an occupation-centered approach to identifying clients' abilities, limitations, and participation restrictions. These documents can directly inform therapists' scope of practice, reimbursement, ethical practices, uniform terminology, and supervision requirements.

Occupational Therapy Practice Framework: Domain and Process

The occupational therapy process is described in detail in the *Occupational Therapy Practice Framework: Domain and Process* (*OTPF;* AOTA, 2014a) as consisting of evaluation and intervention to achieve targeted outcomes. According to the *OTPF,* evaluation is composed of two important elements: (1) the occupational profile and (2) analysis of occupational performance. The description of evaluation in the *OTPF* is geared toward assessing people and their caregiver, family member, significant other, or teacher. Use of the *OTPF* in group-, system-, and program-level evaluations is currently limited.

Occupational profile

The *occupational profile* is a formative, nonstandardized assessment that includes a client's occupational history and experiences, patterns of ADLs, interests, values, and needs (AOTA, 2014b, 2017a; see Appendix A, "AOTA Occupational Profile Template"). The occupational profile is a core component of any occupational therapy evaluation and underscores the collaboration between the client and the practitioner with a strong emphasis on human occupation. The occupational profile's goal is to identify areas of potential occupational disruption, reason for seeking services, strengths, supports, barriers, and priorities.

Administering the entire occupational profile may be unrealistic during an evaluation session (e.g., in the intensive care unit, in which the critical nature of the client's illness may limit participation of both the client and the caregivers). However, it is critical for therapists to gain insight into the client as a person and to understand what is and is not important to him or her. Therefore, administration of the occupational profile may need to be done over time or with input from others, when allowable. The *OTPF*, although effective for most settings, presents minimal guidance for circumstances in which exceptions need to be made during administration of the occupational profile, such as a client who is not able to respond because of condition, illness, or age.

Analysis of occupational performance

The *OTPF* describes the **analysis of occupational performance** as the step in the evaluation process in which the strengths and limitations of the client's performance skills, patterns, context, or environments are assessed using nonstandardized and standardized assessments. In this step, targeted outcomes are identified and, using clinical reasoning, an intervention plan is developed to confirm the planned outcomes. Although *OTPF* describes the intervention plan in a separate intervention phase, in most settings it is an integral part of the evaluation. The intervention plan must be based on data from the evaluation. Moreover, its development must be done in collaboration with the client, and the evaluation should document adequate detail to justify treatment and support implementation.

Scope of Practice

AOTA's scope-of-practice documents are based on the *OTPF* and the *Philosophical Base of Occupational Therapy* (AOTA, 2017), which states that "the use of occupation to promote individual, community, and population health is the core of occupational therapy practice, education, research, and advocacy" (p. S65). AOTA recommends using scope-of-practice documents along with the AOTA Model Practice Act (AOTA, 2007) in developing state-level documents.

AOTA's (2014b) *Scope of Practice* defines *occupational therapy* and provides detailed descriptions of specific client factors, performance skills and patterns, occupations, and environments that occupational therapists can assess across a client's lifespan (Exhibit 1.2). The parameters for decision making are outlined to set commonly accepted limits on practice. The *Scope of Practice* also outlines settings for the practice of occupational therapy and the education and certification requirements for occupational therapists. The *Scope of Practice* does not, however, elaborate on the process of evaluation or provide guidance on the selection of assessments, both areas in which therapists are likely to struggle in a practice setting.

Standards of Practice for Occupational Therapy

Practice standards are the most important responsibilities of a professional organization to its members, the profession, and society (AOTA, 2015b). The minimum requirements for performance of all aspects of the occupational therapy process are outlined in the **Standards of Practice for Occupational Therapy** (AOTA, 2015b). Clients, employers, researchers, peers, and payers use these standards to ascertain the quality of care. Any occupational therapy process that does not adhere to these standards is incompetent practice. The standards also provide a role-based delineation of the duties of occupational therapists and occupational therapy assistants, as shown in Exhibit 1.3. Both occupational therapists and occupational therapy assistants are equally responsible for ensuring that standards are followed, adequate oversight exists for appropriate administration of assessments, and accurate documentation is completed (Arthur & Trotman, 2020; Thomas, 2019).

Although the process is collaborative, supervising occupational therapists are ultimately responsible for selecting

---

EXHIBIT 1.2. Areas Evaluated Across the Lifespan in Occupational Therapy

- ADLs
- IALDs
- Occupations, including education, work, play, leisure, social participation, rest, and sleep
- Client factors and body functions
- Habits, routines, roles, and behavior patterns
- Cultural, physical, environmental, social, and spiritual contexts
- Performance skills

Source. American Occupational Therapy Association (2014b).
Note. ADLs = activities of daily living; IADLs = instrumental activities of daily living.

EXHIBIT 1.3. Evaluation Standards for Occupational Therapy Assistants and Occupational Therapists

The occupational therapy assistant
- Participates in the evaluation and reevaluation process under the direction of the occupational therapist;
- Contributes to the screening, evaluation, and reevaluation process by implementing delegated assessments; and
- Provides verbal and written reports of observations and client capacities to the occupational therapist.

The occupational therapist
- Supervises and may delegate aspects of specific assessments to be administered by the occupational therapy assistant and
- Is responsible for
  - Selecting specific assessments,
  - Initiating and completing the evaluation,
  - Interpreting the data, and
  - Developing the intervention plan.

The occupational therapist and occupational therapy assistant
- Work collaboratively during evaluation;
- Share responsibility for ensuring that the occupational therapy assistant is competent to administer the specific assessment assigned;
- Comply with practice and competency standards;
- Use current assessments and assessment procedures; and
- Comply with federal and state laws, other regulatory and payer requirements, and AOTA documents.

Source. American Occupational Therapy Association (2015a).
Note. AOTA = American Occupational Therapy Association.

EXHIBIT 1.4.	AOTA Standards of Practice for Occupational Therapy: Standard II—Screening, Evaluation, and Reevaluation

1. An occupational therapist is responsible for all aspects of the screening, evaluation, and reevaluation process.
2. An occupational therapist accepts and responds to referrals in compliance with state or federal laws, other regulatory and payer requirements, and AOTA documents.
3. An occupational therapist, in collaboration with the client, evaluates the client's ability to participate in daily life tasks, roles, and responsibilities by considering the client's history, goals, capacities, and needs; the activities and occupations the client wants and needs to perform; and the environments and context in which these activities and occupations occur.
4. An occupational therapist initiates and directs the screening, evaluation, and reevaluation process and analyzes and interprets the data in accordance with federal and state law, other regulatory and payer requirements, and AOTA documents.
5. An occupational therapy assistant contributes to the screening, evaluation, and reevaluation process by administering delegated assessments and by providing verbal and written reports of observations and client capacities to the occupational therapist in accordance with federal and state laws, other regulatory and payer requirements, and AOTA documents.
6. An occupational therapy practitioner uses current assessments and assessment procedures and follows defined protocols of standardized assessments and needs assessment methods during the screening, evaluation, and reevaluation process.
7. An occupational therapist completes and documents the results of the occupational therapy evaluation. An occupational therapy assistant may contribute to the documentation of evaluation results. An occupational therapy practitioner abides by the time frames, formats, and standards established by practice settings, federal and state law, other regulatory and payer requirements, external accreditation programs, and AOTA documents.
8. An occupational therapy practitioner communicates screening, evaluation, and reevaluation results within the boundaries of client confidentiality and privacy regulations to the appropriate person, group, organization, or population.
9. An occupational therapist recommends additional consultations or refers clients to appropriate resources when the needs of the client can best be served by the expertise of other professionals or services.
10. An occupational therapy practitioner educates current and potential referral sources about the scope of occupational therapy services and the process of initiating occupational therapy services.

Source. From "Standards of Practice for Occupational Therapy," by the American Occupational Therapy Association, 2015a, *American Journal of Occupational Therapy, 69*(Suppl 3), pp. 3–4. Copyright © 2015 by the American Occupational Therapy Association. Used with permission.
Note. AOTA = American Occupational Therapy Association.

assessments, initiating and completing the evaluation, interpreting the data, and developing an intervention plan. Occupational therapy assistants can contribute to screening, sections of the evaluation, and the reevaluation process in accordance with federal and state laws, other payer requirements, and other regulatory documents.

Although the *OTPF* does not recognize screening as an occupational therapy process, the standards clearly describe screening as a legitimate aspect of practice. Standard II is dedicated to screening, evaluation, and reevaluation (AOTA, 2015b, pp. 3–4; Exhibit 1.4). Along with the responsibilities of each type of occupational therapy practitioner, this standard further explains that therapists need to follow the protocols of standardized assessments and should communicate the results of the evaluation process or recommended referrals in accordance with confidentiality and privacy regulations to the client and appropriate designated persons or organizations.

Standard IV relates to transition, discharge, and outcome measurement. Occupational therapists are responsible for outcome measurement, which includes selecting, measuring, documenting, and interpreting expected and achieved outcomes. Occupational therapy assistants collaborate in identifying the information necessary for supervising therapists to make an appropriate decision.

Accredited Education Programs

Entry-level occupational therapy students at both the doctoral and the master's levels are required to learn to select, administer, and interpret standardized and nonstandardized assessments according to the 2018 *Accreditation Council for Occupational Therapy Education (ACOTE®) Standards* for educational programs (ACOTE, 2018). Occupational therapy assistant students at both the associate and the baccalaureate level are required to be able to collect assessment data and collaborate with occupational therapists in screening, evaluation, and reevaluation (ACOTE, 2018). The standards emphasize culturally relevant evaluation based on theory and available evidence. The new standards adopted by ACOTE in 2018 went into effect in July 2020 and include several changes that emphasize clinical reasoning and a client-centered approach in all aspects of the evaluation process. The ACOTE standards related to screening, evaluation, and referral are provided in Exhibit 1.5. All occupational therapy practitioners are expected to keep up to date and follow the most current expectations of practice.

Occupational Therapy Code of Ethics

Ethical standards and ground rules for ethical conduct are established during an evaluation, typically a first encounter with a client. Occupational therapy students, occupational therapists, and occupational therapy assistants must all abide by the *Occupational Therapy Code of Ethics* and can be held accountable for their actions as members of AOTA (AOTA, 2015a). The main purpose of the ethical standards is to provide guidance on ethical conduct to AOTA members in their work in paid or volunteer roles. The Code of

EXHIBIT 1.5.   ACOTE Standards Related to Screening, Evaluation, and Referral

OCCUPATIONAL THERAPY ASSISTANT (ASSOCIATE AND BACCALAUREATE LEVEL)

B.4.4. Standardized and Nonstandardized Screening and Assessment Tools
- Contribute to the evaluation process of client(s)' occupational performance, including an occupational profile, by administering standardized and nonstandardized screenings and assessment tools and collaborating in the development of occupation-based intervention plans and strategies.
- Explain the importance of using psychometrically sound assessment tools when considering client needs, and cultural and contextual factors to deliver evidence-based intervention plans and strategies.
- Intervention plans and strategies must be client centered, culturally relevant, reflective of current occupational therapy practice, and based on available evidence

B.4.6. Reporting Data
- Under the direction of an occupational therapist, collect, organize, and report on data for evaluation of client outcomes.

OCCUPATIONAL THERAPIST (MASTER'S AND DOCTORAL LEVELS)

B.4.4. Standardized and Nonstandardized Screening and Assessment Tools
- Evaluate client(s)' occupational performance, including occupational profile, by analyzing and selecting standardized and nonstandardized screenings and assessment tools to determine the need for occupational therapy intervention(s). Assessment methods must take into consideration cultural and contextual factors of the client.
- Interpret evaluation findings of occupational performance and participation deficits to develop occupation-based intervention plans and strategies.
- Intervention plans and strategies must be client centered, culturally relevant, reflective of current occupational therapy practice, and based on available evidence.

B.4.5. Application of Assessment Tools and Interpretation of Results
- Select and apply assessment tools, considering client needs, and cultural and contextual factors.
- Administer selected standardized and nonstandardized assessments using appropriate procedures and protocols.
- Interpret the results based on psychometric properties of tests considering factors that might bias assessment results (e.g., culture and disability status related to the person and context).

B.4.6. Reporting Data
- Collect, analyze, and report data in a systematic manner for evaluation of client and practice outcomes. Report evaluation results and modify practice as needed.

B.4.7. Interpret Standardized Test Scores
- Interpret criterion-referenced and norm-referenced standardized test scores on the basis of an understanding of sampling, normative data, standard and criterion scores, reliability, and validity.

B.4.8. Interpret Evaluation Data
- Interpret the evaluation data in relation to accepted terminology of the profession and explain the findings to the interprofessional team.

B.4.9–B.4.28
- Description of content in these standards: Evaluation specific to certain situations, for example, consultation, orthoses, mobility, and dysphagia. The standards also include referral, discharge plan, and documentation.

Source. From "Accreditation Council for Occupational Therapy Education (ACOTE®) Standards" by Accreditation Council for Occupational Therapy Education, 2018, *American Journal of Occupational Therapy, 72*(Suppl. 2), pp. 44–46. Copyright © 2018 by the American Occupational Therapy Association. Used with permission.

Ethics can be used along with state laws and board regulations. AOTA (2015a) describes six principles and related standards of conduct: beneficence, nonmaleficence, autonomy, justice, veracity, and fidelity (Table 1.1). Evaluation of a client needs to adhere to all six principles.

Beneficence includes appropriate evaluation practices that are intended for the well-being and safety of clients, such as client-centered and evidence-based practices. *Nonmaleficence* prohibits harm to clients and others from internal and external factors that may influence evaluation, such as financial incentives. *Autonomy* dictates respect for the clients' rights by seeking consent before evaluation, collaborating on an intervention plan, and maintaining privacy and confidentiality of the findings. *Justice* promotes fairness to clients with nondiscriminatory behavior and timely response to referrals. *Veracity* seeks truthfulness when representing occupational therapy during evaluation and throughout the occupational therapy process. *Fidelity* includes a commitment to respect for and fairness toward clients and others when conducting an evaluation.

International Classification of Functioning, Disability and Health

Common terminology across different disciplines was facilitated by the *International Classification of Functioning, Disability and Health (ICF)* framework developed by the World Health Organization (WHO) and adopted by several countries as an international standard for measuring health (WHO, 2002). The *ICF* is based on the social model of disability, which broadens the scope of rehabilitation beyond medicine (Hinojosa et al., 2017). Functioning and disability related to health are two parameters described in the *ICF*. The *ICF* parameter of functioning includes body structure and function, activities, and participation, and the corresponding areas of disability are impairments, limitations, and restrictions, respectively. The *ICF* recognizes functioning and

TABLE 1.1.   Ethical Principles and Standards of Conduct as Applied to Occupational Therapy Evaluation

ETHICAL PRINCIPLE	RELATED STANDARD OF CONDUCT	RELEVANCE TO EVALUATION
Beneficence	All forms of action intended for the well-being and safety of clients	Provide appropriate evaluation, intervention plan, reassessment, and reevaluation in a client-centered and evidence-based manner within the scope of occupational therapy practice.
Nonmaleficence	Abstain from causing harm to others	Avoid undue internal and external influences on evaluation that may compromise the occupational therapy process.
Autonomy	Respect clients' right to self-determination, privacy, confidentiality, and consent	Always seek consent before evaluation and maintain privacy and confidentiality of the reports and results.
Justice	Promote fairness and objectivity	Respond to referral in a timely manner as determined by law, regulation, or policy and nondiscriminatory behavior.
Veracity	Be truthful when representing occupational therapy	Refrain from making false claims based on the evaluation.
Fidelity	Commit to treating clients and others with respect, fairness, discretion, and integrity	Treat clients and others with respect, and establish collaborative communication.

disability in the person's own context that includes social, environmental, and spiritual contextual factors.

The *ICF* was later used as the basis for an assessment instrument for individuals and populations, the WHO Disability Assessment Schedule 2.0 (WHODAS 2.0), which has 36-, 24-, and 12-item versions (Üstün et al., 2010). The WHODAS 2.0 covers six domains: cognition (understanding and communicating), mobility (moving and getting around), self-care (hygiene, dressing, eating, staying alone), getting along (interacting with others), life activities (domestic, leisure, work, school), and participation (community activities).

EFFECTIVE EVALUATION AND OCCUPATIONAL THERAPISTS' RESPONSIBILITIES

Simply stated, evaluation is based on what is known about the client and the client's occupations, activities, environment, and resources, combined with an honest, constructive reaction to the client's performance without judgment and based on data and professional knowledge. All occupational therapists should strive to be effective evaluators to provide better care for their clients. This book seeks to guide occupational therapists in this process by expanding on what effectiveness means and how to get there:

> Effective evaluators have a comprehensive knowledge of the domain of concern of the profession, human development and individual variation, statistics, tests and measurements, and the concepts of activities and occupation. (Hinojosa & Kramer, 2014, p. 12)

The responsibilities placed on the evaluator to demonstrate expertise and high competence go beyond the standards discussed in the preceding section; additional standards are proposed to incorporate best practices for effective evaluation. Additional standards align with the advances in standards of organizations such as the American Psychological Association (2017), the American Counseling Association

(2014), the Council for Exceptional Children (2015), and the *Standards for Educational and Psychological Testing* developed by the American Educational Research Association et al. (2014).

Effective occupational therapy evaluators need to closely follow three key domains of the occupational therapy profession: (1) client, (2) occupation, and (3) activities. Discussion during an evaluation should center on the client, and the client's needs and wants must be considered with respect. The occupation of interest and priority to the client should be the focus of the occupational profile and the intervention plan. Occupational therapy is distinctive in that evaluations and interventions are centered on who the client is on a personal level (i.e., being) and what the client wants to do in their life (i.e., doing; Hayward & Taylor, 2011). To that end, the evaluation needs to identify the types of activities that are of interest to the client and view the performance of these activities as objective goals.

Therapists are frequently faced with a dilemma in which the client and therapist see the same situation differently. For example, therapists may encounter situations in which a client wants to be independent in toileting but is content with receiving help with bathing. The therapist can certainly explain the ways in which an intervention plan that includes bathing could be beneficial for the client, but the client's choice and level of readiness to work on toileting needs to be considered and respected. If the therapist has evidence that the client does not have the capacity for decision making, the plan would still consider the client's choices and involve other appropriate members of the client's team to make an informed decision. Clients have the right to accept or refuse evaluation and intervention. They also have the right to know when the therapist is using standardized assessments, what the outcomes are, and how they are being interpreted.

Occupational therapists need to contextualize their overall interpretation of the findings within a client's personal life, developmental stage, roles, habits, interests, and environment. Therapists must review the results of their assessments and the full evaluation with clients and be prepared to present evidence for their decisions to the client and the care team. The evaluation documentation needs to reflect these professional domains of client, occupation, and activities for effective practice.

Skilled evaluators acknowledge and appropriately handle differences in beliefs, gender, socioeconomic status, culture, and language, and they inform their practice by means of professional documents such as position papers. For most skilled evaluators, nondiscrimination and inclusion are part of a deliberate process (AOTA, 2020), and the first step in this process is the acknowledgment of differences. Therapists' awareness of their own life story and that of the client can bring to light some of the similarities, differences, and potential biases that need to be acknowledged. Understanding a client's priorities and removing the bias that the evaluator may bring into the situation is the next step toward inclusion. Because of their client- and occupation-centered practice, occupational therapists are well suited to lead the way toward inclusion and advocate for best practices within a care team.

INFLUENCE OF EVALUATION ON INTERVENTION PLANNING

Once occupational therapists have completed a screening or a thorough review of the client's educational or health records, they decide how to proceed with evaluation. The assessments used in the evaluation process will affect the intervention process and approach. Sometimes therapists know what theory or frame of reference would be appropriate for a client just by reading the client's chart or interviewing the client. Other times, limited information is available to help determine which theoretical approach would be the best to follow. While proceeding with the evaluation, therapists should think about what the proper approach might be, even if it might change their original frame of reference.

During the process of evaluation, occupational therapists continually review the assessment data and make decisions and judgments based on the information. The process, referred to as **data-driven decision making,** is intensive and dynamic, and it requires reflective practice and constant thought and decision making as the client completes each assessment. As therapists review the data from each assessment, they decide how to proceed, and each decision leads to another set of choices regarding the next steps, rather like a decision tree. Experienced therapists' clinical decisions flow smoothly, reflecting that continuous thought process.

To become competent evaluators, entry-level occupational therapists need to become familiar with a wide variety of assessments and develop their skills in using them. Both experienced and entry-level therapists use reflective practice approaches to learn by critically analyzing responses to their interventions. This reflective practice allows them to continually deepen and improve their assessment skills.

Clinical constraints influence clinical decision making during evaluation. Practice settings typically allow little time for evaluation, and at times third-party payers, or certain settings such as educational institutions, prescribe the assessments to be used. In addition, an institution may have a set protocol for evaluation that is required for every client, regardless of the client's individual needs. In such situations, the occupational therapist's evaluation decisions are greatly influenced by outside factors. Despite this, it is imperative that therapists develop their skills and competence so they can adequately justify their actions and decisions in evaluations.

Evaluation Report

The purpose of the evaluation report is to communicate information to others. When constructing the report, occupational therapists need to focus on the target audience. The report may need to be written with an educational focus for a school setting, whereas a physician may need medical data presented in a succinct manner. A third-party payer may require that the report meet the requirement for reimbursement. This sometimes requires therapists to write more than one summary for the same client.

Because the evaluation report may be the first impression the therapist makes on the intended audience, it should be clearly written, professional, and meet the goals for which it was intended. Occupational therapists should proofread the report carefully to make sure that there are no errors and that it is accurately written and legally defensible. All evaluation reports should indicate which assessments were used, whether they are standardized or nonstandardized, and that they are reliable and valid for the specific client or population. In addition, if an assessment is generally used with another population, a clear rationale should be provided for its use in this situation, as well as its strengths or limitations for use with this client or population.

Accountable Evaluation

Accountable evaluation refers to evaluation that can be justified by the clinician. Accountable evaluation begins with an evaluation process based on the occupational profile, followed by the choice of specific assessments that are standardized, reliable, valid, and suitable for the specific client or client group. Moreover, the standardized assessments chosen should be acceptable to other professionals, consumers, and third-party payers. Accountability concerns are reflected through the form and content of the evaluation report and the degree to which the report is evidence based, outcome focused, or both. These assessments or processes are defensible in terms of professional standards and best practice, and they reflect the profession's domain of concern.

Because of the occupation-focused nature of occupational therapy, all evaluations should include an occupational profile that describes the client's meaningful occupations and contextual information and client-defined priorities. When clients are unable to express their ideas, the occupational profile may be generated with information from care providers, significant others, and other professionals. Full accountability requires that an evaluation provide an accurate assessment of the client's performance, skills, and deficits, combined with his or her personal needs and goals, in a manner that is generally acceptable in the context of that client's life.

Evidence-Based Evaluation

Evidence-based evaluation requires occupational therapists to have sufficient facts about the client, the assessments, and the evaluation process to support appropriate decision making. Therapists should use a reflective process to consider what the particular client needs as a starting point for exploring the literature for guidance about best practice. The literature can help therapists identify the most appropriate assessments to use in the relevant situation, as well as the value and rigor of those assessments, including their intended purposes, reliability, and validity.

As part of this process, occupational therapists are required to be personally reflective about their own clinical experiences and integrate them with information gleaned from the literature regarding the assessments, client characteristics, and context of the evaluation. During this reflective process, therapists consider those assessments in which they are knowledgeable and competent and that meet the client's age range and suspected strengths and deficits. This process should result in a well-thought-out plan for evaluation.

Outcome-Focused Evaluation

Outcome-focused evaluation is the process of evaluating a client on the basis of the client's desired outcomes. This process requires occupational therapists to use a client-centered perspective and to begin with the client's identified needs, desires, and limitations. Once the client has identified the preferred outcome of treatment (through an interview or an occupational profile), therapists need to determine what type of additional evaluation tools will measure the achievement of those desired outcomes. The client's desired outcomes guide the therapist's judgment during evaluation and throughout treatment.

Another type of outcome-focused evaluation can take place before discharge from occupational therapy services. The client's level of performance improvement can be determined by comparing the data from the initial evaluation with the discharge evaluation data, exploring changes relative to the stated expectations at the beginning of intervention. Occupational therapists should consider whether the desired outcome was reached and at the same time reflect on whether the initial goals were realistic and whether the process used was effective enough to achieve the desired results. At the end of this process, therapists may reflect that additional assessments should have been used during the initial evaluation or to determine outcome performance. The next client can benefit from this reflection, thus improving the process of outcome-focused evaluation for the clinician in the future.

Team Approach

Interventions are often planned and implemented using a *team approach*, which is the process of involving a team of diverse professionals who bring their own expertise and skills together for a client's common goal, such as rehabilitation, habilitation, discharge, or independence. The occupational therapy evaluation report then becomes part of a comprehensive team evaluation. Sharing hypotheses among the team generally provides an enhanced view of the client. Individual members of the team often contribute a different perspective on the client as a result of their own evaluation processes. This collaborative process often provides a more complete picture of the client's abilities and disabilities. Usually, the team discusses which assessment each member will use and the purpose of that assessment. This ensures that no duplication will occur and that all assessments will provide complementary information regarding the client's skills and abilities.

Generally, it is helpful for team members to keep their findings and interpretations confidential until all members have completed their evaluations. It is helpful for each professional to come to their own conclusions individually before the team meets collectively. Such a strategy can prevent one member from being swayed by the views of another, allowing a comprehensive view of the client to emerge and avoiding any inaccurate conclusions. By operating in this manner, the team can identify variations in the client's performance from one evaluation session to another.

EXTERNAL INFLUENCES ON THE EVALUATION PROCESS

At times, the type and focus of an evaluation are externally determined. The institution may require that an evaluation include one or more specific assessments; for example, a nursing facility may require that all clients on a unit be evaluated using the Section GG (Centers for Medicare and Medicaid Services, n.d.). Alternatively, a service delivery model may require that the evaluation have a specific focus; for example, a school system typically requires an evaluation with a focus on educational relevancy or a screening to provide early identification of students with potential learning difficulties. In other circumstances, a referral may suggest or require a specific type of evaluation, such as a referral for occupational therapy after joint replacement surgery.

In these examples, the evaluation focuses on a specific area rather than an overall perspective on the client's skills and abilities. Regardless of whether occupational therapists have a choice in the evaluation process or the assessments used, they have a professional responsibility to make certain that the overall evaluation meets the client's needs, reflects the domain of concern of occupational therapy, and is relevant to the programming and intervention services that will be offered.

When completing an occupational profile, knowledgeable clients often bring their own concerns, ideas, and expectations about what the evaluation process will include and what outcomes they expect. Occupational therapists may agree with a client's perspective or may have differing views about what the evaluation should entail. It is critical that therapists always consider the client's point of view. Open discussion about the evaluation process, the concerns of both parties, and how evaluation results will be used is critical to developing a rapport, which serves as the basis for a positive therapeutic relationship. Therapists should inform clients that the results of the evaluation will not be available immediately because it takes time to review all assessment results. Through a collaborative process, therapists and clients work toward a consensus on the evaluation process—what it will include and its focus. It is important for therapists and clients to be open and to consider each other's perspective to ensure that a trusting relationship can develop because this will be an important part of the foundation for future intervention.

SUMMARY

Evaluation is a major aspect of the occupational therapy process. It is complex, starting with screening and moving on to a more comprehensive assessment of aspects of the profession's domain of concern as it relates to the individual client. In occupational therapists' role as evaluators, they must comply with AOTA's current standards of practice and code of ethics and use sound professional judgment. Occupational therapy assistants participate in the evaluation process under the direction of occupational therapists.

The process of evaluation is complex and challenging, requiring both knowledge and skills on the part of therapists. Entry-level academic education provides a core understanding of evaluation in general, but clearly this is just the beginning. To gain proficiency in evaluation, occupational therapists must continually learn new assessments, develop mastery of a variety of assessments, reflect on the relevancy of generally used assessments, understand the various roles that the client plays in the evaluation process, and examine the literature regarding all aspects of evaluation. This text provides the foundational knowledge on evaluation to competently engage in test and measurement processes as an occupational therapist.

QUESTIONS

1. What is the difference between screening and evaluation? Will an occupational therapist always perform both with a client? Why or why not?
2. Define *formative* and *summative* as they relate to evaluation. What is the importance of each?
3. What is the relationship between *Standards of Practice for Occupational Therapy* and an occupational therapy evaluation?
4. What is the relationship between evaluation and the *Occupational Therapy Code of Ethics*?
5. Define the terms *accountable evaluation*, *evidence-based evaluation*, and *outcome-focused evaluation*. What is the importance of each?

REFERENCES

Accreditation Council for Occupational Therapy Education. (2018). Accreditation Council for Occupational Therapy Education (ACOTE®) standards. *American Journal of Occupational Therapy, 72*(Suppl. 2), 7212410005. https://doi.org/10.5014/ajot.2018.72S217

American Counseling Association. (2014). 2014 *ACA code of ethics*. Retrieved from https://www.counseling.org/Resources/aca-code-of-ethics.pdf#tizra-target%3A_blank

American Educational Research Association, American Psychological Association, & National Council on Measurement in Education. (2014). *Standards for educational and psychological testing*. Washington, DC: American Educational Research Association.

American Occupational Therapy Association. (2007). *Model Occupational Therapy Practice Act*. Retrieved from https://www.aota.org/~/media/Corporate/Files/Advocacy/State/Resources/PracticeAct/MODEL%20PRACTICE%20ACT%20FINAL%202007.pdf

American Occupational Therapy Association. (2014a). Occupational therapy practice framework: Domain and process (3rd ed.). *American Journal of Occupational Therapy, 68*(Suppl. 1), S1–S48. https://doi.org/10.5014/ajot.2014.682006

American Occupational Therapy Association. (2014b). Scope of practice. *American Journal of Occupational Therapy, 68*(Suppl. 3), S34–S40. https://doi.org/10.5014/ajot.2014.686S04

American Occupational Therapy Association. (2015a). Occupational therapy code of ethics (2015). *American Journal of Occupational Therapy, 69*(Suppl. 3), 6913410030. https://doi.org/10.5014/ajot.2015.696S03

American Occupational Therapy Association. (2015b). Standards of practice for occupational therapy. *American Journal of Occupational Therapy, 69*(Suppl. 3), 6913410057. https://doi.org/10.5014/ajot.2015.696S06

American Occupational Therapy Association. (2017a). AOTA occupational profile template. *American Journal of Occupational Therapy, 71*(Suppl. 2), 7112420030. https://doi.org/10.5014/ajot.2017.716S12

American Occupational Therapy Association. (2017b). The philosophical base of occupational therapy. *American Journal of Occupational Therapy, 71*(Suppl. 2), S65. 7112410045. https://doi.org/10.5014/ajot.2017.716S06

American Occupational Therapy Association. (2018). Guidelines for documentation of occupational therapy. *American Journal of Occupational Therapy, 72*(Suppl. 2), 7212410010. https://doi.org/10.5014/ajot.2018.72S203

American Occupational Therapy Association. (2020). Occupational therapy's commitment to diversity, equity, and inclusion. *American Journal of Occupational Therapy, 74*(Suppl. 3), 7413410030. https://doi.org/10.5014/ajot.2020.74S3002

American Psychological Association. (2017). *Ethical principles of psychologists and code of conduct with the 2010 and 2016 amendments*. Retrieved from https://www.apa.org/ethics/code/index#tizra-target%3A_blank

Arthur, P., & Trotman, T. (2020). The occupational therapy assistant. In K. M. Matuska (Ed.), *Ways of living: Intervention strategies to enable participation* (5th ed., pp. 25–33). Bethesda, MD: AOTA Press.

Asaba, E., Nakamura, M., Asaba, A., & Kottorp, A. (2017). Integrating occupational therapy specific assessments in practice: Exploring practitioner experiences. *Occupational Therapy*

International, 2017, 7602805. https://doi.org/10.1155/2017/7602805

Centers for Medicare and Medicaid Services. (n.d.). *Coding Section GG self-care and mobility activities included on the post-acute care item sets: Key questions to consider when coding.* Retrieved from https://www.cms.gov/Medicare/Quality-Initiatives-Patient-Assessment-Instruments/IRF-Quality-Reporting/Downloads/GG-Self-Care-and-Mobility-Activities-Decision-Tree.pdf

Clemson, L., & Fitzgerald, M. H. (1998). Understanding assessment concepts within the occupational therapy context. *Occupational Therapy International, 5*, 17–33. https://doi.org/10.1002/oti.65

College of Occupational Therapists. (2017). *Professional standards for occupational therapy practice.* London: Author.

Council for Exceptional Children. (2015). *What every special educator must know: Professional ethics and standards.* Retrieved from https://www.cec.sped.org/Standards/Ethical-Principles-and-Practice-Standards#tizra-target%3A_blank

Cronin, A., & Graebe, G. (2018). *Clinical reasoning in occupational therapy.* Bethesda, MD: AOTA Press.

Davies, P. L., Soon, P., Young, M., & Clausen-Yamaki, A. (2004). Validity and reliability of the School Function Assessment in elementary school students with disabilities. *Physical and Occupational Therapy in Pediatrics, 24*(3), 23–43. https://doi.org/10.1300/J006v24n03_03

Donohue, M. V. (2013). *Social Profile: Assessment of social participation in children, adolescents, and adults.* Bethesda, MD: AOTA Press.

Fisher, A. G., & Bray Jones, K. (2014). *Assessment of Motor and Process Skills: Vol. 2. User manual* (8th ed.). Fort Collins, CO: Three Star Press.

Fisher, A. G., Bryze, K., Hume, V., & Griswold, L. A. (2007). *School Assessment of Motor and Process Skills.* Fort Collins, CO: Three Star Press

Hayward C., & Taylor, J. (2011). Eudemonic well-being: Its importance and relevance to occupational therapy for humanity. *Occupational Therapy International, 18*, 133–141. https://doi.org/10.1002/oti.316

Hinojosa, J., & Kramer, P. (2014). *Evaluation in occupational therapy: Obtaining and interpreting data* (4th ed.). Bethesda, MD: AOTA Press

Hinojosa, J., Kramer, P., Royeen, C. B., & Luebben, A. J. (2017). The core concept of occupation. In P. Kramer, J. Hinojosa, & C. B. Royeen (Eds.), *Perspectives in human occupation: Theories underlying practice* (2nd ed., pp. 23–38). Philadelphia: F. A. Davis.

Longest, B. B., Jr. (2014). *Health program management from development to evaluation* (2nd ed.). San Francisco: Jossey-Bass

Newcomer, K. E., Hatry, H. P., & Wholey, J. S. (2015). *Handbook of program evaluation* (4th ed.). Hoboken, NJ: Jossey-Bass

Occupational Therapy Australia. (2017). *Position paper: Occupational therapy scope of practice framework.* Fitzroy, Victoria, Australia: Author. Retrieved from https://otaus.com.au/publicassets/725829df-2503-e911-a2c2-b75c2fd918c5/Occupational%20Therapy%20Scope%20of%20Practice%20Framework%20(June%202017).pdf

Swearingen, R. (2002). *A primer: Diagnostic, formative, and summative assessment.* Retrieved from http://www.ewcupdate.com/userfiles/assessmentnetwork_net/file/A%20Primer_%20Diagnostic,%20Formative,%20&%20Summative%20Assessment.pdf

Thomas, H. (2019). Working with occupational therapy assistants. In K. Jacobs & G. L. McCormack (Eds.), *The occupational therapy manager* (pp. 385–391). Bethesda, MD: AOTA Press.

Townsend, E., & Polatajko, H. (2007). *Enabling occupation II: Advancing an occupational therapy vision for health, well-being & justice through occupation.* Ottawa: CAOT Publications.

Üstün, T. B., Kostanjsek, N., Chatterji, S., & Rehm, J. (Eds). (2010). *Measuring health and disability: Manual for WHO Disability Assessment Schedule (WHODAS 2.0).* Geneva: World Health Organization. Retrieved from https://apps.who.int/iris/bitstream/handle/10665/43974/9789241547598_eng.pdf;jsessionid=68C29E47F8C1A34184EA737053FEA34C?sequence=1

Wales, K., Clemson, L., Lannin, N. A., & Cameron, I. D. (2012). Functional assessments used by occupational therapists with older adults at risk of activity and participation limitations: A systematic review and evaluation of measurement properties. *Systematic Reviews, 1*, 45. https://doi.org/10.1186/2046-4053-1-45

World Health Organization. (2002). *Towards a common language for functioning, disability and health.* Geneva: Author. Retrieved from https://www.who.int/classifications/icf/icfbeginnersguide.pdf

Philosophical and Theoretical Influences on Evaluation

Paula Kramer, PhD, OTR, FAOTA

CHAPTER HIGHLIGHTS

- Philosophical influences on evaluation
- Beginning the evaluation process
- Choosing the frame of reference
- Occupational therapist perspectives, theory, and practice

KEY TERMS AND CONCEPTS

- Assessment stage
- Being
- Bias
- Bottom-up approach
- Clear choice
- Concepts
- Contextual approach
- Contextual factors
- Evaluation process
- Evaluation report
- Evaluation summary
- Exploratory approach
- Frame of reference
- Idiosyncratic approach
- Perspective
- Philosophical beliefs
- Population
- Postulates
- Reassessment
- Screening stage
- Theories
- Top-down approach

INTRODUCTION

Each occupational therapist has a set of philosophical assumptions and beliefs based in part on those of the profession, acquired through education, and in part on personal experiences gained in their professional career. These assumptions and beliefs influence the way therapists conduct evaluations, the assessments they choose, the theories they use, and the approaches they apply to intervention. Some therapists follow particular models, others use distinct paradigms, and still others use specific frames of reference. No matter which particular perspective or approach is used, evaluation is an essential part of practice. This chapter focuses on the links among philosophy, theory, and practice as they influence evaluation and provides an overview of the evaluation process.

PHILOSOPHICAL INFLUENCES ON EVALUATION

Fundamental philosophical beliefs influence what occupational therapists and occupational therapy assistants consider important and guide their actions. ***Philosophical beliefs*** refer to values and beliefs that are accepted throughout the profession. These philosophical beliefs collectively form the unique philosophical foundations of the profession. Therefore, occupational therapy's philosophical beliefs have a strong influence on therapists' actions, including how they perform evaluation and provide intervention. The following foundational beliefs of occupational therapy were first attributed to William Rush Dunton, Jr. in a retrospective article (American Occupational Therapy Association [AOTA], 1967):

- Occupation is as necessary to life as food and drink.
- Every human being should have both physical and mental occupations.
- All should have occupations that they enjoy or hobbies—at least two, one outdoor and one indoor.
- Sick minds, sick bodies, and sick souls may be healed through occupation (p. 261).

Although several authors have updated these basic beliefs (e.g., Kielhofner, 2009; Mosey, 1996), the core is still the same: Occupation is necessary to a healthy, meaningful life (AOTA, 2012, 2018; Baum & Christiansen, 2005; Baum et al., 2015).

One conceptualization of the profession's philosophy reflects this belief in terms of its view of the person and their rights (Mosey, 1996). Occupational therapists and occupational therapy assistants believe that a person

- Has the right to a meaningful existence;
- Is influenced by the biological and social nature of the human species;
- Can be understood only within the context of family, friends, community, and cultural group membership;

https://doi.org/10.7139/2020.978-1-56900-596-5.002

- Has the need to participate in a variety of social roles and to have periodic relief from participation;
- Has the right to seek their potential through personal choice in the context of accepted social constraints; and
- Is able to reach his or her potential through purposeful interaction with the human and nonhuman environments.

These beliefs about a person's rights are reinforced in the most recent iteration of the *Philosophical Base of Occupational Therapy* (AOTA, 2017):

All individuals have an innate need and right to engage in meaningful occupations throughout their lives. Participation in these occupations influences their development, health, and well-being across the lifespan. Thus, participation in meaningful occupations is a determinant of health and leads to adaptation. . . . The focus and outcome of occupational therapy are clients' engagement in meaningful occupations that support their participation in life situations. (p. 1)

Occupational therapists believe in a *client-centered approach*, which means that clients have the right to make choices and to be active participants in the therapeutic process. The importance of the client's collaboration in the evaluation process is discussed throughout this book. Evaluation begins with the client and considers the client's life experiences, life roles, interests and occupations, age, cultural background, and context. The client's own view of what is important to them and the client's own perceived strengths and limitations are essential to the evaluation process in occupational therapy.

In addition, occupational therapists have strong beliefs about the importance of occupations and activities, including that people are naturally active beings (i.e., have an occupational nature) and that occupation is necessary to society and culture. Kielhofner (2009) proposed that occupation is a basic need for people, a source of meaning in their lives, and a domain of human behavior. These constructs influence the ways occupational therapists look at people, the ways they evaluate clients, and the areas in which they intervene. Thus, an occupational therapy evaluation always considers the person's

- Biological and individual development,
- Cultural and social context,
- Relationships with family and significant others,
- Engagement in meaningful occupations,
- Quality of occupational performance, and
- Unique occupations in relationship to their physical and psychological development.

A fundamental belief of the profession is the importance of occupation and occupational performance. In refining the Occupational Therapy Intervention Process Model, Fisher (2013) and Fisher and Bray Jones (2017) discussed the importance of evaluation focusing on occupation. Fisher (2013) made a clear distinction among the following terms: *occupation centered, occupation based*, and *occupation focused*. Exhibit 2.1 includes Fisher's definitions of each term. Fisher maintained that although the initial assessment may not be occupation focused, it is occupation based. During the interview, occupational therapists focus on the person's occupations and how they are realized

in the person's life. According to Fisher, the performance analysis component of the evaluation, which may use standardized assessments, should be both occupation based and occupation focused.

Basic philosophical beliefs influence the way occupational therapists conduct an evaluation. Therapists operationalize their beliefs, professional values, and perhaps biases when evaluating clients. However, to perform an effective client-centered evaluation, therapists should consider best practice and keep personal values and biases in check. Personal beliefs, values, and biases that influence individual therapists are separate from the beliefs and values of the profession. Therapists should develop an awareness of their beliefs, values, and biases so that they do not interfere with their choice of assessments and interpretation of the results.

The following six principles are proposed as best practices reflecting the philosophy of the occupational therapy profession regarding evaluation and as being fundamental to an effective *evaluation process*:

1. Evaluation, in the form of screening, starts when occupational therapists first receive information about the client or population and continues until the client is discharged from therapy.
2. Evaluation of a client always considers the client's perspective as well as those of the family, significant others, and caregivers with the client's permission.
3. Specific meaningful information about the client or population is best acquired through interviews, assessments, and observation of occupational performance.
4. Therapists need to be aware that assessments have potential biases that may influence their usefulness and appropriateness with clients, groups of people, or populations and these biases may affect assessment results.
5. Contextual factors may influence a client's performance on assessments.
6. Evaluation is an ongoing process in which therapists continually gather information about a client.

EXHIBIT 2.1. Summary of the Definitions of the Terms *Occupation Centered, Occupation Based,* and *Occupation Focused*

How we guide our reasoning and our subsequent actions

- *Occupation centered:* To adopt a profession-specific perspective—a world view of occupation and what it means to be an occupational being—where occupation is placed in the center and ensures that what we do is linked to the core paradigm of occupational therapy.

What we do and how we do it in research, education, and practice

- *Occupation based:* To use occupation as the foundation—to engage a person in occupation (i.e., the performance of chosen daily life tasks that offer desirable levels of pleasure, productivity, and restoration and unfold as they ordinarily do in the person's life) as the method used for evaluation and/or intervention
- *Occupation focused:* To focus one's attention on occupation—to have occupation as the proximal (i.e., immediate) focus of the evaluation or the proximal intent of the intervention

Source. From "Occupation-Centered, Occupation-Based, Occupation-Focused: Same, Same or Different?" by A. G. Fisher, 2013, *Scandinavian Journal of Occupational Therapy, 20,* p. 167. Copyright © 2013 by Taylor & Francis. Used with permission.

Beginning the Evaluation Process

When the occupational therapist first receives a referral for a potential client, the evaluation process has begun. The first step of the evaluation process is to screen the client using data collected from referral information, recorded observations, and knowledge of the possible sequelae of the client's diagnosis. If the occupational therapist determines that occupational therapy services may be needed, the process continues with a thorough review of available data.

Occupational therapists begin this dynamic interactive process with the client through an interview with the client to gain foundational information about the client's occupational focus. The interview usually involves the use of the occupational profile (AOTA, 2014) and is a critical part of the assessment because it helps therapists understand the client. The interview process relates to a concept that Hayward and Taylor (2011) referred to as the *being* of the client, which refers to the individual's subjective experience of who they are as a person. The interview also aids in determining the most appropriate assessments for use in the client's particular situation. The administration of assessments and the data collected continue to be part of the process between therapist and client. Both parties shape the evaluation through their input, interaction, and responses to each other and to the assessments or activities. Although therapists may start with a formalized assessment, the process is fluid and may take many different directions.

Occupational therapists expend much effort in evaluating their clients, striving to do so effectively and efficiently to obtain all the information necessary with optimal reliability and validity. The formal evaluation provides a baseline measurement of the client's performance. Using this baseline, the therapist determines the client's specific needs for intervention. Once an initial evaluation is done, *reassessment* takes place throughout the intervention. With ongoing reassessment, the therapist continually observes whether the client is making progress and whether a change in programming is needed. The therapist conducts a reevaluation at regular intervals to ensure that the intervention plan is meeting the identified goals.

This overview of evaluation emphasizes that evaluation begins with the referral and first contact with the client and continues until the client is discharged from therapy. The *evaluation report,* which is sometimes referred to as the *evaluation summary,* should include a comprehensive description of the client's occupational roles, client factors, performance skills, performance patterns, context and environment, and activity demands that influence the client's occupational performance, as well as the standardized assessments used, the scores obtained, and the performances observed.

The occupational therapy philosophy provides a continued underpinning for practice, making the profession's contribution to society unique. This philosophy defines who the occupational therapist is and the therapist's focus. The profession's philosophical belief in the importance of occupation-based, client-centered care should guide the therapist's practice, determining what the therapist will assess and how the therapist will intervene.

Perspective of Clients, Families, Significant Others, and Caregivers

An essential element of the evaluation is to address the client's *perspective* and the client's desired outcomes for intervention. This is an area in which occupational therapy differs from other professions. The profession puts an emphasis on being client centered. A client cannot be evaluated in isolation, however, and it is important in a client-centered approach to consider the client's wishes regarding the involvement of family members, significant others, and caregivers. These people are additional sources of data and may give the therapist another view of the client and the client's ability to engage in meaningful activities, as long as the therapist has the client's permission. The therapist interprets information from these sources using clinical reasoning and judgment to gain a total picture of the client.

Written evaluations need to be complete enough to provide others with all-important information about the total person, the person's lifestyle, and the occupations and activities that are meaningful to the person. Evaluation reports and summaries should not discuss just one client factor, performance skill, performance pattern, or contextual factor that influences a person's occupational performance. They must be complete and discuss all performance skills, patterns, and contextual factors evaluated. Moreover, evaluation reports should reflect the client's strengths and any limitations. Occupational therapy evaluation narratives should reflect the values of the profession in providing an integrated snapshot of the client's life.

Reassessments throughout the intervention process should capture the focus of intervention and the functional changes that occur as the intervention progresses. Reassessment data may be routinely gathered through various sources, including observations, family members, significant others, and other professionals who interact with the client. The goal of intervention—progress toward meaningful, relevant goals—will be reflected in the data about the client's daily life activities.

Client or Population Assessment

The data collected from assessments are specific to the client or population. Client data offer insight into who the client is, what occupations are important to the client, and what the client's performance skills are. Data collected from client assessments are personalized, reflecting the fact that no two people have the same strengths, needs, or expected outcomes from intervention.

For a *population,* assessments offer a greater understanding of a group as consisting of members, the unique characteristics that identify it as a population, the health needs and life patterns of group members, and the specific activities in which members engage. Assessments and interpretation of population data should also provide some insight into the activity needs of the population and the supports needed to participate in society. Some characteristics may be common across groups, but the data will also reflect the unique identity of each group, including differing values, strengths, limitations, and performance goals.

The data that occupational therapists collect should be within the occupational therapy scope of practice and should shed light on how to facilitate engagement in personally meaningful activities and occupations that will fulfill life roles. Once therapists interpret the data, they may find that they need more information from additional assessments or from other professionals and team members. Because the area of assessing populations is relatively new, it is discussed further in Chapter 14, "Evaluation in Emerging Practice Settings."

Assessment Biases

Assessments have potential biases that may influence their applicability to, usefulness with, and appropriateness for selected groups of people. *Bias* refers to preference given to certain areas related to the assessments or certain groups of individuals that results in unfair interpretations. All assessments have some degree of bias. The most obvious biases are based on culture, gender, age, lifestyle, health status, geographical area, and socioeconomic status. With standardized assessments, the bias may result from the use of a homogeneous population when the assessment was standardized. It may also come from certain items that are specific to one cultural group or gender or to a particular region of the country. For example, assessments developed for daily activities in United States may be biased toward the common activities encountered in this country and may not apply to individuals from other countries.

Another type of bias is personal or *examiner bias*, resulting from personal beliefs or feelings of the evaluator that are conscious or unconscious (Goldyne, 2007; King-Thomas, 1987). One type of examiner bias is based on expectations. If the client is wearing soiled clothing, for example, the examiner may expect that the client will not do well on the evaluation, and the examiner's unconscious actions or attitudes may influence the results. All people have some prejudices, but they may not be aware of them and how these prejudices affect the way they view others. Although it is difficult to acknowledge and explore one's own prejudices, it is important to do so to prevent these prejudices from interfering with one's professional judgment (Campinha-Bacote, 2003; Jeffreys, 2006).

In addition, occupational therapists may have preconceived notions about client characteristics based on their professional background and experiences. When therapists read a diagnosis in a chart, for example, they may expect to see certain characteristics that may or may not be present. Therapists need to be aware of what they are actually observing to guard against being deceived by expectations. Although reading a chart and becoming familiar with the client's history are part of good practice, therapists need to avoid letting that information influence their own data gathering and conclusions.

Influence of Contextual Factors on Assessment

Occupational therapy is concerned with clients' functional performance in their daily lives, including not only what clients can or cannot do but also how they function in the context of their environment. When using assessments, occupational therapists must think about the *contextual factors*—the physical, social, cultural, and temporal influences of the context on clients' performance.

Occupational therapists must also examine potential contextual supports for and barriers to clients' performance (Dunn, 2017). As Dunn (2017) noted, a person reacts to contextual variables in unique ways. For one person, background music might be distracting, whereas for another, it might be relaxing. A group setting might be stimulating for one adolescent but might be contributing to social anxiety for another. When interpreting data from assessments, therapists must consider whether contextual factors affected the client's performance.

Ongoing Data Gathering Through Reassessment

Occupational therapy practitioners continually monitor clients' responses to intervention and gather data about any changes in behavior or performance. The ongoing reassessment that continues throughout intervention is more informal than the initial evaluation, adjusting to the needs and demands of the intervention process. Data from various sources are used to ascertain whether the intervention is assisting the client in achieving the established short-term goals. Progress is identified by comparing the baseline evaluation data with any ongoing reassessment data obtained. Family, significant others, and additional professionals may provide valuable reassessment data, if the client approves.

The principle of reassessment requires that occupational therapists and occupational therapy assistants continually reflect on what happens during the intervention and identify changes in the client's behaviors or performance skills. When the therapist and assistant determine that reassessment data indicate that the intervention program needs to be changed or modified, they should engage in a collaborative discussion to modify the plan. At that point, a formal reevaluation might be necessary.

THEORY'S ROLE IN EVALUATION

In addition to understanding the influence of philosophical beliefs on the evaluation process, it is critical to explore the effect of theory on this process. Philosophical beliefs guide, to some extent, those theories that are applicable to or appropriate for the profession to use. The theories that an occupational therapist chooses to guide practice must be congruent with the philosophical perspective of the profession.

Theories are a collection of concepts, definitions, and postulates that help professionals make predictions about relationships between events. *Concepts* are labels describing phenomena that have been observed; the meanings of concepts are their definitions. The stated relationships between two or more concepts are *postulates* (Hinojosa et al., 2020; Kramer & Hinojosa, 2010). The person or people who develop a theory identify and define the concepts and state the postulates, thus determining the scope and parameters of the theory. A theory organizes information and explains the relationships between ideas and observed events in a logical, understandable manner. A theory links the various concepts, definitions, and principles in a coherent way around a central theme or organizing principle. Theories are critical to the foundation of any type of intervention and are therefore basic to evaluation.

Occupational therapists treat deficits in occupational performance. Theories guide intervention, and when occupational therapists choose assessments, they are guided by theory as well. Many assessments are developed around a particular theory. Some examples of the use of theory in intervention are obvious.

For example, during the screening process of observing a child, the therapist might see behaviors indicative of a sensory processing problem. This observation would lead the therapist to consider the possibility of using a sensory processing theory and then choose assessments related to a sensory dysfunction, such as the Sensory Profile (Dunn, 1999), the Sensory Integration and Praxis Tests–Revised (Ayres, 2003), the Bruininks–Oseretsky Test of Motor Proficiency (Bruininks & Bruininks, 2005), or the Miller Function and Participation Scale (Miller, 2006). On the basis of the screening findings, the therapist would then decide exactly which theory to use to develop an appropriate intervention for the child.

In another example, when an occupational therapist is observing a male adult with tremors, the therapist might have a more general idea of which theory to use. The clinical reasoning process might be that tremors are usually neurological and therefore may not be remediated in treatment; therefore, the theory used for intervention would be compensatory rather than remedial. The assessments chosen would be related to determining the client's specific occupational performance deficits and desires for improved functioning. There are various assessments the therapist might use; for example, for tremors related to Parkinson's disease, the Unified Parkinson's Disease Rating Scale items related to different types of tremors seen in Parkinson's disease can be used (Movement Disorder Society Task Force on Rating Scales for Parkinson's Disease, 2003).

Regardless of what theories are used in intervention, therapists need to select assessments that measure some aspects of occupational performance. Occupational therapists could choose assessments that are applicable to the client and would fit the contextual factors that influence the client's occupational performance. In reality, some assessments focus on specific areas that fit neatly with the theories and philosophical beliefs important to occupational therapy, whereas many others relate to the profession's concerns but were developed using other theoretical orientations.

Although theory is important in the choice of assessments, other factors also influence which assessments are used. Some assessments are used because they are popular. Other assessments are used because other professions value them. Some are used because they are standardized, and standardized data are required in certain settings. Some are used because an institution, regulations, or particular service delivery models require that they be used. Under these circumstances, occupational therapists have the additional responsibility to translate the assessment results into the domain of concern of the profession.

The application of theory to practice is a complex process. Occupational therapists are obliged to take ideas that are abstract and apply them at a level at which they can be used functionally. There are several acceptable ways of conceptualizing occupational therapy practice. In each, evaluation is an important component and serves as the basis for intervention. Some of the more common conceptualizations are frames of reference (Hinojosa et al., 2020; Kramer & Hinojosa, 2010; Mosey, 1970, 1996), conceptual models of practice (Dunn, 2011; Ikiugu, 2007; Kielhofner, 2008), and occupation-based frameworks for practice (Baum & Christiansen, 2005; Baum et al., 2015; Brown et al., 2011). All of these approaches allow therapists to use theory as the basis for their evaluations and interventions. In this book, frames of reference are used as the way of conceptualizing practice to illustrate the evaluative process.

A *frame of reference* is an acceptable vehicle for organizing theoretical material in occupational therapy and translating it into practice through a functional perspective. A frame of reference provides a linking structure between theory and practice (Dunn, 2011; Hinojosa et al., 2020; Kramer & Hinojosa, 2010; Mosey, 1996) and draws from one or more theories to provide a basis for what will occur throughout the intervention process. On the basis of theoretical information, a frame of reference addresses specific behaviors or physical signs that are considered functional and specific behaviors or physical signs that are considered dysfunctional (Mosey, 1992, 1996). Occupational therapists often use more than one frame of reference to address a client's distinctive therapeutic needs.

Inherent in a theoretical perspective or frame of reference may be a *top-down approach,* which looks at the person's occupations first; a *bottom-up approach,* which looks at the components of tasks that are interfering with performance first; or a *contextual approach,* which looks at the contextual effects on performance. The theory and the available assessments that are consistent with the theory then help to define the evaluation process. Therapists' personal predilections should not guide the choice of assessments. Currently, many more assessments are driven by task components than are driven by occupations or contextual issues. However, as the profession becomes more occupation focused, more assessments are being developed that have a top-down approach, such as the Assessment of Motor and Process (Fisher & Bray Jones, 2014a, 2014b).

Regardless of whether occupational therapists select a top-down, bottom-up, or contextual approach, it is incumbent on them to explore all of these areas to gain a comprehensive view of the client. One perspective is generally primary during the intervention process, but effective intervention usually combines all three approaches to some degree.

CHOOSING A FRAME OF REFERENCE

Theory and practice need to be continually linked and related to the client. Screening provides the first opportunity to decide which theory or theories will guide practice with a particular person. If the screening provides enough information to decide on a theoretical approach, then the occupational therapist has a theoretical direction for evaluation and intervention. However, if the screening does not yield sufficient information to choose a theoretical perspective, then the therapist may need to use additional assessments to gain more information about the client and determine an appropriate approach. Whenever a therapist develops an intervention plan, it must be based on sound evidence and guided by theory. The theory selected predicts the consequences of intervention to some degree.

Screening Stage

The *screening stage* is the first opportunity for an occupational therapist to gather data about a client that may result in a clear direction toward a frame of reference. Screening plays a critical role in the choices that therapists make in evaluating a client. Data from the screening process have an ongoing effect on the evaluation and intervention process. Sometimes, just by reading a chart or interviewing a client, therapists know which theoretical perspective or frame of reference would be appropriate for the client. When therapists determine during a screening that a specific frame of reference is appropriate, they proceed to administer assessments that are consistent with that frame of reference. For example, if a therapist screens a report on a young man with a fracture of his nondominant hand caused by a fall from a bicycle, the therapist may decide to use a biomechanical frame of reference. On the basis of this decision, the therapist proceeds to administer assessments consistent with this approach (e.g., range of motion and manual muscle testing).

When a frame of reference is not immediately apparent, occupational therapists can use specific screening assessments or data collection strategies to gather more information about the client and the client's occupational performance needs. The purpose of screening is to obtain an overview of the person's needs, strengths, limitations, and environment; it is not meant to be a comprehensive evaluation. Screening may involve an observation of the client, a chart review, a medical and developmental history, information gained from the parents or care providers, or data gathered by other professionals involved with the client. The following are examples of standardized and nonstandardized screening assessments that can help therapists identify an appropriate frame of reference:

- Screening Test for Evaluating Preschoolers (FirstSTEP™; Miller, 1993)
- Miller Function and Participation Scales (Miller, 2006)
- Denver II Developmental Screening Test (Frankenburg et al., 1991)
- Clinical Observations of Neuromuscular Integration (Ayres, 1976, 2005)
- Family Observation Guide (Hinojosa & Kramer, 2008)
- Activity Configuration (Mosey, 1986)
- Model of Human Occupation Screening Tool (Parkinson et al., 2006)
- Occupational Performance History Interview (Kielhofner, 2004).

A screening is usually complete when therapists have enough information to recommend whether the client needs to receive occupational therapy services and, if services are required, to determine an intervention approach with an appropriate frame of reference.

Screening data provide therapists with a preliminary picture of the client and a potential view of what occupational therapy might offer. While reflecting on the screening data, the therapist decides whether the client's needs relate to the occupational therapy's domain of concern and, if so, how to

proceed with the evaluation using the assessments that will be most appropriate for the setting and to obtain the data needed. If the therapist decides that occupational therapy is not necessary, the client is discharged from occupational therapy and, if indicated, the therapist refers the client to another service.

Assessment Stage

The *assessment stage* is the next stage; therapists use nonstandardized and standardized tests to gather relevant data to plan an intervention. When selecting the assessments to use in the comprehensive evaluation, there are three possibilities (Figure 2.1):

1. The occupational therapist has enough information from the screening to choose a frame of reference to guide evaluation and intervention;
2. The therapist needs to use an exploratory approach to determine which way to proceed with evaluating the client; or
3. The therapist decides, given the client's specific problems, that an idiosyncratic approach to evaluation must be used.

The occupational therapist chooses assessments that will identify the presence of functional and dysfunctional behaviors and physical signs as described by the selected frame of reference. Some frames of reference are associated with specific assessments; with other frames of reference, it is up to the therapist to determine which assessment will best be able to identify the presence of behaviors or physical signs. The same theory or theories should underlie both the assessments and the treatment approach to ensure that they are congruent.

FIGURE 2.1. Three approaches to evaluation that lead to theoretically based intervention.

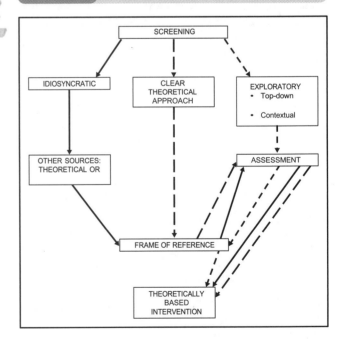

Source. From "Philosophical and Theoretical Influences on Evaluation," by P. Kramer & J. Hinojosa. In J. Hinojosa & P. Kramer (Eds.), *Evaluation in Occupational Therapy: Obtaining and Interpreting Data, 4th Ed.*, p. 27. Bethesda, MD: AOTA Press. Copyright © 2014 by the American Occupational Therapy Association. Used with permission.

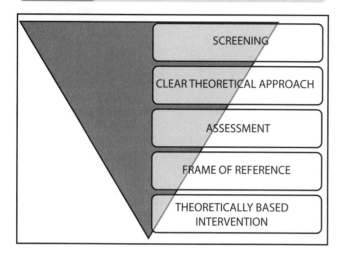

FIGURE 2.2. Occupational therapy process when presented with a clear choice of a frame of reference.

SCREENING

CLEAR THEORETICAL APPROACH

ASSESSMENT

FRAME OF REFERENCE

THEORETICALLY BASED INTERVENTION

Source. From "Philosophical and Theoretical Influences on Evaluation," by P. Kramer & J. Hinojosa. In J. Hinojosa & P. Kramer (Eds.), *Evaluation in Occupational Therapy: Obtaining and Interpreting Data, 4th Ed.*, p. 27. Bethesda, MD: AOTA Press. Copyright © 2014 by the American Occupational Therapy Association. Used with permission.

Clear choice of a frame of reference

When a clear theoretical approach is evident from the screening data, the occupational therapist has a ***clear choice*** of a frame of reference and chooses an assessment based on that approach (Figure 2.2). Many frames of reference or theoretical approaches are associated with one or more assessments that are consistent with that theoretical perspective (see Case Example 2.1).

Exploratory approach to evaluation

After screening, if the occupational therapist does not have a clear theoretical direction for how to proceed in the evaluation process, the therapist might consider taking an ***exploratory approach.*** This broad approach to evaluation includes, if possible, a more in-depth interview with the client to determine specific personal goals and to explore physical, psychosocial, and environmental issues (and their component parts) that may prevent those goals from being met. It is essential to understand the client's perspective on why these goals cannot be met at this time.

With the exploratory approach, the occupational therapist may start in many places: from the top down, by exploring the client's meaningful occupations (see Case Example 2.2); from the bottom up, by exploring the underlying

---

CASE EXAMPLE 2.1. CARMEN: CLEAR CHOICE OF A FRAME OF REFERENCE

Carmen is an 18-month-old who has been diagnosed with quadriplegic cerebral palsy. She exhibits high distal tone in all extremities and severely delayed developmental milestones. A review of Carmen's medical chart provided the occupational therapist with extensive information. The therapist also observed Carmen for a period of time and then held her, finding low proximal tone and high distal tone. After this screening, the therapist selected a postural control approach with handling and decided to use the neurodevelopmental frame of reference (Barthel, 2020). During the assessment, along with a more extended observation of Carmen's ability to interact with toys and other aspects of her environment, the therapist used the Alberta Infant Motor Scale (Piper & Darrah, 1994) and the Bayley Scales of Infant and Toddler Development (Bayley, 2006), to assess Carmen's gross motor abilities. Once the therapist determined the specific delays, she could proceed to develop a plan for intervention.

CASE EXAMPLE 2.2. DON: TOP-DOWN APPROACH

Don, age 55 years, is 1 week post–cerebrovascular accident. His physician has determined that he is medically stable. He was referred to occupational therapy for a complete evaluation and potential intervention. The occupational therapist read the medical documentation as part of the screening process and met with Don. Don's concerns and the data the therapist collected from the screening directed her to focus on ADLs. The evaluation explored Don's ability to feed, bathe, toilet, and dress himself. Through functional activities and specific assessments, including the Canadian Occupational Performance Measure (Law et al., 2019) and the occupational profile (AOTA, 2014), the therapist determined that Don had a problem with the performance area of ADLs. Being independent in his self-care activities was very important to him. She evaluated specific components of his performance (i.e., bottom-up approach), such as manual muscle testing and range of motion, to gain more information about how a body structure deficit might be affecting this area of occupation. Although the therapist's approach for Don is primarily from the top down, bottom-up assessments can occasionally be helpful as a supplemental evaluation. Then, with consideration of the context, the therapist was able to develop a plan for intervention, focusing on the occupations that were critically important to Don.

components of meaningful tasks (see Case Example 2.3); or from a contextual perspective, by exploring environmental issues (see Case Example 2.4; Hinojosa & Kramer, 1998; Ideishi, 2003; Weinstock-Zlotnick & Hinojosa, 2004). The therapist's intent is to understand the client and the identified problems and to determine a theoretical approach or frame of reference for intervention (Figure 2.3).

Although therapists might begin an evaluation with one approach, a comprehensive evaluation requires that they continually analyze the data and consider all approaches—top down, bottom up, and contextual—before a comprehensive evaluation is complete. Their clinical reasoning skills may indicate that a change in focus is warranted to address the issues that arise from the individual client. Using the data that they have collected, therapists select an appropriate theoretical perspective to guide intervention.

Idiosyncratic approach

Occupational therapists with advanced knowledge and expertise sometimes screen a client who presents with problems that are unusual and unique. The presenting picture of these clients is not consistent with known frames of reference or problems traditionally seen in occupational therapy.

FIGURE 2.3.   Exploratory approach to evaluation.

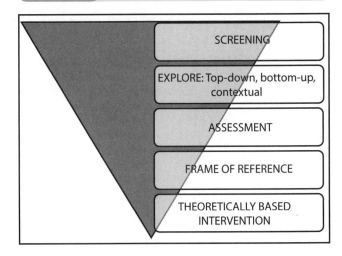

SCREENING

EXPLORE: Top-down, bottom-up, contextual

ASSESSMENT

FRAME OF REFERENCE

THEORETICALLY BASED INTERVENTION

Source. From "Philosophical and Theoretical Influences on Evaluation," by P. Kramer & J. Hinojosa. In J. Hinojosa & P. Kramer (Eds.), *Evaluation in Occupational Therapy: Obtaining and Interpreting Data*, 4th Ed., p. 29. Bethesda, MD: AOTA Press. Copyright © 2014 by the American Occupational Therapy Association. Used with permission.

CASE EXAMPLE 2.3. SUMAN: BOTTOM-UP APPROACH

Suman, age 4 years, was referred to occupational therapy because of suspected developmental delay. She has limited speech and does not make eye contact, and her gross and fine motor skills are delayed. After reading the referral documentation and getting an overview of the child as a person through a discussion with her care providers, the occupational therapist decided to assess Suman's gross and fine motor skills, muscle tone, movement patterns, and manipulation skills using a standardized assessment, the Screening Test for Evaluating Preschoolers

(Miller, 1993) and Clinical Observations of Neuromuscular Integration (Ayres, 1976, 2005). The therapist also referred Suman for a speech evaluation. Once the therapist identified those components of performance that were interfering with Suman's functional abilities through clinical observation and the data obtained from the two assessments, the therapist ascertained the areas of occupation that were affected. After this step, and considering the context, the therapist was able to develop a plan for intervention.

CASE EXAMPLE 2.4. MOHAMMAD: CONTEXTUAL APPROACH

Mohammad, age 72 years, was recovering from a head trauma resulting in an aneurysm. He presented with mild motor deficits. He was referred to occupational therapy for an evaluation of ADLs before being discharged to an assisted living facility. After reading the referral documentation, the occupational therapist decided to assess Mohammad's performance of ADLs, considering in the process both his wants and what he would need to do independently in the assisted living facility. The therapist interviewed Mohammad and observed the assisted living facility. The therapist found that before his hospitalization, Mohammad lived alone and was now fearful of returning to his apartment. Given his age and lifestyle, along with his

newly acquired disability, he felt that he would be more comfortable in the assisted living residence, where he could get help if he needed it. He chose this particular setting because he believed that it was respectful of his cultural background and he would feel comfortable with the people around him.

The therapist used the data from the assessment of the context as the background for the assessment of the areas of occupation and the components of performance. Using all of the data, the therapist was able to develop an intervention plan for Mohammad that focused on developing his ability to function in the assisted living facility and identified areas in which he might need ongoing help after his move.

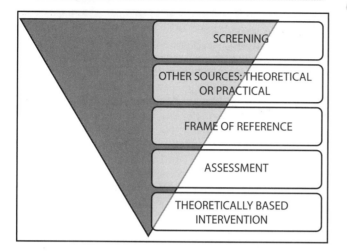

FIGURE 2.4. Idiosyncratic approach to evaluation.

SCREENING

OTHER SOURCES: THEORETICAL OR PRACTICAL

FRAME OF REFERENCE

ASSESSMENT

THEORETICALLY BASED INTERVENTION

Source. From "Philosophical and Theoretical Influences on Evaluation," by P. Kramer & J. Hinojosa. In J. Hinojosa & P. Kramer (Eds.), *Evaluation in Occupational Therapy: Obtaining and Interpreting Data, 4th Ed.,* p. 29. Bethesda, MD: AOTA Press. Copyright © 2014 by the American Occupational Therapy Association. Used with permission.

Therapists may encounter such clients when they move into nontraditional or emerging areas of practice, develop a new program area, or begin work with a new population not generally seen in occupational therapy. This situation may also occur when new phenomena are seen in a clinical environment, such as postpolio syndrome or the aging process in extended life. The type of evaluation approach needed for such clients is an ***idiosyncratic approach.*** Rather than starting with traditional assessments, therapists may need to look to other sources and professions for theoretical perspectives to use as a basis for developing an appropriate theoretical base to guide intervention. Once a theoretical base can be articulated, it will provide the foundation for selecting appropriate assessments for the evaluation of these clients.

In some cases, other professions and disciplines have already dealt with this problem or have theories that relate to this problem that will allow occupational therapists to combine that knowledge with occupational therapy's unique view (Figure 2.4). This type of evaluation is complex and should not be the role or responsibility of a novice therapist (see Case Example 2.5).

THEORY IN INTERVENTION PLANNING AND IMPLEMENTATION

Throughout the course of evaluation, occupational therapists interpret data and draw conclusions. This reasoning process is ongoing throughout the evaluation process. Once the evaluation is complete, therapists have a wealth of information to use in developing an intervention plan. If they have not already chosen a particular frame of reference, therapists must at this time choose a theoretical approach to lay the foundation for the development of goals and creation of a comprehensive intervention plan for the client.

When planning the intervention, occupational therapists are generally heavily influenced by the context of care and payers for services. However, therapists must ensure that the completed evaluation is consistent with the frame of reference they have chosen. They must develop goals and interventions based only on the data they have gathered. In addition, therapists have to ensure that the client's needs, the therapist's professional responsibilities, and the ethics of the therapist's actions are consistent with the requirements of the setting and the availability of payment.

An enormous amount of information is collected during the evaluation of a client, and its scope and complexity can be overwhelming. The occupational therapist's goal is to synthesize the data and interpret them to develop appropriate goals consistent with the frames of

CASE EXAMPLE 2.5. MARIANNE: IDIOSYNCRATIC APPROACH

Marianne, age 16 years and with obesity, was having difficulty relating to her peer group, resulting in depression, social isolation, and acting-out behaviors. She also has a history of suicidal ideation. She had been receiving ongoing psychological help for 3 years and had been involved in an occupational therapy group, but she showed little response and stopped receiving treatment. Marianne was referred again to occupational therapy to try a different approach involving exploration of her self-image and obesity to promote more appropriate social behaviors.

Because there is no articulated frame of reference identified with working with adolescent obesity combined with depression, the occupational therapist needed to search for theoretical information outside of occupational therapy. The therapist explored literature on lifestyle reengineering, cognitive–behavioral therapy, and theories related to locus of control. Once the therapist identified particular constructs that might relate to Marianne, she proceeded to identify assessments that would provide information to develop a plan for intervention. Although the therapist was not using occupational therapy literature or assessments, she was able to develop an idiosyncratic approach to providing occupational therapy evaluation of this client.

Once the occupational therapist chose several theories to contribute to a frame of reference, she explored the evaluation data to determine appropriate goals for Marianne. These goals provided the foundation of the intervention plan. Although the idiosyncratic approach sounds different and complex, occupational therapists have addressed unique client issues in this way for years. When occupational therapists first started working with clients with HIV/AIDS, postpolio syndrome, and autism spectrum disorder, they used an idiosyncratic approach to evaluation.

reference. Therapists often use more than one frame of reference to address a client's distinctive therapeutic needs to enhance occupational performance. Interpretation of evaluation data requires that therapists bring all the findings together to create a profile of the client as an occupational being in their life context. With this visualization of the client, therapists conscientiously select key long- and short-term goals that reflect an integration and synthesis of all the evaluation data and, when possible, the needs and aspirations of the client. The goals should be realistic, functional, and achievable, based on clear baseline data. Finally, the number of goals should be limited to major goals that are reasonable given the intervention approach and the frequency of sessions. It is recommended that a therapist develop at least one long-term goal and no more than six long-term goals.

The initial evaluation is complete when the therapist writes the evaluation report. The report should have a complete description of the evaluation, including all assessments used and any standardized scores obtained, because they support the therapist's interpretation. Evaluation reports should document findings, not serve as a lecture on the selected frame of reference. Reports should be as concise as possible and provide a sound argument for occupational therapy services based on the synthesis of the evaluation data. Moreover, they should be clear and describe observed behaviors, and they should always include the client's strengths and limitations. Therapists should be careful not to overinterpret data and should check all scores for accuracy. Reports should include clear descriptions of baseline data that describe the client's behaviors and performance deficits.

Hinojosa and Foto (2004) described the importance of evaluation reports in communicating information in a succinct and effective manner. They suggested that all evaluation reports should avoid jargon and be proofread for misspellings, grammatical errors, and awkward sentences. They described a comprehensive evaluation summary as one that identifies key information considered when preparing the report, including age, diagnosis, and referral information. The summary should

- List all tests administered and report how they were administered;
- Identify factors influencing the client's performance;
- Record actual test scores and interpretation of the data, disclosing any concerns about cultural issues or test bias;
- Present a clear description of the client's performance and behaviors;

- Report findings that provide an objective baseline of the client's performance deficits and abilities; and
- Document baseline data that provide a clear picture of the client's overall functional level and that can be used to assess the efficacy of the intervention plan.

In addition, the evaluation report should include a clear, concise evaluation summary. An evaluation summary is important to both the client and the third-party payer. It briefly reviews all pertinent data from the report in a clear, concise manner. This is a critical piece of the report; sometimes it is the only section that is read by the other team members.

THERAPIST PERSPECTIVES, THEORY, AND PRACTICE

Other factors important throughout the evaluation process are occupational therapists' skills and perspective. All people acquire a different set of skills based on what they have been formally and informally taught, what they have learned, what their experiences have been, and who they are as professionals. Although most occupational therapists have been taught a consistent body of knowledge, it may have been presented from different orientations and organized in different manners. For example, all professional educational programs base their content on the 2018 Accreditation Council for Occupational Therapy Education (ACOTE®) Standards (ACOTE, 2018), but this content may be taught using different orientations (ACOTE, 2018) and emphasizing different areas. Some programs may focus on specific treatment techniques, whereas others may emphasize the clinical reasoning process.

In addition, although occupational therapists may be taught the same content, individual differences mean that therapists learn and interpret material differently. On the basis of individual experiences and training, therapists may identify a favorite frame of reference that they prefer to use more frequently. Finally, therapists' practice setting also influences the choice of frame of reference. For example, some frames of reference may be impossible to implement in a home-based, school-based, or community setting or hospital. Although all the factors mentioned may influence the choice of a frame of reference, the client's needs should be given primary consideration. Frames of reference provide a vehicle for theory-directed interventions.

QUESTIONS

1. Identify three personal philosophical beliefs about human development and performance. Are they consistent with those found in this chapter? In what ways are they similar or different?
2. Review the "Philosophical Influences on Evaluation" section in this chapter. In what ways is it different from previous statements made by the leaders of the profession or other therapists with whom you have had contact?
3. When would you, as an evaluator, want to include data from a significant other or care provider as part of an evaluation? What should you do in these cases? What factors might include the involvement of a significant other in the evaluation process?

4. Think back on an experience in which you were evaluated. Can you identify any biases (positive or negative) that you experienced or sensed during the evaluation that might have affected the outcome?
5. Can you identify any times when you have felt a bias when interacting with another person? Do you think that you have any biases that might affect your ability to evaluate another person? How can you overcome or change this in the future?
6. The author purports that theory should influence the choice of an assessment. Identify two assessments—What are the theories, frames of reference, or models of practice that provide the foundation for these assessments?
7. Explain the difference between a top-down approach and a bottom-up approach to evaluation. In what ways are they similar and in what ways are they different?
8. What can the profession do to increase the number of top-down evaluations?

REFERENCES

Accreditation Council for Occupational Therapy Education. (2018). 2018 Accreditation Council for Occupational Therapy Education (ACOTE®) standards. *American Journal of Occupational Therapy, 72*(Suppl. 2), 7212410005. https://doi.org/10.5014/ajot.2018.72S217

American Occupational Therapy Association. (1967). Presidents of the American Occupational Therapy Association (1917–1967). *American Journal of Occupational Therapy, 21,* 290–298.

American Occupational Therapy Association. (2012). *Policy manual.* Bethesda, MD: American Occupational Therapy Association.

American Occupational Therapy Association. (2014). Occupational therapy practice framework: Domain and process (3rd ed.). *American Journal of Occupational Therapy, 68*(Suppl. 1), S1–S48. https://doi.org/10.5014/ajot.2014.682006

American Occupational Therapy Association. (2017). Philosophical base of occupational therapy. *American Journal of Occupational Therapy, 71*(Suppl. 2), 7112410045. https://doi.org/10.5014/ajot.2017.716S06

American Occupational Therapy Association. (2018). *The reference manual of the official documents of the American Occupational Therapy Association.* Bethesda, MD: AOTA Press.

Ayres, A. J. (1976, March). *Clinical observations of neuromuscular integration: Administration of the Southern California Sensory Integration Tests* [Certification course]. Presented at a conference sponsored by the Center for the Study of Sensory Integrative Dysfunction, Valhalla, NY.

Ayres, A. J. (2003). *Sensory Integration and Praxis Test manual.* Los Angeles: Western Psychological Services.

Ayres, A. J. (2005). *Sensory integration and the child: 25th anniversary edition.* Los Angeles: Western Psychological Services.

Barthel, K. A. (2020). A frame of reference for neurodevelopmental treatment. In P. Kramer, J. Hinojosa, & T. S. Howe (Eds.), *Frames of reference for pediatric occupational therapy* (4th ed., pp. 205–246). Philadelphia: Lippincott Williams & Wilkins.

Baum, C. M., & Christiansen, C. (2005). Person–environment–occupation–performance: An occupation-based framework for practice. In C. Christiansen, C. M. Baum, & J. Bass-Haugen (Eds.), *Occupational therapy: Performance, participation, and well-being* (3rd ed., pp. 243–266). Thorofare, NJ: Slack.

Baum, C. M., Christiansen, C., & Bass, J. (2015). Person–environment–occupation–performance: An occupation-based framework for practice. In C. Christiansen, C. M. Baum, & J. Bass (Eds.), *Occupational therapy: Performance, participation, and well-being* (4th ed., pp. 243–266). Thorofare, NJ: Slack.

Brown, C., Stoffel, V., & Munoz, J. P. (2011). *Occupational therapy in mental health: A vision for participation.* Philadelphia: F. A. Davis.

Bruininks, R., & Bruininks, B. (2005). *Bruininks–Oseretsky Test of Motor Proficiency* (2nd ed.). Minneapolis: Pearson.

Campinha-Bacote, J. (2003). *The process of cultural competence in the delivery of healthcare services: A culturally competent model of care.* Cincinnati: Transcultural C.A.R.E. Associates.

Dunn, W. (1999). *Sensory Profile: User's manual.* San Antonio: Psychological Corporation.

Dunn, W. (2011). Using frames of reference and practice models to guide practice. In W. Dunn (Ed.), *Best practice occupational therapy for children and families in community settings* (2nd ed., pp. 39–72). Thorofare, NJ: Slack.

Dunn, W. (2017). Ecological model of occupation. In J. Hinojosa, P. Kramer, & C. B. Royeen (Eds.), *Perspectives in human occupation: Theories underlying practice* (pp. 207–236). Philadelphia: Lippincott Williams & Wilkins.

Fisher, A. G. (2013). Occupation-centred, occupation-based, occupation-focused: Same, same or different? *Scandinavian Journal of Occupational Therapy, 20,* 162–173. https://doi.org/10.3109/11038128.2012.754492

Fisher, A. G., & Bray Jones, K. (2014a). *Assessment of motor and process skills: Vol. 1. Development, standardization and administration manual* (8th ed.). Fort Collins, CO: Three Star Press.

Fisher, A. G., & Bray Jones, K. (2014b). *Assessment of motor and process skills: Vol. 2. User manual* (8th ed.). Fort Collins, CO: Three Star Press.

Fisher, A. G., & Bray Jones, K. (2017). *Occupational therapy intervention process model.* In J. Hinojosa, P. Kramer, & C. B. Royeen (Eds.), *Perspectives in human occupation: Theories underlying practice* (pp. 237–286). Philadelphia: Lippincott Williams & Wilkins.

Frankenburg, W. K., Dodds, J., Archer, P., Bresnick, B., Maschka, P., Edelman, N., & Shapiro, H. (1991). *The Denver II Developmental Screening Test.* Denver: Denver Developmental Materials.

Goldyne, A. J. (2007). Minimizing the influence of unconscious bias in evaluations: A practical guide. *Journal of the American Academy of Psychiatry and the Law, 35,* 60–66.

Hayward, C., & Taylor, J. (2011). Eudaimonic well-being: Its importance and relevance to occupational therapy for humanity. *Occupational Therapy International, 18,* 133–141. https://doi.org/10.1002/oti.316

Hinojosa, J., & Foto, M. (2004). Occupational therapy documentation for reimbursement: Sensory integration. *Sensory Integration Special Interest Section Quarterly, 27*(4), 1–3.

Hinojosa, J., & Kramer, P. (1998). Evaluation: Where do we begin? In J. Hinojosa & P. Kramer (Eds.), *Evaluation: Obtaining and interpreting data* (pp. 1–15). Bethesda, MD: American Occupational Therapy Association.

Hinojosa, J., & Kramer, P. (2008). Integrating children with disabilities into family play. In D. L. Parham & L. S. Fazio (Eds.), *Play in occupational therapy for children* (2nd ed., pp. 321–334). St. Louis: Mosby Year Book.

Hinojosa, J., Kramer, P., & Howe, T. H. (2020). Structure of the frame of reference: Moving from theory to practice. In P. Kramer, J. Hinojosa, & T. S. Howe (Eds.), *Frames of reference for pediatric occupational therapy* (4th ed., pp. 3–19). Philadelphia: Lippincott Williams & Wilkins.

Ideishi, R. I. (2003). The influence of occupation on assessment and treatment. In P. Kramer, J. Hinojosa, & C. B. Royeen (Eds.), *Perspectives in human occupation: Participation in life* (pp. 278–296). Baltimore: Lippincott Williams & Wilkins.

Ikiugu, M. N. (2007). *Psychosocial conceptual practice models in occupational therapy: Building adaptive capacity.* St. Louis: Mosby/Elsevier.

Jeffreys, M. R. (2006). *Teaching cultural competence in nursing and health care: Inquiry, action and innovation.* New York: Springer.

Kielhofner, G. (2004). *A user's manual for the Occupational Performance History Interview (Version 2.1), OPHI–II.* Chicago: Model of Human Occupation Clearinghouse, University of Illinois, Department of Occupational Therapy.

Kielhofner, G. (2008). *Model of Human Occupation: Theory and application.* Baltimore: Lippincott Williams & Wilkins.

Kielhofner, G. (2009). *Conceptual foundations of occupational therapy practice* (4th ed.). Philadelphia: F. A. Davis.

King-Thomas, L. J. (1987). Responsibilities of the examiner. In L. J. King-Thomas & B. J. Hacker (Eds.), *The therapist's guide to pediatric assessment* (pp. 11–18). Boston: Little, Brown.

Kramer, P., & Hinojosa, J. (2010). *Frames of reference for pediatric occupational therapy* (3rd ed.). Baltimore: Lippincott Williams & Wilkins.

Law, M., Baptiste, S., Carswell, A., McColl, M., Polatajko, H. & Pollock, N. (2019). *Canadian Occupational Performance Measure* (5th ed., rev.). Altona, MB: COPM Inc.

Miller, L. J. (1993). *Screening Test for Evaluating Preschoolers (FirstSTEP™).* San Antonio: Psychological Corporation.

Miller, L. J. (2006). *Miller Function and Participation Scale.* San Antonio: Harcourt Assessment.

Mosey, A. C. (1970). *Three frames of reference for mental health.* Thorofare, NJ: Slack.

Mosey, A. C. (1986). *Psychosocial components of occupational therapy.* New York: Raven Press.

Mosey, A. C. (1992). *Applied scientific inquiry in the health professions: An epistemological orientation.* Rockville, MD: American Occupational Therapy Association.

Mosey, A. C. (1996). *Applied scientific inquiry in the health professions: An epistemological orientation* (2nd ed.). Bethesda, MD: American Occupational Therapy Association.

Movement Disorder Society Task Force on Rating Scales for Parkinson's Disease. (2003). The Unified Parkinson's Disease Rating Scale (UPDRS): Status and recommendations. *Movement Disorders, 18,* 738–750. https://doi.org/10.1002/mds.10473

Parkinson, S., Forsyth, K., & Kielhofner, G. (2006). *User's manual for the Model of Human Occupation Screening Tool (MOHOST) (Version 2.0).* Chicago: University of Illinois, Department of Occupational Therapy.

Piper, M. C., & Darrah, J. (1994). Alberta Infant Motor Scale: Construction of a motor assessment tool for the developing infant. In M. C. Piper & J. Darrah (Eds.), *Motor assessment of the developing infant* (pp. 25–35). Philadelphia: W. B. Saunders.

Weinstock-Zlotnick, G., & Hinojosa, J. (2004). Bottom-up or top-down evaluation: Is one better than the other? *American Journal of Occupational Therapy, 58,* 594–599. https://doi.org/10.5014/ajot.58.5.594

Assessment Identification and Selection

Julie D. Bass, PhD, OTR/L, FAOTA

CHAPTER HIGHLIGHTS

- Identifying assessments
- Describing the need for an assessment
- Locating existing assessments that meet current needs
- Analyzing the quality of an assessment: Formal method assessment
- Ethical issues related to selection and use of assessments

KEY TERMS AND CONCEPTS

- Characteristics of interest
- Classification systems
- Conceptual and practice perspectives
- Databases
- Documentation
- Ethical issues
- Expert critiques
- Intended purposes
- Locating existing assessments
- Methodological approach
- Need for an assessment
- Population of clients
- Practical needs
- Qualifications
- Resources
- Selecting assessments

INTRODUCTION

This chapter introduces a process for identifying and selecting assessments for occupational therapy practice. Sources of information on assessments in occupational therapy and other disciplines are identified. This chapter also includes a summary of assessment criteria and a discussion of practical and ethical issues related to the use of assessments.

Identifying and selecting the best assessments for evaluation is an important step in the occupational therapy process. Using a formal process to choose assessments is one of the best mechanisms for ensuring that the outcome of an evaluation and intervention is efficient and effective and that the use of an assessment is fair (American Psychological Association [APA], Joint Committee on Testing Practices, 2004).

Identifying assessments that meet the purpose of an evaluation requires a ***methodological approach*** that includes knowing what you are looking for, where to look, and how to look. Many strategies can help in this process, and selecting a specific assessment requires a careful examination of existing tools and instruments. This examination includes determining the strengths and weaknesses of the assessment in terms of specific criteria and finding a recommendation for how the assessment should be used in a particular setting.

Occupational therapists need to be cautious and rigorous when ***selecting assessments***. They should not simply use what is currently available in the setting. They must be confident that the specific assessment is appropriate for assessing the client. When they decide that they need to adapt an existing assessment or develop an instrument, they need to follow sound test construction design to ensure the instrument's credibility. If test construction guidelines are not followed when an instrument is adapted or modified, therapists are not providing best practice in occupational therapy. In addition, use of such an instrument may jeopardize occupational therapy's professional standing.

IDENTIFYING ASSESSMENTS

Occupational therapists can identify and select instruments in multiple ways. A systematic process of assessment identification for therapists and their facilities can support efficiency and rigor. To identify and select an assessment that meets the needs of an evaluation, describe your needs, find existing assessments that meet those needs, and analyze the quality of the available assessments as described in these steps:

- Determine the need for a specific assessment in the evaluation process.
- Locate and examine information about existing assessments that describes their intended purpose, characteristics, quality, and use in evaluation.
- Identify a few assessments that seem to match the practice need, and draw up a plan to analyze and compare them in a more deliberate manner. This last step results in the selection of a specific assessment for the evaluation process.

https://doi.org/10.7139/2020.978-1-56900-596-5.003

DESCRIBING THE NEED FOR AN ASSESSMENT

In almost every practice setting, there comes a time when an occupational therapist needs to select an assessment as part of an evaluation process. Before reviewing available assessments, therapists must reflect on the overall **need for an assessment** in a particular situation. Therapists should consider several broad areas of need:

- The person–environment–occupation (PEO) characteristics of interest and importance
- Intended uses for or purposes of the assessment
- Population of clients to be evaluated using this assessment
- Qualifications or characteristics of the user of the assessment
- Other practical considerations.

Characteristics of Interest and Importance in the Assessment

There are several approaches to describing the characteristics of interest and importance in an assessment. **Characteristics of interest** refer to the qualities that are needed in the assessment, such as an appropriate match with the frame of reference, practical issues with administration, or psychometric integrity. Several chapters in this text introduce ideas to help occupational therapists reflect on the characteristics and purposes of evaluation. For example, Chapter 2, "Philosophical and Theoretical Influences on Evaluation," provides more guidance on frames of reference; Chapter 4, "Practical Aspects of the Evaluation Process," discusses the practical considerations for evaluation; and Chapter 9, "Psychometric Properties Related to Standardized Assessments," provides guidance on psychometric properties of interest. The PEO and other occupational therapy practice models may serve as organizing frameworks for evaluation (Hinojosa et al., 2017; Reed & Sanderson, 1999). Other classification systems such as the *International Classification of Functioning, Disability and Health* (*ICF*; World Health Organization [WHO], 2001) are intended to provide an international language that is helpful in describing individual status.

Person–environment–occupation models

Models that address person, environment, and occupation as essential constructs (Baum et al., 2015; Kielhofner, 2007; Law et al., 1996; Mathiowetz & Bass-Haugen, 2008; Trombly Latham, 2014) and other occupational therapy practice models provide an important foundation for identifying factors that therapists must consider when selecting an assessment. The characteristics of interest and importance in an assessment generally include a description of the person's characteristics, the contextual and environmental characteristics, and the person's occupations or occupational performance.

PEO models and other occupational therapy practice models also provide the necessary terminology for accessing the literature, and they may suggest related terms or key words found in other sources. For example, an occupational therapist might be interested in measuring performance of ADLs for a given client in a given situation.

One PEO model might include the concept of ADLs in its description, and another conceptual model might use different terms while still emphasizing the importance of this occupation. Terms such as *self-care, daily living skills, self-maintenance,* and *functional performance* may also be used to describe basic occupations of everyday life.

Conceptual and practice perspectives

Conceptual and practice perspectives also provide guidelines for evaluation. Occupational therapy uses concepts, models, theories, and frames of reference to describe ideas that influence the conceptual and practice foundations of the profession. Individual therapists, and most practice settings, adopt beliefs or perspectives that guide clinical reasoning and the occupational therapy process. Regardless of the perspective adopted, therapists must always remember that occupational therapy's unique contribution is a focus on occupational performance (Baum & Law, 1997).

Conceptual and practice perspectives may originate either outside occupational therapy or within the domain of occupational therapy. Reed and Sanderson (1999) described 10 models of health commonly used in occupational therapy practice: biomedical, biopsychosocial, chronicity, holistic, milieu, health education and prevention, health development, wellness, normality, and rehabilitation. Models of occupational therapy are often organized by domains of concern (Reed & Sanderson, 1999), including adaptation, context or ecology, occupation or activity, occupational performance and competence, developmental, prevention, productivity, play or leisure, sensorimotor, cognitive, psychosocial, and professional development.

For example, an occupational therapist may be interested in evaluating the biomechanical characteristics (a sensorimotor domain of concern) that support or limit a person's occupational performance after a hand injury. An examination of this perspective on performance may lead to assessments related to joint range of motion and physical endurance.

Classification systems

Classification systems provide another option for describing the characteristics measured by an assessment. The *ICF* (WHO, 2001) has become an important tool for characterizing people and the environments in which they live. The primary classification areas of the *ICF* are body structure, body function, activity, participation, and contextual factors of the person and environment.

For example, an occupational therapist who needs to assess support systems for occupational performance might find it helpful to look at the *ICF* subcategories under "Support and Relationships." Other classification systems used by occupational therapy practitioners include the *Occupational Therapy Practice Framework: Domain and Process* (American Occupational Therapy Association [AOTA], 2014). The Institute of Medicine (IOM) introduced an alternative classification and model to characterize the complex characteristics of the PEO relationship called the *Modified IOM Model* (Committee on Assessing Rehabilitation Science and Engineering, 1997, p. 68). Enacting any one of these systems in practice guides therapists' choice of an assessment, focusing the identification and selection process.

Assessment Intended Purposes or Uses

After identifying the characteristics of interest and importance, the next step in describing the need for an assessment is determining its *intended purposes* or uses. Initially, it may help to think about the purposes or uses in words that depict a specific situation. For example, one occupational therapist might need an assessment of functional and community mobility for the purpose of discharge planning with a client. In another scenario, an occupational therapy researcher might need an assessment of executive cognitive function to support theory development in Alzheimer's research.

A broad summary of the intended purposes or uses of an assessment will help identify the need in a given situation (Dunn, 2017). Three purposes of assessments are often described in the literature:

1. Description
2. Decision making
3. Theory building.

Assessments used for description clarify and define a person's current needs or performance abilities. If an assessment is needed for decision making, the purpose may be to select interventions, predict future performance, or demonstrate outcomes of services, along with an array of other decisions based on assessment and evaluation results. Theory-building assessments may be part of larger research agendas that support development of the occupational therapy and occupational science knowledge base.

When the intended purpose or use of an assessment involves decision making, the occupational therapist should consider the nature of the decisions that will be made using the assessment (Law & MacDermid, 2017). In some situations, the results of an assessment may be part of decisions that greatly affect people's lives. In occupational therapy, the outcomes of evaluation may contribute to decisions about where a person should live, the driving status of an older person, classroom placement for a child, qualification for specific services, the ability to return to work after an injury, or a person's need for guardianship. In such cases, it is critical to uphold high standards in selecting assessments (Plake, 2002; Tannenbaum & Kane, 2019).

Description of Populations or Clients

Along with identifying the personal characteristics of interest in the evaluation process, it is also important to describe the general *population of clients* who will be evaluated. The population may be described in terms of age, certain demographic characteristics, clinical conditions, special needs, or all of these. This step in defining the needs for a practice setting is necessary because most assessments have been developed for specific populations. When trying to locate assessments, information on the characteristics of the population or functional performance to be evaluated will help in identifying more targeted assessments.

User Qualifications

When examining the need for an assessment in a specific setting, it is important to consider the *qualifications* of the occupational therapist or therapists who will be using the assessment. Users of occupational therapy evaluations have four primary responsibilities:

1. Administration
2. Scoring
3. Interpretation
4. Reporting.

These responsibilities may be carried out by one person or by different people who contribute to the evaluation process.

Several questions can be asked to clarify the user's qualifications:

- What is the therapist's training and educational background with respect to the assessment?
- What experience does the therapist have in the specific evaluation area?
- What level of expertise does the therapist have in administration, scoring, and interpretation in general, as well as with the specific selected assessment
- What professional standards have been established for evaluation in this area?
- What resources are available to obtain additional training in these assessments, if needed?

Some professional associations and test publishers have specific standards related to user qualifications for assessments (College of Occupational Therapists of Ontario, 2016; Turner et al., 2001). Occupational therapists should refer to these standards when describing their qualifications in a specific setting. In addition, some tests require special certification to administer them accurately. Therapists will not be using best practice if they use such tests without the appropriate certification.

Practical Considerations

When selecting an assessment, occupational therapists must consider all the *practical needs* of the setting in which the assessment will be administered, including the format, cost, and time available for an assessment. The options available for the format of an assessment may include observation or performance-based tests, self-report, and written or verbal questionnaires. Some assessments may not cost anything, requiring only the permission of the author for their use. Other assessments may require the purchase of the test itself and an ongoing budget for the training of test users or the acquisition of test booklets, assessment kits, and software.

The time required for the overall evaluation process must also be considered. Some assessments can be completed in a single session, whereas others include an extensive battery of subtests to obtain a complete picture of a person's performance and therefore take a more extended period of time. Also, some assessments might need to be completed over several sessions to get the most accurate picture of a client.

LOCATING EXISTING ASSESSMENTS THAT MEET CURRENT NEEDS

The description of the need for an assessment, as discussed earlier, should be documented and should guide the strategies used for the next step: *locating existing assessments* that meet this need. Several strategies are available for locating information on assessments relevant to occupational therapy.

Investigate Occupational Therapy and Interprofessional Resources

One strategy is to consider disciplines or professions that may have an interest in measuring the identified characteristics. Occupational therapists should always consider instruments within their own profession first and then expand to exploring assessments from related professions that have an interest in the area. OT Search (a database available through the American Occupational Therapy Foundation and AOTA), OTseeker (an Internet site and database that focuses on evidence-based practice in occupational therapy), occupational therapy sourcebooks (e.g., Asher, 2014; Hemphill-Pearson, 2008; Law et al., 2017; Mulligan, 2013; Vroman & Stewart, 2014), and textbooks in occupational therapy are important tools for finding occupational therapy assessments.

Psychology, education, and medicine are secondary areas that may have assessments relevant to occupational therapy. A second strategy is to consider the sources of information on assessments themselves. Libraries have reference books (e.g., *Mental Measurements Yearbook* (Carlson et al., 2017)), databases (e.g., *Health and Psychosocial Instruments* from Behavioral Management Database Services), journals, textbooks, and other materials that can help in locating and critiquing assessments. The Internet has a wide array of sites that provide information on assessment tools (APA, 2019). There are also publishers who specialize in tests and assessments and have developed a reputation for marketing measurement tools with a certain focus, such as Western Psychological Services (Torrance, CA) and Pearson Education (Upper Saddle River, NJ).

Explore Professional Associations and Networks

A third strategy is to use professional connections and networks to keep abreast of changes in assessment and evaluation; these resources may include professional associations, governmental agencies, professional colleagues, and experts in the field. A good identification strategy includes using more than one resource to compare independent reviews.

Reed and Sanderson (1999) reported that occupational therapists use more than 300 assessments in occupational therapy practice. Despite this large number, it is critical that occupational therapists explore sources outside of occupational therapy and occupational science. Reed and Sanderson (1999) have also described knowledge resources for occupational therapy as including biological sciences, social sciences, humanities and the arts, applied sciences (medicine, nursing, physical therapy, social work, and speech pathology), engineering and technology, orthotics and prosthetics, business and management, government, and vocational rehabilitation. *The AOTA Blueprint for Entry-Level Education* (AOTA, 2010) and *The Occupational*

EXHIBIT 3.1.   Sources of Information About Assessments

Occupational Therapy

- *Assessments in Occupational Therapy Mental Health: An Integrative Approach* (Hemphill-Pearson, 2008, 2019)
- CanChild Centre for Childhood Disability Research (http://www.canchild.ca/en/)
- *Measuring Occupational Performance: Supporting Best Practice in Occupational Therapy* (Law et al., 2017)
- *Asher's Occupational Therapy Assessment Tools: An Annotated Index* (Asher, 2014)
- *Occupational Therapy Evaluation for Children: A Pocket Guide* (Mulligan, 2013)
- *Occupational Therapy Assessments for Older Adults: 100 Instruments for Measuring Occupational Performance* (Bortnick, 2017)
- OT Search (American Occupational Therapy Foundation; https://www.aotf.org/Programs/Wilma-L-West-Library-OT-Search)
- OTseeker (http://www.otseeker.com/)

Psychology

- APA Science Directorate (https://www.apa.org/science/programs/testing/find-tests)
- *Mental Measurements Yearbook* (http://buros.unl.edu/buros/jsp/search.jsp)
- PsycINFO (https://www.apa.org/pubs/databases/psycinfo/index)
- PsycTESTS (http://www.apa.org/pubs/databases/psyctests/)

Education

- ERIC/AE Digest (https://www.ericdigests.org/1996-1/test.htm)
- Educational Testing Service Test Collection (http://www.ets.org/test_link/about)

Medicine and Rehabilitation

- CINAHL (https://www.ebscohost.com/nursing/products/cinahl-databases/cinahl-complete)
- Cochrane Library (https://www.cochrane.org/)
- Health and Psychosocial Instruments (https://www.ovid.com/product-details.866.html)
- ISCMR Outcomes Database (https://www.iscmr.org/content/outcomes-database)
- National Quality Forum (http://www.qualityforum.org/Home.aspx)
- NIH Toolbox (http://www.healthmeasures.net/explore-measurement-systems/nih-toolbox)
- PubMed (http://www.ncbi.nlm.nih.gov/pubmed)
- Patient Reported Outcomes Measurement Group (http://phi.uhce.ox.ac.uk/home.php)
- Rehabilitation Measures Database (https://www.sralab.org/rehabilitation-measures)

Competence Model (Polatajko, 1992) also suggest searching within disciplines relevant to

- The person (e.g., psychology, biology, kinesiology and human movement, philosophy, neuroscience, human ethnology),
- The environment (e.g., architecture, forestry, ecology, geography, sociology, political science, economics, social policy, public health), and
- An occupation's interaction with the person, environment, or both (e.g., career development, leisure studies, psychology of play, sports psychology, anthropology, archeology, human geography, human ecology, sociology).

Identify Major Databases or Resources to Locate Assessments

Numerous databases or resources may be helpful in locating assessments. Exhibit 3.1 provides a summary of the most common *resources* in occupational therapy, psychology, education, and medicine. In most disciplines, reference books or databases contain lists and brief descriptions of tests and assessments for relevant domains. These reference books and *databases* are important tools for obtaining both general and specific information on existing assessments. The information provided often includes a description of the assessment, the publisher, supporting research studies, measurement characteristics, and critiques by experts in the field. These resources are helpful for both novice and experienced practitioners who want an efficient and effective way of obtaining key information on assessments. For example, the Rehabilitation Measures Database at the Shirley Ryan Ability Lab (https://www.sralab.org/rehabilitation-measures) has documentation on more than 400 measures used in rehabilitation.

Occupational therapists unfamiliar with these sources of information should initially consult a reference librarian to access these sources and identify other strategies for finding assessments. Some institutions have medical libraries with reference librarians to assist with information location and access. Most academic libraries provide instructions, guides, and website addresses that are helpful for a new user of these sources.

The ability to access information will change rapidly in the future with general access through library databases and search engines such as Google Scholar. Some library databases have specific limiters that may be selected when conducting a search. For example, PsycINFO (TM: Tests and Measures) and ERIC (Tests/Questionnaires) limiters restrict the results of the search to include publications on specific measures used in studies. When using databases that do not have these limiters, consider including a string of assessment keywords (e.g., assessment OR measur* OR test OR outcome) along with the topic keywords when conducting a search. Tutorials on library databases are available and can help develop advanced skills in searching for assessments in peer-reviewed publications.

ANALYZING ASSESSMENT QUALITY: FORMAL METHOD ASSESSMENT

A search for existing assessments may often lead to several matches that meet the needs of a specific situation. The next stage in the selection process is to analyze the overall quality of each assessment using standards and criteria associated with good measurement tools. The *Standards for Educational and Psychological Testing* (American Educational Research Association et al., 2014) provide guidelines for evaluating the quality of tests and testing practices. Although occupational therapists may find it difficult to meet all of these guidelines, they present a model toward which the profession should strive. Most assessment ratings, or critique forms and guidelines, are similar to or based on these standards (Boyt Schell et al., 2019; CanChild Centre for Childhood Disability Research, 2004; Coster, 2013; Law, 2014; Tickle-Degnen, 2014). The standards typically include four parts:

1. Technical standards for test construction and evaluation
2. Professional standards for test use
3. Standards for particular applications (including a section on testing people with disabilities)
4. Standards for administrative procedures (including scoring and interpretation).

To critique an assessment, consider test construction and evaluation, test use, particular applications, and administrative procedures.

Assessment analysis begins with the acquisition of available *documentation* on the assessment. Several resources should be obtained before beginning a critique of an assessment: the technical manual (if available), published summaries and critiques of the assessment, and published research on the assessment. Documentation of the resources used to analyze the quality of an assessment is important because the quality and utility of an assessment may change over time as it is developed further. An assessment may not be selected at one point in time because of its overall quality, but if it evolves into an assessment that meets the specific needs of the evaluation, the occupational therapist may decide to use it.

A formal method of analysis involves two primary steps: (1) description of the assessment as it relates to practice needs and (2) evaluation of the assessment's overall quality (see Exhibit 3.2). The description of the assessment includes the characteristics of interest and importance, the purpose, the population or clients, user qualifications, and practical considerations. Evaluation of the overall quality of the assessment requires the examination of

- The technical manual,
- The method of assessment development and administration,
- Scoring and scales and norms used for interpretation,
- Reliability evidence, and
- Validity evidence.

The *Standards for Educational and Psychological Testing* (American Educational Research Association et al., 2014) and other guidelines provide specific criteria for each of these analysis areas. For example, the National Center for Education Statistics (2002) has stated that the development of an assessment must abide by an explicit set of specifications. These specifications must be clearly documented so that the development of the assessment can be replicated. Examples of specifications include the purpose of the assessment, domain and constructs, outline of the format, number of items, time requirements, context, participant characteristics, psychometric properties, administration and scoring procedures, and reporting of results.

EXHIBIT 3.2.	Formal Method for Analyzing an Assessment			
	SOURCES OF INFORMATION	CHARACTERISTICS AND SUMMARY	CRITIQUE	RECOMMENDATIONS AND COMMENTS
Name and publication information				
Characteristic				
Purpose				
Population or clients				
User qualifications				
Practical considerations				
Technical manual				
Development and administration				
Scores, scales, and norms				
Reliability				
Validity				
Overall				

Testing standards are especially important when high-stakes decisions are made on the basis of the assessment. For such uses, especially in educational settings, it is critical that the assessment be evaluated in terms of its alignment with test specifications, the opportunity to learn, freedom from bias and sensitive situations, developmental appropriateness, score consistency and reliability, and appropriateness of mastery-level cutpoints (Plake, 2002).

Occupational therapists should make good use of *expert critiques* to complete an analysis of the assessment, evaluate its technical standards, and determine its proper and improper use. Sourcebooks and critical reviews in the literature provide expert critiques of commonly used assessments. These critiques summarize the quality of an assessment in key areas and provide recommendations on how the therapist should use the assessment in practice. Tracking the dates of published critiques and more recent studies can give practitioners an indication of an assessment's stage of development, how it has been used in practice, theory development, and outcomes research.

Completing formal analyses of several assessments can help occupational therapy practitioners identify the best assessment for a given situation or setting. It also makes therapists aware of the appropriate uses for an assessment and the cautions that must be taken, given its limitations. These types of summary statements and recommendations about an assessment should be incorporated into the information given during the evaluation process and shared in appropriate ways with both the health care team and the client.

ETHICAL ISSUES RELATED TO ASSESSMENT SELECTION AND USE

Ethical dilemmas occur at every stage of the evaluation process, which is why professional associations adopt and enforce codes of ethics and standards of practice that guide evaluation and practice (AOTA, 2015a, 2015b). Three *ethical issues* are noted here as they relate to the selection and use of assessments. Other responsibilities and values related to ethics and best practice in evaluation are described in Chapter 15, "Ethical Issues in Evaluation."

Unauthorized Use

One pertinent ethical issue relates to the unauthorized use of published and copyrighted assessments. In the past, it was common practice in many health care and education settings to simply copy test manuals and test scoring forms from original publications. It is the responsibility of the assessment user to purchase published assessments directly from the publisher. If an assessment is copyrighted but is not available through a publisher, the user must contact the author and obtain written permission to use the assessment (APA, 2004).

Assessment Users' Qualifications

A second ethical issue relates to the selection of assessments that may not be a good match with the assessment users' qualifications. Some organizations (American Counseling Association, 2003, 2014) provide specific criteria on the qualifications of test users, including knowledge and skills in the following areas:

- Professional practice and relevant theory supporting an assessment
- Testing theory
- Measurement concepts and statistics
- Ability to review, select, and administer appropriate assessments
- Administration and scoring in relation to specific assessments' purposes
- Impact of diversity on accuracy

- Responsible use of assessments and evaluation in diagnosing, predicting future ends, and planning intervention. If the occupational therapist's current qualifications for a given assessment are not adequate, several options may be considered. Therapists may obtain and maintain the additional knowledge and skills required to use the assessment. Sometimes qualifications include earned academic degrees, professional credentials, or certification to administer a specific assessment, so this may not be an effective short-term solution. Alternatively, another assessment with similar characteristics and fewer user restrictions may be chosen, or the assessment may be used for only limited purposes (e.g., screening) with clearly identified cautions against misuse and as part of a larger evaluation process.

Adapting Assessments to Fit Needs

A third ethical dilemma arises when no existing assessments are found in the literature for the needs of a specific practice setting. Unfortunately, a common practice is to create or adapt an assessment that seems to fit the situation. Routinely adopting this approach can set in motion dangerous practices for administering, scoring, and interpreting assessments.

Adapting a standardized assessment will not yield a standard score and may not give the user appropriate information. Keep in mind that assessment and evaluation are powerful tools that either support or refute occupational therapy outcomes, occupational therapy recommendations to clients and other professionals, and the credibility of occupational therapy practice in the larger health care, social service, and educational systems in which practitioners work. The creation or use of "homegrown" assessments, or the adaptation of existing assessments, should be rare in occupational therapy practice and should be accompanied by disclaimers that warn others against inappropriate application and caution in interpreting the results. It is important that major decisions and recommendations regarding clients are never based on these types of assessments alone.

SUMMARY

Assessment identification and selection is an important component of the evaluation process. It is a critical step in the effort to ensure that the results of evaluation are accurate and that the outcomes of interventions are effective and efficient. This chapter introduced a three-stage process for selecting assessments: (1) reflection on the needs in practice, (2) identification of existing assessments that meet those needs, and (3) critical analysis to evaluate the strengths and limitations of assessments and to determine the best assessment for a given situation. Using a formal method to identify and select assessments is one of the best ways to develop confidence in the assessments chosen for evaluation and to gain a professional reputation for excellence in evaluation.

QUESTIONS

1. When planning an assessment of a particular client with stroke. what parameters would you use to choose an assessment? What parameters would be different if the client were a 3-year-old child with Down syndrome?
2. How does the setting or context influence assessment selection?
3. Three purposes of assessment are description. decision making, and theory building. Explain each of these and how they relate to occupational therapy.
4. Go to an online assessment database and select a performance area. What are three appropriate tools for use with an adolescent client?
5. What are the ethical issues related to creating your own assessment method to meet a particular situation? How could you avoid this ethical dilemma?
6. A therapist has suggested that you use a particular assessment for an evaluation. How would you analyze the quality of this assessment? How would you handle the situation if you determined that it was not a quality assessment?

REFERENCES

American Counseling Association. (2003). *Standards for qualifications of test users*. Alexandria, VA: Author. Retrieved from https://www.nbfe.net/resources/Documents/ACA%20Standard%20for%20Qualififications%20of%20Test%20Users.pdf

American Counseling Association. (2014). *2014 ACA code of ethics*. Alexandria, VA: Author. Retrieved from https://www.counseling.org/docs/default-source/ethics/2014-code-of-ethics.pdf?sfvrsn=2d58522c_4

American Educational Research Association, American Psychological Association, & National Council on Measurement in Education. (2014). *Standards for educational and psychological testing*. Washington, DC: American Educational Research Association.

American Occupational Therapy Association. (2010). Blueprint for entry-level education. *American Journal of Occupational Therapy, 64*, 186–203. https://doi.org/10.5014/ajot.64.1.186

American Occupational Therapy Association. (2014). Occupational therapy practice framework: Domain and process (3rd ed.). *American Journal of Occupational Therapy, 68*(Suppl. 1), S1–S48. https://doi.org/10.5014/ajot.2014.682006

American Occupational Therapy Association. (2015a). Occupational therapy code of ethics (2015). *American Journal of Occupational Therapy, 69*, 6913410030. https://doi.org/10.5014/ajot.2015.696S03

American Occupational Therapy Association. (2015b). Standards of practice for occupational therapy. *American Journal of Occupational Therapy, 69*, 6913410057. https://doi.org/10.5014/ajot.2015.696S06

American Psychological Association. (2019). *FAQ: Finding information about psychological tests.* Retrieved from https://www.apa.org/science/programs/testing/find-tests

American Psychological Association, Joint Committee on Testing Practices. (2004). *Code of fair testing practices in education.* Washington, DC: Author. Retrieved from https://www.apa.org/science/programs/testing/fair-testing.pdf

Asher, I. E. (Ed.). (2014). *Asher's occupational therapy assessment tools: An annotated index* (4th ed.) Bethesda, MD: AOTA Press.

Baum, C. M., Christiansen, C. H., & Bass, J. D. (2015). The Person–Environment–Occupation–Performance (PEOP) Model. In C. H. Christiansen, C. M. Baum, & J. Bass (Eds.), *Occupational therapy: Performance, participation, and well-being* (4th ed., pp. 49–55). Thorofare, NJ: Slack.

Baum, C. M., & Law, M. (1997). Occupational therapy practice: Focusing on occupational performance. *American Journal of Occupational Therapy, 51,* 277–288. https://doi.org/10.5014/ajot.51.4.277

Bortnick, K. (2017). *Occupational therapy assessments for older adults: 100 instruments for measuring occupational performance.* Thorofare, NJ: Slack.

Boyt Schell, B. A., Gillen, G., & Scaffa, M. E. (Eds.). (2019). *Willard and Spackman's occupational therapy* (13th ed.). Philadelphia: Wolters Kluwer.

CanChild Centre for Childhood Disability Research. (2004). *Critical review forms and guidelines.* Hamilton, Ontario, Canada: Institute of Applied Health Sciences, McMaster University. Retrieved from https://www.canchild.ca/en/resources/137-critical-review-forms-and-guidelines

Carlson, J. F., Geisinger, K. F., & Jonson, J. L. (2017). *The twentieth mental measurements yearbook.* Lincoln, NE: Buros Institute of Mental Measurements.

College of Occupational Therapists of Ontario. (2016). *Standards for occupational therapy assessments.* Retrieved from https://www.coto.org/docs/default-source/default-document-library/standards_for_occupational_therapy_assessments.pdf?sfvrsn=2

Committee on Assessing Rehabilitation Science and Engineering, Brandt, E. N., & Pope, A. M. (Eds.). (1997). *Enabling America: Assessing the role of rehabilitation science and engineering.* Washington, DC: National Academies Press.

Coster, W. J. (2013). Making the best match: Selecting outcome measures for clinical trials and outcome studies. *American Journal of Occupational Therapy, 67,* 162–170. https://doi.org/10.5014/ajot.2013.006015

Dunn, W. (2017). Measurement concepts and practices. In M. Law, C. Baum, & W. Dunn (Eds.), *Measuring occupational performance: Supporting best practice in occupational therapy* (3rd ed., pp. 17–28). Thorofare, NJ: Slack.

Hemphill-Pearson, B. (2008). *Assessments in occupational therapy mental health: An integrative approach* (2nd ed.). Thorofare, NJ: Slack.

Hemphill-Pearson, B. (2019). *Assessments in occupational therapy mental health: An integrative approach* (3rd ed.). Thorofare, NJ: Slack.

Hinojosa, J., Kramer, P., & Royeen, C. B. (Eds.). (2017). *Perspectives on human occupation: Theories underlying practice* (2nd ed.). Philadelphia: F. A. Davis.

Kielhofner, G. (2007). *Model of human occupation: Theory and application* (4th ed.). Baltimore: Lippincott Williams & Wilkins.

Law, M. (2014). Appendix B—Outcomes measures review: Form and guidelines. In M. Law & J. MacDermid (Eds.), *Evidence-based rehabilitation: A guide to practice* (3rd ed., pp. 339–356). Thorofare, NJ: Slack.

Law, M., Baum, C., & Dunn, W. (Eds.). (2017). *Measuring occupational performance: Supporting best practice in occupational therapy* (3rd ed.). Thorofare, NJ: Slack.

Law, M., Cooper, B. A., Strong, S., Stewart, D., Rigby, P., & Letts, L. (1996). The Person–Environment–Occupation Model: A transactive approach to occupational performance. *Canadian Journal of Occupational Therapy, 63,* 9–22. https://doi.org/10.1177/000841749606300103

Law, M., & MacDermid, J. (2017). Guiding therapist decisions about measuring outcomes in occupational therapy. In M. Law, C. Baum, & W. Dunn (Eds.), *Measuring occupational performance: Supporting best practice in occupational therapy* (3rd ed., pp. 43–58). Thorofare, NJ: Slack.

Mathiowetz, V., & Bass-Haugen, J. (2008). Assessing abilities and capacities: Motor behavior. In M. V. Radomski & C. A. Trombly Latham (Eds.), *Occupational therapy for physical dysfunction* (6th ed., pp. 186–211). Baltimore: Lippincott Williams & Wilkins.

Mulligan, S. (2013). *Occupational therapy evaluation for children: A pocket guide* (2nd ed.). Baltimore: Lippincott Williams & Wilkins.

National Center for Education Statistics. (2002). *NCES statistical standards.* Retrieved from http://nces.ed.gov/statprog/2002/stdtoc.asp

Plake, B. (2002). Evaluating the technical quality of educational tests used for high-stakes decisions. *Measurement and Evaluation in Counseling and Development, 35,* 144–152. https://doi.org/10.1080/07481756.2002.12069059

Polatajko, H. (1992). Naming and framing occupational therapy: A lecture dedicated to the life of Nancy B. *Canadian Journal of Occupational Therapy, 59,* 189–199. https://doi.org/10.1177/000841749205900403

Reed, K. L., & Sanderson, S. N. (1999). *Concepts of occupational therapy* (4th ed.). Baltimore: Lippincott Williams & Wilkins.

Tannenbaum, R. J., & Kane, M. T. (2019). *Stakes in testing: Not a simple dichotomy but a profile of consequences that guides needed evidence of measurement quality* (Research Report No. RR-19-19). Princeton, NJ: Educational Testing Service. Retrieved from https://onlinelibrary.wiley.com/doi/pdf/10.1002/ets2.12255

Tickle-Degnen, L. (2014). Communicating evidence to clients, managers, and funders. In M. Law (Ed.), *Evidence-based rehabilitation: A guide to practice* (3rd ed.). Thorofare, NJ: Slack.

Trombly Latham, C. (2014). Conceptual foundations for practice. In M. V. Radomski & C. A. Trombly Latham (Eds.), *Occupational therapy for physical dysfunction* (7th ed., pp. 1–23). Baltimore: Lippincott Williams & Wilkins.

Turner, S. M., DeMers, S. T., Fox, H. R., & Reed, G. M. (2001). APA's guidelines for test user qualifications: An executive summary. *American Psychologist, 56,* 1099–1113. https://doi.org/10.1037/0003-066X.56.12.1099

Vroman, K., & Stewart, E. (2014). *Occupational therapy evaluation: A pocket guide* (2nd ed.). Philadelphia: Lippincott Williams & Wilkins.

World Health Organization. (2001). *International classification of functioning, disability and health.* Geneva: Author. Retrieved from https://www.who.int/classifications/icf/en/

Practical Aspects of the Evaluation Process

Denise Chisholm, PhD, OTR/L, FAOTA

4

CHAPTER HIGHLIGHTS

- Screening
- Referral
- Assessments
- Environment
- Time
- Teamwork

- Materials
- Documentation
- Accountability
- Participation of occupational therapy assistants
- Professional development

KEY TERMS AND CONCEPTS

- Accountability
- Assessments
- Competence
- Confidentiality
- Documentation
- Effective communication
- Emotional factors
- Employees
- Environment
- Fair treatment

- Independent contractors
- Journal club
- Laws
- Materials
- Mentor
- Mood
- Occupational therapy assistants
- Physical factors
- Preparing clients
- Professional development

- Referral
- Regulations
- Reimbursement models
- Right to privacy
- Screening
- State laws
- Team
- Time-related factors

INTRODUCTION

The increased demands of today's practice environments require that occupational therapists perform evaluations more effectively and efficiently. Evaluation is a complex process that guides occupational therapy intervention and, as such, is an essential component in the provision of high-quality services. Many practical issues related to performing an occupational therapy evaluation can either facilitate or challenge the efficacy and efficiency of the process.

This chapter outlines practical information for the occupational therapist to use to evaluate clients that comprehensively focuses on the priority issues, using quality assessments in the shortest amount of time. Unfortunately, there is no magic recipe; however, occupational therapists with a working knowledge of the evaluation process can use strategies that maximize efficacy and efficiency. This chapter addresses "real-world" practical aspects that affect the evaluation process, including screening, referral, assessments, environment, time, teamwork, materials, documentation, accountability, participation of occupational therapy assistants, and professional development. Most of these issues are applicable across practice environments; however, when appropriate, information related to the unique aspects of specific occupational therapy practice settings is provided.

SCREENING

Many practice settings (e.g., acute care, skilled nursing, long-term-care facilities, schools) include screening before or as a component of the evaluation process. *Screening* is a process that involves review of referrals, available records, observations, and screening tools to determine the need for further, more comprehensive evaluation. Although screening a potential client is typically not a reimbursable service, it can be highly valuable in determining the need for referrals for clients requiring occupational therapy evaluation and intervention, which are reimbursable services. For these reasons, occupational therapists must carefully consider the amount of time and effort dedicated to screening, with the goal of performing screening as efficiently as possible.

The first step is to determine the reasonable or approved time frame for completing the screening of a potential

---

EXHIBIT 4.1. Helpful Hints for Screening

- Screening determines the need for evaluation.
- Screening is typically not a reimbursable service.
- Screening can be highly valuable in generating referrals for reimbursable services.
- Screening is usually no more than one unit of service (about 15 minutes).

---

client for the specific practice setting or facility. Many facilities have a guideline of one unit of service, which is 15 minutes.

The next step is to review available data and interview, observe, or administer a screening instrument to the potential client to determine the need for an occupational therapy evaluation. If obtaining and reviewing data takes longer than 15 minutes, the client almost certainly needs a comprehensive evaluation for occupational therapy services (see Exhibit 4.1). A general rule is if the therapist cannot unequivocally determine that the client could not benefit from occupational therapy services through the screening, then they should initiate a comprehensive evaluation. *State laws* and regulatory codes may address screening, so it is essential that occupational therapists know the rules and regulations set forth by payers in their state. Therapists should have a copy of or quick access to the state laws and regulatory requirements applicable to their facility and practice setting.

REFERRAL

The implementation of occupational therapy services for most practice settings is based on receipt of a *referral,* which is a written order for a specific service. Referral procedures vary on the basis of state and federal laws and the regulatory and payer requirements of the facility or practice setting. Occupational therapists must accept and respond to referrals in compliance with state laws and regulatory codes. Therefore, therapists must have a working knowledge of the laws and regulatory codes that affect practice and understand the interpretation of the rules. Often, the definitions and rules are different for direct services versus indirect services, such as consultation and screening. For example, in Pennsylvania, a referral is not required for an evaluation:

> An occupational therapist may enter a case for the purposes of providing indirect services, consultation, evaluating an individual as to the need for services and other occupational therapy services for conditions such as perceptual, cognitive, sensory integration and similar conditions. Implementation of direct occupational therapy to an individual for a specific medical condition shall be based on a referral from a licensed physician, licensed optometrist, licensed podiatrist, licensed certified registered nurse practitioner or licensed physician assistant (Pennsylvania Occupational Therapy Practice Act of 1982, P. L. 502-140, p. 9).

Occupational therapists must be familiar with the current laws and regulations of the state where they practice. Laws and regulations are distinct. Legislative bodies pass *laws* whereas **regulations** are developed by agencies to implement these laws. Therapists' awareness of the current state of laws and regulations is important because they may change or be revised, and changes in other laws affect current laws. For example, when the Pennsylvania Occupational Therapy Practice Act was originally written, occupational therapists were able to accept referrals only from licensed physicians and podiatrists. However, over the years, the law was amended to include licensed optometrists, and in 2012 licensed nurse practitioners and physician assistants were added to the list of professionals who may refer patients for occupational therapy services in Pennsylvania. Similar licensure changes have occurred in other states. Therefore, therapists should be aware of the laws in their state.

When examining the laws, rules, and regulations, therapists should identify those sections related to the evaluation process (i.e., screening, referral, evaluation, occupational therapy assistants, and supervision of others). Because of the complexity of the language, it is often helpful to discuss these documents with members of professional associations and colleagues, including those within the therapist's own facility and those in the same or similar practice settings.

Occupational therapists need to have a working knowledge of the documents that govern occupational therapy practice. They must establish a system for obtaining updates and revisions. When therapists are unsure about the meaning or interpretation of the content, they should address questions to the boards or agencies overseeing the laws and regulations.

A licensed physician usually writes referrals for occupational therapy services. State laws may also address oral orders (i.e., if and when a referral in the form of an oral order can be accepted) and identify other professionals from whom occupational therapists can accept a referral (e.g., licensed optometrist, licensed podiatrist, certified registered nurse, physician assistant). Occupational therapists need to read each referral form carefully and ensure they address all pertinent areas in the evaluation process and associated documentation.

Occupational therapists also need to ensure that the professionals ordering services understand the unique focus of occupational therapy. It is the responsibility of each therapist to ensure that referral sources understand that the focus of occupational therapy services is on occupations—that is, the "every day activities that people do as individuals, in families and with communities that occupy time and bring meaning and purpose to life" (World Federation of Occupational Therapists, 2012). Referrals must accurately reflect the services being ordered. When they do not, occupational therapists need to identify education opportunities and implement strategies to facilitate the ordering of appropriate services (see Exhibit 4.2).

In pediatric practice settings, a child's parents or guardians must give permission for an occupational therapy evaluation. In the educational setting, a referral usually addresses education issues. Occupational therapists have to be in compliance with the federal law, and the state rules and regulations may differentiate between the need for services to address an educational issue, on the one hand, and a medical need, on the other, and may not require a referral to address problems related to educational issues.

ASSESSMENTS

Occupational therapists can use many assessments in the evaluation process. The difficulty is finding the best ones to address the needs of the client and practice setting. The specific **assessments**—the tools, instruments, or systematic interactions (e.g., observation, interview protocol) used in the evaluation process—should address occupational therapy's unique focus on occupational performance and factors that support occupational performance. Occupational therapists select assessments on the basis of the demographic (e.g., diagnoses, ages, discharge destinations) and occupational performance needs of the client population by considering and prioritizing the relevant occupations, client factors (e.g., body functions, body structures), performance skills and patterns, and contextual and environmental factors.

Additionally, occupational therapists consider the influence of factors related to the practice setting, including reimbursement sources. From this combined information, therapists identify a list or inventory of potential assessments that measure the occupational performance needs of the typical client. From the multitude of possible assessments, they determine the best assessment or assessments to use with a specific client (see Exhibit 4.3).

Occupational therapists need to examine a range of factors when determining the best assessments to use during the evaluation process with clients in their practice setting. The most effective assessment selection method is for two or more therapists to reach agreement through analyzing, discussing, and carefully considering the following information for each assessment:

- Purpose (i.e., what the assessment is intended to measure),
- Theoretical basis,
- Psychometric integrity (e.g., test–retest and interrater reliability; internal consistency; face, criterion-related, construct, and content validity; responsiveness),
- Population (e.g., age, diagnosis, abilities, limitations),
- Setting (e.g., environmental requirements for use and maintenance),

- Degree of measurable objective data obtained,
- Costs (e.g., purchase, training, use, maintenance),
- Time issues (e.g., training and administration, set-up and clean-up, documentation of results),
- Client perception of assessment, and
- Utility (in conjunction with assessments used by other disciplines on the team).

Resources

The process for selecting the most appropriate assessments for a particular client becomes more intuitive and proficient with increased clinical experience; however, both novice and expert occupational therapists can benefit from using assessment resources. The fourth edition of *Asher's Occupational Therapy Assessment Tools: An Annotated Index* (Asher, 2014), which contains profiles of nearly 600 assessments, is useful to therapists choosing appropriate assessments for clinical practice or research purposes. A few other resources are *Occupational Therapy Evaluation for Children: A Pocket Guide* (Mulligan, 2013), *Occupational Therapy Evaluation for Adults: A Pocket Guide* (Vroman & Stewart, 2013), *Measuring Occupational Performance: Supporting Best Practice in Occupational Therapy* (Law et al., 2017), and *Willard & Spackman's Occupational Therapy* (Schell & Gillen, 2018).

Another valuable resource that connects occupational therapists to other occupational therapists in their practice areas is the American Occupational Therapy Association's (AOTA) Special Interest Sections (SISs). The *SIS Quarterly Practice Connections* compendium (a supplement to *OT Practice*), discussion forums on CommunOT (https://communot.aota.org/), and professional networking communities are resources for identifying assessment tools in specific practice areas (e.g., Developmental Disabilities, Children & Youth, Home & Community Health, Mental Health, Productive Aging, Rehabilitation & Disability, Sensory Integration & Processing, Work & Industry).

AOTA also offers publications (e.g., *American Journal of Occupational Therapy, OT Practice*) and an extensive collection of products that occupational therapists can easily search by type (e.g., assessments, books, continuing education, electronic publications, workshops) or topic (e.g., assessment and evaluation, geriatrics, vision, mental health, pediatrics). Multiple databases have also emerged in recent years; Chapter 3, "Assessment Identification and Selection," outlines them in detail.

Occupational therapy educational programs are also an excellent resource for exploration and choice of assessments, because they typically have a wide range of assessments for teaching purposes. Members of the faculty are generally willing to assist their students, alumni, and fieldwork educators with clinical issues, including investigating assessments. Additionally, most faculty members are familiar with the psychometric integrity of the assessments, so they can assist in the interpretation of information. Faculty may also be able to connect therapists who are interested in using the assessments with a network of professional resources.

Psychometric Properties

Reading the assessment manual is paramount to successfully administering and appropriately using the instrument for clinical or research purposes. It is beneficial for occupational therapists to read and reread the assessment manual and relevant literature (i.e., research articles addressing the reliability and validity of the assessment) and to analyze and discuss the information to understand the utility of the instrument for their practice setting. When investigating assessments, therapists should carefully consider the following for each assessment:

- *Purpose of the assessment:* What does the instrument measure?
- *Theoretical approach of the assessment:* Does it match the theoretical approach of the practice setting and facility?
- *Clinical (or research) utility of results:* How can the results be used?
- *Populations for which the assessment was developed:* Do these match the populations to whom the instrument will be administered in the clinical or research setting?
- *Reliability:* How repeatable or consistent is the instrument? To what degree does it yield the same results or measures the same way each time it is administered under the same condition with the same population?
- *Validity:* Does the instrument measure the specific concept it is intended to measure? Are the conclusions, inferences, or propositions correct?

Just because an assessment is published and the authors report good psychometric integrity does not necessarily mean that it actually has good psychometric integrity. Occupational therapists should use resources, including the assessment manual and *Buros Mental Measurements Yearbook* (Carlson et al., 2017), to interpret and better understand the psychometric properties of assessments. Chapter 9, "Psychometric Properties Related to Standardized Assessments," provides detailed information on psychometrics and selecting assessments.

An effective method of learning about the psychometric integrity of assessments is to establish a *journal club* in your practice setting or facility to review publications related to the evaluation process and assessments. The journal club can include staff members and students. It is important to designate specific meetings to address the evaluation process. For example, if the journal club meets monthly, consider having 4 out of the 12 meetings each year address evaluation. The articles selected can address the evaluation of particular diagnostic categories (e.g., stroke, brain injury, developmental disabilities) related to your client population, or they could address a particular assessment.

Participation in a journal club can build the evidence-based skills of those participating. Participants should not merely read and repeat what the author reports but instead should discuss and interpret the assessments' psychometric properties. Practice Guidelines set forth by AOTA (e.g., Wolf & Nilsen, 2015) can also be helpful resources because their condition-specific set of guidelines include recommendations on assessment scales and related literature. Students can be important contributors to and facilitators of journal clubs because of their access to university libraries, time to assess the literature, current evidence-based practice knowledge from coursework, access to faculty who can help them further understand the literature, and access to recent editions of books from their curriculum.

Format

Another consideration is the format of the assessment, which ranges from interviews to paper-and-pencil tests, performance-based tasks, and computerized tests. Occupational therapists should consider which format is best for their population and practice setting. Additionally, therapists must consider which format best measures occupational performance and the components that support the client's occupational performance. Although performance-based measures may take therapists more time to administer, these measures yield objective data related to occupational performance. When choosing assessments, occupational therapists should consider both the quality and the quantity of measurable objective data the assessment yields.

Time

Occupational therapists must be knowledgeable about the time it takes to administer the assessment. This factor is particularly important in evaluation of younger children or people with low endurance or cognitive limitations. Therapists must also consider the amount of time required to set up and clean up the assessment, as well as the time needed to score and interpret it. Ideally, the assessment selected provides the best objective and most useful information in the shortest amount of time. Other time considerations include the amount of time required for both formal and informal training, depending on the requirements of the assessment. Time factors are discussed in greater detail later in this chapter.

Practice Setting Considerations

Although most occupational therapists commonly use particular assessments in their practice setting, they should go through a thoughtful process to select the most appropriate assessments for their clinical population, rather than simply using tools historically used by the facility. It is helpful to have a summary of available assessments.

One effective way of compiling assessment summaries is for occupational therapists to create user-friendly one-page handouts on the best assessment tools (from their "short list") for their client population. Include the complete reference for the assessment and a brief description of the assessment's format, purpose (i.e., what it is intended to measure), populations, length of time for administration, setup and testing criteria, required materials, psychometric properties (i.e., reliability, validity), scoring, and helpful hints or considerations for administration. Additionally, a summary chart of the best assessments used to evaluate a specific area (e.g., basic ADLs, work, perception, strength, fine motor skills) can guide therapists in the selection of the most appropriate assessments for a specific client. A summary chart can include categories such as title of the assessment, purpose, description of the assessment, population or type of clients, method of rating, source, and training.

Facilities and occupational therapists should have the current edition of the assessments they use when evaluating a client. Current editions may have revised normative data that will provide the most up-to-date information on the client. If an outdated version of the assessment is used, the results may not be an accurate measure of the patient's skills.

The facility also should have an established method for obtaining and maintaining literature and resources relevant to using the assessment. For example, a staff member or pair of staff members can provide a staff development session on updates, revisions, or new evidence related to a specific assessment. An evidence-based library of assessments relevant to the practice of the department can be created and maintained (i.e., updated at least annually). Evidence-based activities are great learning assignments for students during fieldwork experiences. As a rule, assessments that obtain objective, clearly defined, quantifiable data are most effective to include in the evaluation process for all populations; however, they are essential when the evaluation helps to determine placement decisions (e.g., school-based programs, discharge planning; see Exhibit 4.4).

The process of creating an evidence-based library of the assessments used in a clinical practice or work site begins with identification of an appropriate organizational structure. The information could be organized by type

of assessment (e.g., performance based, interview, questionnaire), the domain addressed by the assessment (e.g., occupations, performance skills, body functions and body structures, performance patterns, contextual and environmental factors), or age group for which the assessment is designed (e.g., 0–3 years, 3–7 years, 7–12 years, adolescent, adult, older adult). Remember to establish a system for adding new evidence related to the evaluation process and assessments to your library.

ENVIRONMENT

Occupational therapists must carefully consider the environment when selecting appropriate assessments for their facility and when administering the assessments in their clinical practice. *Environment* includes both physical factors (e.g., space, seating, sound, temperature, people, and tasks) and emotional factors (i.e., involve both the client and the therapist).

Physical Environment

Occupational therapists must consider *physical factors,* such as the size and type of space needed and available for administering the assessment. Some assessments may require a large space so the client can perform gross motor movements, whereas other assessments may require tasks to be performed in a kitchen or need a table surface for administration. Occupational therapists must also take into account the type and number of objects and materials needed and available.

Additionally, the arrangement of the objects and materials, including seating, is important. Some assessments require specific objects to be positioned in a precise order. Some assessment manuals state the recommended or required positioning of the therapist and client; for example, the occupational therapist needs to sit across from the client, at a 90° angle, or next to the client.

Occupational therapists must know the environmental requirements of the assessment and identify the optimal environment for administering it. Often, the therapist must modify the clinical setting to create the most favorable environment for administration of the assessment. If the clinical environment does not match the environmental requirements of the assessment, the therapist needs to determine whether modification is permissible. Occupational therapists must be aware that administering an assessment in an alternative or modified environment may result in skewed data and invalidate the results of the evaluation.

Occupational therapists also must attend to the temperature and sound of the environment. The client's perception, needs, and comfort should be the determining factors in adjusting temperature and monitoring sound. Eliminating excess noise and distractions is optimal for administering most, if not all, assessments but is essential for conducting an evaluation with a pediatric client or client with a cognitive disability.

The location of the evaluation depends on the type of practice setting. In some practice settings the evaluation process occurs in a small room, whereas in other settings occupational therapists administer assessments in the client's room or in a clinic area. Ideally, therapists conduct evaluations in a private location to support the client's best

---

EXHIBIT 4.4. Helpful Hints for Assessments

- Use your resources.
  - Peer-reviewed journals
  - Textbooks
  - Professional organization magazines and forums
  - Educational programs and faculty members
  - Establish a journal club
- Determine the best assessments for your client populations and setting.
- Create user-friendly one-page handouts for the best assessments
- Develop a summary chart of assessments related to your client populations.
- Create an evidence-based library.

EXHIBIT 4.5.	Helpful Hints for the Physical Environment

Refer to the assessment manual when considering

- Size and type of space;
- Objects and materials, and their arrangement;
- Seating and positioning of the therapist and the client;
- Temperature;
- Sound;
- People; and
- Complexity, structure, and order of the tasks.

---

performance. Therapists should avoid environments where other people (e.g., practitioners, clients, parents, teachers) are in the area or passing through.

Occupational therapists often have to be creative in selecting a location for the evaluation. For example, a therapist who works in a school environment may consider using the hallways, cafeteria, gymnasium, playground, auditorium stage, or a classroom not in use. Other clinical environments may have a specified area for conducting evaluations.

The number of people present in the environment and their roles can affect the evaluation process and the client's performance. In busy environments, therapists might not obtain the client's best or optimal performance. If a parent or caregiver is present during the evaluation, it may be helpful to ask them to leave the room temporarily, so the therapist can observe the client interact with the environment independently. Therapists should consider the use of a two-way mirror that allows parents (or others) to observe the child (or the client) during the evaluation process without creating undue distractions. Unfortunately, this setup is not always available.

Occupational therapists who work in clients' homes have unique challenges. For example, a therapist who works in early intervention or with older adults often needs to evaluate clients in their homes. If possible, the therapist should request clarification of the evaluation site location before conducting the evaluation. Home environments have many variations that can both positively and negatively affect the evaluation process. Administering assessments in the home requires more spontaneous decision making and flexibility, because therapists do not have the opportunity to preplan or familiarize themselves with the environment before the evaluation session.

Occupational therapists must consider the tasks or items required by the assessment and their relationship with the environment. Therapists should ask,

- How complex are the tasks?
- Are there time limits and restrictions?
- Are the tasks highly structured or loosely organized?
- Do the tasks require a serious atmosphere or encourage a playful mood?
- Is there a social dimension to the tasks?
- Are the tasks more cooperative or competitive?

Occupational therapists must consider the order in which the assessment tasks or items are administered. First and foremost, the therapist must refer to the assessment manual to determine whether there is a standardized format for administration of the tasks. If the assessment specifies the order, the occupational therapist must adhere to

it so that the results are valid. If the order is flexible, then the therapist must determine the most favorable order of administration for the client while taking into account the environmental constraints (see Exhibit 4.5).

Emotional Environment

In addition to the physical factors of the environment, occupational therapists must give special consideration to the environment's *emotional factors*—the mood of both the client and the occupational therapist. Therapists cannot control the mood of the client; however, they can promote and facilitate desired affective behaviors using effective communication strategies. As health care professionals, occupational therapists may need to modify their natural communication style and learn more effective communication techniques. The challenge is for the therapist to change communication styles on the basis of the needs and styles of the client.

Occupational therapists' clinical effectiveness in the evaluation process is directly related to their communication skills. Therapists can learn communication techniques and incorporate effective techniques into their interpersonal style through ongoing self-evaluation, practice, and feedback. All communication has a nonverbal message (i.e., how the therapist conveys the information) in addition to the verbal message (i.e., the information the therapist gives).

Preparing clients and their family members or significant others for the evaluation process is essential. The initial contact with the client at the start of the evaluation session is key to creating a therapeutic atmosphere that communicates trust and caring. Occupational therapists must make sure to provide a thorough, user-friendly orientation to both occupational therapy services and the evaluation process. Clients must understand what the therapist is going to do and what the therapist expects them to do. Clients are typically more involved and invested in the process if they understand how the services and evaluation connect with their health goals.

Regardless of the practice setting, occupational therapists have a tendency to use medical and therapy jargon. Occupational therapists should transform their jargon into user-friendly language for clients and their families. For example, therapists working in an educational setting need to define clearly words such as *proprioception, vestibular, sensory integration, sensory processing,* and *kinesthetic* using plain, nonmedical language. Clear, simple language in this situation will ensure that parents and team members (e.g., teachers, school administrators) understand what the therapist says or writes. Therapists need to accept that preparing the client (including the family and significant others) is an ongoing process and that it is their responsibility to do so to provide high-quality, individualized services.

The *mood* of the occupational therapist is the other half of the emotional factor of the environment. Mood includes the therapist's temperament, how they convey it, and how it influences communication with the client. Therapists' mood can facilitate or hinder desired affective behaviors of the client. Therapists must be aware of their mood, the message they are conveying through their mood, and the effect it has on the therapeutic relationship. Mood is interrelated

EXHIBIT 4.6.	Helpful Hints for the Emotional Environment

- Consider the mood of the client.
- Be aware of your mood as a therapist and its effect on the therapeutic relationship.
- Modify your communication style to facilitate desired affective behaviors in the client.
- Use self-evaluation, practice, and feedback to improve your communication techniques.
- Prepare clients and their families or significant others for the evaluation process.
- Create an atmosphere of trust and caring.
- Avoid the use of medical and therapy jargon when speaking with clients and their families or significant others.

EXHIBIT 4.7.	Helpful Hints for Time

- Know the "time" rules (i.e., state and federal laws and regulatory and payer codes, facility or setting policies) for responding to referrals and for completing evaluations and reevaluations.
- The total time needed for an evaluation includes both the hands-on time for administering the assessment and the time for documentation.

with communication techniques, and the same ongoing process of self-evaluation, practice, and feedback applies to incorporating effective techniques into one's interpersonal style. See Exhibit 4.6 for helpful hints for improving the emotional environment.

TIME

Occupational therapists need to consider *time-related factors*, including the time requirements for responding to the referral for an evaluation, the time it takes to administer the assessments, and the time needed to become proficient in documenting the evaluation results. In today's practice settings, time demands are great and many, so efficiency is essential.

Occupational therapists need to complete the evaluation process in a timely manner. Doing so requires that therapists know the "time" rules (i.e., state and federal laws and regulatory codes, facility or practice setting policies) for evaluations. The timeline for the evaluation process varies by practice setting and facility. Occupational therapists may have 24 hours to respond to and complete the evaluation of a client in an intensive care unit, whereas the timeline for a client in another unit (e.g., acute, skilled, rehabilitation), facility, or practice setting may be within 48 hours, 3 working days, 1 week, or longer. For example, most school-based services have a 60-calendar-day timeline for initial evaluations to be completed and for the interdisciplinary team meeting to be held.

Occupational therapists often complete the evaluation in one session; however, it may be acceptable in some practice settings for an evaluation to take more than one session. Facilities may have a policy regarding the time allotted for the completion of the evaluation. The policy of one facility may be for the evaluation to be completed within a 45-minute session, whereas the policy of another facility may allow up to 1.5 hours.

Additionally, facilities may have policies regarding the time allotted for the occupational therapist to interpret and document the assessment data, as well as to develop and document objective and measurable goals that address targeted outcomes. The documentation format affects the time needed for documenting the evaluation. The time needed to complete electronic documentation is different than the time needed to complete a written narrative or to dictate the evaluation findings.

There are also time differences within formats. The electronic documentation procedure at one facility may be more or less time intensive than that of another facility. Occupational therapists must include both the hands-on time for administering the assessment and the time for documentation when determining the total time needed for the evaluation. For example, if the hands-on component of a pediatric evaluation takes approximately 1.5 hours, including parental consultation time, followed by documentation time of approximately 1 hour, the total time of the evaluation is 2.5 hour. The more complex the assessment is, the more time typically is required for administration and documentation. However, the yield of data regarding the client's occupational performance is typically also greater.

Occupational therapists also need to know the rules and regulations regarding reevaluation. The time frame for reassessment and reevaluation of the plan may vary from weekly to monthly to every 6 months or annually, depending on the practice setting (e.g., outpatient reevaluations are typically completed every 2 to 4 weeks; school-based re-evaluations may be yearly or every 2 or 3 years, with quarterly progress reports). Occupational therapists must be aware that the laws, regulations, and facility policies change, sometimes frequently, so being up to date on the rules that affect one's practice is essential. As previously stated, occupational therapists need to have a working knowledge of the current state and federal laws, regulatory and payer requirements, and facility policies relevant to their practice setting. It is important to consider all of these time factors when determining the total time the occupational therapist needs to perform an evaluation, which is necessary information when coordinating the therapist's and departmental schedule (see Exhibit 4.7).

TEAMWORK

Occupational therapists must remember they are part of a *team.* They do not work with the client in isolation but are members of a team of professionals, each contributing unique services but all focusing on maximizing the health and wellness of the client. Team members may include a physician, nurse, physical therapist, speech–language pathologist, audiologist, psychologist, recreational therapist, dietitian, respiratory therapist, neurologist, or other specialized physicians. In the school setting, the team typically includes a teacher, guidance counselor, case manager, principal, and sometimes the director of special education, in addition to therapy providers.

> **EXHIBIT 4.8.** Helpful Hints for Teamwork
>
> - Each member of the team contributes unique services.
> - All team members focus on maximizing the health and wellness of the client.
> - The client and family are central members of the team.
> - Effective communication is essential.
> - Know the unique contributions of each team member.
> - Ensure that all members of the team understand the unique focus of occupational therapy.

> **EXHIBIT 4.9.** Helpful Hints for Materials
>
> - Determine the materials (general and assessment specific) needed to complete the evaluation.
> - Remember that occupation-based materials usually reflect real-world materials.
> - Organize evaluation materials for efficient access and use.

Central to the team, and also members of the team, are the client and their family (e.g., parent, guardian, spouse, adult child). The communication skills discussed earlier apply not only to interactions with the client and family but also to interactions with all of the team members. Communication among team members may occur in person, in writing, by email, or by phone. Regardless of the format, communication is essential for completion of a comprehensive evaluation. Occupational therapists need to ensure that all members of the team understand the unique focus of occupational therapy and its relevance to the client and other services. No matter how indirect or brief the interaction is, occupational therapists should make sure that everyone with whom they come in contact understands that the focus of occupational therapy services is on occupations.

Each team member needs to know the unique contributions that the other team members add to the comprehensive evaluation of the client. Occupational therapists must ensure that the evaluation process, including the assessments administered, focuses on the client's occupational performance and the underlying factors that affect performance. The evaluation documentation also needs to reflect the unique focus of occupational therapy. See Exhibit 4.8 for helpful hints for fostering teamwork.

MATERIALS

Occupational therapists need to determine the *materials* needed to complete the evaluation, including general materials and materials specifically required for an assessment. Typically, the assessment manual provides a list of required equipment and supplies. The more occupation based the assessment is, the more likely it is that the materials will reflect real-world materials (i.e., objects available in people's homes and for purchase in local retail stores). Examples of these materials include dishes, pots and pans, clothing, banking forms, job applications, and medication bottles. Additionally, clients often use their own materials for occupation-based assessments (e.g., hygiene supplies, clothing, medications).

The evaluation process usually involves general materials, such as paper, pencil, pen, clipboard, watch or stopwatch, tape measure, and magnifying glass. Materials may also relate to the practice setting. For example, when conducting an evaluation in a pediatric practice setting, occupational therapists may use a child-size desk and chair, therapy mat, therapy ball, variety of writing implements (e.g., crayons, pencils, markers, colored pencils), pencil grips, sensory items (e.g., Koosh™ balls, sand, rice, dry beans), paper (e.g., construction, lined, unlined), manipulatives (e.g., stress balls, small objects), scissors (e.g., child sized, right- and left-handed, easy grip), and various age-appropriate toys.

Occupational therapists should organize evaluation materials for the most efficient access and use. In a setting where several occupational therapists use the same assessments, give careful thought to methods for storing and maintaining assessment materials. As with all equipment and supplies, it is beneficial to establish a system for determining who currently has an assessment and its materials, how the assessment and materials are maintained, and who is responsible for monitoring the system.

Evaluation equipment and materials are often stored in plastic bins, canvas or lightweight portable bags, or small rolling upright suitcases. Occupational therapists working in settings that require them to transport materials from site to site (e.g., home or school settings) often use lightweight portable file boxes to keep files and equipment organized in a car trunk. Some therapists organize supplies alphabetically by the days of the week, whereas other therapists use different colors for each school or program site. Additionally, accordion file folders organized by month, Excel spreadsheets, and book or smartphone calendars are all helpful in keeping track of evaluation due dates and assessment materials. General and organizational supplies and storage containers are available at many retail, sporting goods, discount, and office supply stores. Before starting an evaluation, therapists need to make sure that all the necessary materials are available (see Exhibit 4.9).

DOCUMENTATION

When occupational therapists provide a skilled service to a client, they must document the services provided. *Documentation* in the form of a well-written and comprehensive evaluation report is essential because it articulates the rationale for providing occupational therapy services and connects the services to the client's targeted outcomes. Chapter 11, "Interpretation and Documentation of the Evaluation Process," provides a more in-depth discussion on documentation.

In practical considerations for documentation, occupational therapists need to know and understand the state and federal laws, the regulatory and payer requirements of the practice setting, and the facility policies regarding documentation. Therapists also need to be mindful of the type of practice setting, service model, and theoretical perspective of the facility or setting when writing evaluation reports. Knowing the focus of the practice setting is important because it directs the focus and language of the report. Hospital-based and outpatient settings are typically more medically driven, whereas community and school-based settings usually focus on social, family, and education issues.

Service Model Considerations

The link between documentation and the service model is particularly important in pediatric practice settings. For example, occupational therapists providing early intervention services need to know whether the services in their state are medical based or education based, because the service model varies from state to state. Early intervention services are both family driven and family focused; thus, the family is the primary service model, and the early intervention evaluation focuses on issues that affect both the child and the family (Nanof & Schefkind, 2008).

Occupational therapists who evaluate preschool children (ages 3–5 years) generally administer the assessments in a preschool setting, although occasionally they may administer them in the child's home. When services occur in a setting outside of the home, the family is no longer the primary area of concentration but instead is now a secondary service area. The family always remains important, but when writing the evaluation report, therapists must recognize this shift of evaluation and service philosophy, because the evaluation content now focuses primarily on educational issues, and family issues become secondary.

Another example is the need for therapists evaluating school-age children (ages 6–21 years) to focus their documentation on facilitating educational access to the school environment. An appropriate evaluation in a school setting addresses how the student can successfully access the educational environment (in accordance with the Individuals With Disabilities Education Improvement Act of 2004; P. L. 108-446). Parental input is always important, because parents are vital members of the team; however, concentration on school-based issues remains the top priority in school-based evaluations. Sometimes therapists provide supplemental school services in addition to education-based programs; however, they should get clarification from the school-based work site program supervisor regarding the roles of private outpatient and medical-based services before completing an evaluation.

Recommendations, including frequency and duration of services, are also dependent on the type of practice setting. In a pediatric practice setting, it is helpful to begin by asking the work site supervisor about

- The service philosophy regarding treatment frequency;
- Consultation in addition to direct service;
- Involvement of professionals external to the practice setting;
- Parental involvement;
- Team members and their collaborative roles;
- Potential use of instructional aides; and
- The need for nurses if dealing with a child's medical condition, assistive devices, and supplemental equipment and training needs.

It is important that therapists understand all of these issues before writing the evaluation report and providing recommendations. Parents are often confused when they concurrently receive a report from a medical-based outpatient facility and another report from a school-based program. The two sites have differing service philosophies, and billing practices and legal mandates must be explained clearly to the parents and team when service needs are determined for the child. Having a clear understanding of the roles and responsibilities of the evaluating occupational therapists before the evaluation is completed helps make the process smooth and manageable.

Evaluation Reports

The *Guidelines for Documentation of Occupational Therapy* (AOTA, 2018) is a good resource for determining what information to include in an evaluation report. According to the AOTA guidelines, an evaluation report should include client information; referral information; the client's occupational profile; the assessments used and results; an analysis of occupational performance; analysis, interpretation, and summary of the findings; identification of targeted areas of occupation and occupational performance to be addressed; and recommendations regarding necessity for skilled occupational therapy services.

Occupational therapists need to consider the people who read their evaluation reports. The readers likely include a range of health professionals on the team (e.g., physician, nurse, physical therapist, speech–language pathologist, audiologist, psychologist, recreational therapist, dietitian, respiratory therapist, neurologist, other specialized physician); in school-based practice, readers also include numerous education staff (e.g., teacher, guidance counselor, case manager, principal, director of special education). Other readers are the client and family. Another important reader in most practice settings is the payer source. Readers review the evaluation report from their perspective, looking for elements relevant to their specific role in the client's services.

Occupational therapists need to ensure the evaluation report addresses the content the readers expect to see in an occupational therapy evaluation. The challenge is to complete the evaluation report in the most efficient yet comprehensive manner. Therapists need to read their documentation through the eyes of those who will be reading it—people who are not occupational therapists. Therapists need to consider how these readers will interpret the

---

EXHIBIT 4.10. Helpful Hints for Documentation

- Understand that the evaluation report must articulate the rationale for occupational therapy services and connect the services to the client's targeted outcomes.
- Know the laws and regulatory requirements of the practice setting and facility policies regarding documentation.
- Consider the service model when documenting. This is particularly important in pediatric practice settings.
- Use the *Guidelines for Documentation of Occupational Therapy* (AOTA, 2018), which is a good resource.
- Consider the people who read the evaluation report (e.g., other health professionals on the team, education staff, client, family, reimbursement sources).
- Use user-friendly language (i.e., avoid or clearly define medical and educational jargon and acronyms).

information. Just because the report seems clear to the writer and is likely to be clear to other occupational therapists does not mean that the information is understandable to other readers of the report. Similar to when therapists verbally communicate with other team members, when they communicate in writing they need to use user-friendly language by avoiding or clearly defining medical and educational jargon and acronyms. See Exhibit 4.10 for helpful hints regarding documentation.

ACCOUNTABILITY

Accountability means that each occupational therapist is responsible for the services they provide. Accountability includes promoting and maintaining high standards of conduct (AOTA, 2015a). Practical considerations related to accountability apply to a range of professional behaviors, including, but not limited to, truthfulness and honesty, respect, communication, competence, confidentiality, and reimbursement (AOTA, 2015a). Occupational therapists must provide services that are within their level of competence and scope of practice.

Truthfulness

The occupational therapy evaluation may reveal needs of the client that are not within the scope of occupational therapy practice or the expertise of the therapist. If so, and when appropriate, a therapist needs to refer the client to other health care providers. The evaluation report must accurately describe the type and duration of the services provided. Additionally, therapists must inform the client truthfully of the results of the evaluation and the risks and benefits associated with the recommendations.

Communication

Effective communication is an important professional behavior. Occupational therapists need to be truthful, candid, and honest in all aspects of communication, including written, verbal, and electronic forms. *Effective communication* includes honest statements; adherence to applicable laws, guidelines, and regulations; accurate documentation; and avoidance of biased or derogatory language.

Competence

Competence includes maintaining and increasing proficiency and also recognizing the therapist's current level of skill (AOTA, 2015b). Occupational therapists need to take responsibility for maintaining high standards by taking responsible steps through appropriate education and training to ensure their competency when incorporating new assessments into their practice.

Privacy

Occupational therapists are accountable for ensuring that *confidentiality* and the *right to privacy* are respected and maintained for recipients of their services. Information obtained during or associated with the evaluation process is protected information, and therapists must maintain its confidentiality. They must maintain the confidentiality of

all verbal, written, electronic, augmentative, and nonverbal communication, as required by the Health Insurance Portability and Accountability Act of 1996 Privacy Rule (P. L. 104-191) and the Family Educational Rights and Privacy Act of 1974 (P. L. 93-380), also known as the Buckley Amendment.

Occupational therapists working in pediatric settings must be mindful that privacy rules prohibit them from communicating with professionals outside the immediate service agency unless a parent has given specific written permission. As a rule, therapists should consult with their supervisor or administrator to ensure an understanding of the privacy restrictions related to initiating communication with other professionals.

It is important to maintain the privacy of clients (e.g., keeping names covered on files left on a desk in an office or on a table in the clinic). Therapists working in school-, home-, and other community-based practice settings may be required to transport client files in their own car. These confidential files must be protected by being concealed and locked in the vehicle. Additionally, electronic communication must be protected (e.g., using only initials in the subject line of an email rather than the client's full name).

Occupational therapists need to follow their work site's privacy procedures regarding the deletion of electronic files. Therapists must consider privacy rules when responding to or acknowledging clients both within and outside of the therapy setting. It can be helpful to ask clients during the evaluation session how they would like to be recognized (or not recognized) when seen outside of therapy. For example, some older children do not like their therapists to acknowledge them when they are with their peers.

Fair Treatment

Accountability also includes guaranteeing *fair treatment.* Occupational therapists need to ensure that the evaluation services provided are fair and equitable and that the fee for an evaluation is reasonable and commensurate with the service performed. To ensure fair treatment, therapists need to be accountable for their time. They need to keep track of evaluation time, including direct hands-on time and indirect documentation time. Depending on the practice setting, therapists also may be required to keep track of the time spent in consultation with parents, family, and team members as well as the travel time associated with an evaluation. Therapists should record their time daily, typically in 5- to 15-minute increments, depending on the setting.

Paperwork Submission

Submitting paperwork, including the paperwork associated with billing, is an essential professional task. Paperwork may need to be submitted daily, weekly, or monthly. Regardless of the time requirement, therapists need to submit paperwork on time. There are federal, state, agency, and facility rules regarding the length of time copies of client records, including evaluation reports and associated time and billing reports, must be retained. The typical standard for retaining records is a minimum of 3 years; however, therapists should confirm the appropriate length of time to retain records with their work site supervisor or administrator and follow the procedures accordingly. Although this chapter focuses on the evaluation process, the practical considerations associated with accountability relate to services across the occupational therapy process, not just the evaluation.

Employment Role

In addition to being accountable for the services provided, occupational therapists are also accountable for understanding their employment role. Two basic *reimbursement models* of services are (1) employee and (2) independent contractor. The Internal Revenue Service has specific rules regarding these two reimbursement models. Essentially, *employees* receive a salary and benefits and work a prescribed number of hours each week, whereas independent contractors determine their own schedule. *Independent contractors* have flexibility regarding their caseload and traditionally receive a higher hourly reimbursement rate than employees because independent contractors are responsible for their own benefits and tax payments.

In each employment role scenario, it is important that occupational therapists be clear about how they are being reimbursed for services. Occupational therapists must know and understand the implications if being paid by the hour for providing direct and indirect occupational therapy services (which includes evaluations) or if being paid a flat sum for an all-inclusive evaluation session.

Travel Reimbursement

Another employment consideration for which occupational therapists are accountable is reimbursement for travel. This is an important issue, particularly in pediatric and home-care practice settings. Therapists need to clarify travel reimbursement before they engage in the evaluation process. Typically, agencies do not reimburse therapists' travel when they drive to and from their home, because this type of travel is considered commuting to and from the work site. However, agencies may reimburse travel time or mileage if a therapist is driving between evaluation or intervention sessions on the same day and for the same agency. Therapists in practice settings requiring travel to and from multiple work sites should keep track of travel time by using a paper or electronic travel log.

Occupational therapists who work as independent contractors should consult with a certified public accountant to assist with appropriate tax and expense filing requirements. Independent contractors should also ask their agency supervisor or administrator about the availability and type of assessment tools available for use, on-site equipment and supplies, evaluation formats and content requirements, mentoring for evaluation education and training, and documentation requirements (Margow, 2019). Independent contractors may be responsible for purchasing and maintaining their own assessment tools, whereas for employees, the facility generally provides all the required materials for the evaluation process. However, independent contractors may be able to deduct some

of their expenses from their taxes. Consideration of these issues can assist therapists in determining the most appropriate employment reimbursement model for their needs (see Exhibit 4.11).

PARTICIPATION OF OCCUPATIONAL THERAPY ASSISTANTS

Occupational therapy assistants are valuable members of the team. Occupational therapists and occupational therapy assistants must know their roles and their contribution to each component of the occupational therapy process, including the evaluation process. AOTA's (2015c) *Standards of Practice for Occupational Therapy* states that

> an occupational therapy assistant contributes to the screening, evaluation, and reevaluation process by administering delegated assessments and by providing verbal and written reports of observations and client capacities to the occupational therapist in accordance with federal and state laws, other regulatory and payer requirements, and AOTA documents. (p. 664)

Occupational therapists and occupational therapy assistants need to know and adhere to the state and federal laws and the regulatory and payer requirements of their facility and practice setting, including the rules governing the involvement of occupational therapy assistants in the evaluation process and the supervision requirements for occupational therapy assistants. Chapter 1, "Evaluation: Where Do We Begin?" discusses this in detail.

PROFESSIONAL DEVELOPMENT

Occupational therapists need to pursue *professional development* activities to ensure their own competency in performance of the evaluation process (Davis, 2019). Mentorship is a valuable professional development activity, especially for entry-level occupational therapists or therapists new to a practice setting (Gilfoyle et al., 2011). A *mentor* can assist a therapist in identifying strategies to obtain education and training in the evaluation process, including

---

EXHIBIT 4.11. Helpful Hints for Accountability

- Provide services within your level of competence and scope of practice.
- When appropriate, refer clients to other health care providers.
- Write reports that accurately describe the type and duration of services provided.
- Be truthful, candid, and honest in all aspects of communication.
- Ensure your competency by seeking out appropriate education and training.
- Ensure the client's confidentiality and right to privacy.
- Guarantee fair treatment to all clients.
- Know the time factors related to the services you provide, and keep track of them, as needed.
- Understand your employment role (employee vs. independent contractor).

the administration of specific assessments. The strategies may include review of specific evaluation guidelines and opportunities to observe the evaluation process. The mentor does not need to have expertise in the administration of a specialized evaluation, such as a sensory processing evaluation, that the therapist wants or needs to learn; however, the mentor can connect the therapist with other occupational therapists with expertise in that area. Mentors also can provide support for managing clients with challenging behaviors during the evaluation process.

Occupational therapists may request mentorship many times throughout their career, including when they are entry level; when transitioning to a new practice setting, facility, or agency; and when learning a new evaluation process or assessment. Mentoring is an effective professional development activity to enhance a therapist's knowledge and skills. Remember that mentoring is advantageous for both the mentee and the mentor, because both grow professionally.

Being a member of AOTA and a state occupational therapy association can offer therapists many opportunities for continued professional development and updates on regulations. If one uses the resources provided by these organizations, further professional development can be promoted. Therapists can also attend national and state education events, including annual conferences, which typically offer presentations in all practice areas and workshops for specialized content areas. Association members typically receive a reduced registration rate. Additionally, professional associations offer a range of continuing education opportunities, including a variety of publications and online courses. These resources address a variety of practice areas and issues, including topics related to the evaluation process. Therapists can also consider pursuing specialty certifications in a practice area.

EXHIBIT 4.12.	Helpful Hints for Professional Development

- Know that you are responsible for your own competency.
- Understand that mentorship is valuable and advantageous for both the mentee and the mentor.
- Be an active member in professional organizations.
- Use your resources, such as attending conferences and continuing education events, reading publications, and participating in a discussion form.

Another example is the use of discussion forums related to practice areas on CommunOT (https://communot.aota.org). Such discussions are a great place to post questions related to the evaluation process and assessments. These forums give occupational therapists the opportunity to receive feedback from therapists across the country and are a great resource for finding a mentor and connecting with experts in the field. See Exhibit 4.12 for helpful hints for maximizing professional development.

SUMMARY

The goal of occupational therapists is to provide high-quality evaluation services in the most effective and efficient manner. To do so, they must be aware of the current laws and regulatory requirements of their practice area and specific facility policies. They also need to seek out and use professional resources to enhance their competence in performing evaluations. Therapists with an understanding of the practical aspects associated with the evaluation process are better able to identify and implement strategies to maximize proficiency in the evaluation process.

QUESTIONS

1. What would you do if you had questions regarding a rule or regulation related to a referral for an occupational therapy evaluation?
2. What specific steps would you include in the identification, selection, and analysis of assessment tools? What resources are available to assist you in identifying, selecting, and analyzing potential assessments for your practice setting?
3. Describe the teaching methods you would use to ensure that you are competent in administering, scoring, and documenting the results of a new assessment. What strategies would you implement on an ongoing basis to maintain current knowledge about the assessment?
4. Identify two positive features and two negative features of the physical environment that affect the evaluation process. How can you improve the physical environment during an evaluation?
5. What can you do to positively influence the emotional environment during the evaluation process?
6. Describe the unique focus of occupational therapy in the evaluation process and its relevance to the services provided in client care. How would your description of the occupational therapy evaluation process change when speaking with a nurse, a physical therapist, a teacher, or a family member?
7. Identify at least three readers of your evaluation report and the content each reader expects to see in it. Review an occupational therapy evaluation report through the eyes of those reading it. What are two aspects of the documentation that could be changed to make the information more understandable to readers of the report?
8. Identify at least two professional development activities you can pursue to maintain your competency in performance of the evaluation process. What strategies could you use to find a mentor?

REFERENCES

American Occupational Therapy Association. (2015a). Occupational therapy code of ethics (2015). *American Journal of Occupational Therapy, 69*(Suppl. 3), 6913410030. https://doi.org/10.5014/ajot.2015.696S03

American Occupational Thearpy Association. (2015b). Standards for continuing competence. *American Journal of Occupational Therapy, 69*(Suppl. 3), 6913410055. https://doi.org/10.5014/ajot.2015.696S16

American Occupational Therapy Association. (2015c). Standards of practice for occupational therapy. *American Journal of Occupational Therapy, 69*(Suppl. 3), 6913410057. https://doi.org/10.5014/ajot.2015.696S06

American Occupational Therapy Association. (2018). Guidelines for documentation of occupational therapy. *American Journal of Occupational Therapy, 72*(Suppl. 2), 7212410010. https://doi.org/10.5014/ajot.2018.72S203

Asher, I. E. (Ed.). (2014). *Asher's occupational therapy assessment tools: An annotated index* (4th ed.). Bethesda, MD: AOTA Press.

Carlson, J. F., Geisinger, K. F., & Jonson, J. L. (Eds.). (2017). *Buros mental measurements yearbook* (20th ed.). Lincoln, NE: University of Nebraska Press.

Davis, S. (2019). Professional development. In K. Jacobs & G. L. McCormack (Eds.), *The occupational therapy manager* (6th ed., pp. 659–667). Bethesda, MD: AOTA Press.

Family Educational Rights and Privacy Act of 1974, Pub. L. 93–380, 20 U.S.C. § 1232g; 34 CFR Part 99.

Gilfoyle, E., Grady, A., & Nielson, C. (2011). *Mentoring leaders: The power of storytelling for building leadership in health care and education.* Bethesda, MD: AOTA Press.

Health Insurance Portability and Accountability Act of 1996 (HIPAA), Pub. L. 104–191, 42 U.S.C. § 300gg, 29 U.S.C §§ 1181–1183, and 42 U.S.C. §§ 1320d–1320d9.

Individuals With Disabilities Education Improvement Act of 2004, Pub. L. 108–446, renamed the Individuals With Disabilities Education Improvement Act, codified at 20 U.S.C. §§ 1400–1482.

Law, M., Baum, C., & Dunn, W. (2017). *Measuring occupational performance: Supporting best practice in occupational therapy* (3rd ed.). Thorofare, NJ: SLACK.

Margow, S. (2019). Becoming a successful contractor. In K. Jacobs & G. L. McCormack (Eds.), *The occupational therapy manager* (6th ed., pp. 651–658). Bethesda, MD: AOTA Press.

Mulligan, S. (2013). *Occupational therapy evaluation for children: A pocket guide* (2nd ed.). Philadelphia: Lippincott Williams & Wilkins.

Nanof, T., & Schefkind, S. (2008). *IDEA overview and early intervention practice.* Paper presented at the American Occupational Therapy Association Annual Conference & Expo, Long Beach, CA.

Pennsylvania Occupational Therapy Practice Act of 1982, Pub. L. 502–140, S.G. §174.1.

Schell, B. A., & Gillen, G. (Eds.). (2018). *Willard and Spackman's occupational therapy* (13th ed.). Philadelphia: Lippincott Williams & Wilkins.

Vroman, K. G., & Stewart, E. (2013). *Occupational therapy evaluation for adults: A pocket guide* (2nd ed.). Philadelphia: Lippincott Williams & Wilkins.

Wolf, T. J., & Nilsen, D. M. (2015). *Occupational therapy practice guidelines for adults with stroke.* Bethesda, MD: AOTA Press.

World Federation of Occupational Therapists. (2012). *WFOT definition of occupational therapy.* Retrieved from https://www.wfot.org/resources/definitions-of-occupational-therapy-from-member-organisations

Evaluation in the Intervention Planning Process

5

Lou Ann Griswold, PhD, OTR/L, FAOTA

CHAPTER HIGHLIGHTS

- Evaluation process focusing on occupation
- Evaluation leading to intervention planning
- Reassessment throughout the intervention process
- Documentation of evaluation results
- Types of assessments
- Evaluation in context: Pragmatic issues of evaluation
- Learning a new assessment
- Therapeutic use of self during evaluation

KEY TERMS AND CONCEPTS

- Arena assessment
- Compensatory approach
- Criterion-referenced assessment
- Documentation
- Evaluation
- Intervention plan
- Intervention process
- Nonstandardized assessments
- Norm-referenced assessment
- Occupational performance analysis
- Occupational profile
- Occupational roles
- Reassessment
- Reimbursement
- Restorative approach
- Review phase
- Skill acquisition approach
- Standardized assessments
- Therapeutic use of self

INTRODUCTION

Occupational therapists strive to enhance clients' occupational performance and participation in activities that are important to them. Therapists determine where to begin and how best to support a client through evaluation. The evaluation process answers many of the questions occupational therapists have about their clients and enables them to plan the intervention. Evaluation guides therapists in considering what is important to the client, reflecting client-centered services. Furthermore, evaluation establishes a baseline for performance against which therapists can measure the effectiveness of intervention. Occupational therapists emphasize occupation throughout evaluation, highlighting the unique contribution of occupational therapy to improve clients' participation in occupations.

This chapter describes how evaluation informs decision making from the first contact with a client through the intervention process. In particular, the chapter helps occupational therapists

- Focus evaluation on occupation,
- Use evaluation results to plan intervention,
- Identify how frames of reference and pragmatic reasoning influence the evaluation process,
- Differentiate types of assessments, and
- Maintain a focus on occupation when documenting evaluation results.

The chapter introduces assessment options in the context of intervention planning, particularly the purpose of assessments and the intended use of the information gathered. Several case examples illustrate the relationship between evaluation and intervention and allow for examination of the pragmatic issues, determined by the context, that influence evaluation and intervention. Occupational therapists are then encouraged to continue to update their knowledge and skills in assessments, and a process for learning administration of new assessments is suggested. The chapter concludes with a discussion of therapeutic use of self during evaluation.

EVALUATION PROCESS FOCUSING ON OCCUPATION

Occupational therapists evaluate clients' occupational performance, which centers on clients' ability to engage in desired occupations. *Evaluation* refers to the process of gathering information about a client. Mulligan (2014) also recognized that evaluation is a thought process. This point

---

https://doi.org/10.7139/2020.978-1-56900-596-5.005

is important because it reflects the occupational therapist's clinical reasoning used throughout the evaluation process.

One might logically assume that evaluation precedes intervention. The *Occupational Therapy Practice Framework: Domain and Process* (OTPF; American Occupational Therapy Association [AOTA], 2014) identified evaluation as the first phase in the occupational therapy intervention process. In reality, occupational therapists continue to gather information about their clients throughout all phases of the intervention process, as they learn more about the client and their needs, desires, and abilities and observe the client's performance and response to intervention (Vroman & Stewart, 2014).

The purpose and timing of the evaluation determine the type of data collected and the assessment instruments or measures used (Ideishi, 2003; Weinstock-Zlotnick & Hinojosa, 2004). When conducted at the beginning of a therapeutic relationship with a client, evaluation provides information to guide decision making regarding occupational therapy services and leads to intervention, beginning with planning and continuing through implementation of intervention and review of the client's progress. Evaluation is also connected clearly to outcomes; during the evaluation process, the client identifies desired outcomes, which are then revisited at the conclusion of therapy.

EVALUATION LEADING TO INTERVENTION PLANNING

Occupational therapists synthesize evaluation findings to develop an *intervention plan,* which is a series of steps or a program designed to advance the client toward achievement of goals. Therapists develop a plan by considering evaluation data with information about clients' motivation, prognosis, resources, and personal goals. Evaluation data serve as the groundwork upon which therapists develop an appropriate evaluation plan.

Getting to know the client as a person is a critical step in the evaluation process (AOTA, 2014; Brown, 2009; Fisher & Marterella, 2019; Hocking, 2001; Mulligan, 2014; Vroman & Stewart, 2014). Identifying the activities the client likes to do currently, enjoyed doing in the past, and would like to do in the future enables the therapist to know what is important to the client. Learning the client's history gives the therapist information about patterns of behavior and strengths or interests that might be useful in therapy.

Understanding the client as an occupational being and the occupations that are important to them focuses intervention and identifies goals that are meaningful to the client (Brown, 2009). Knowing the client as an occupational being also enables therapists to predict more accurately the outcome of occupational therapy intervention (Simmons et al., 2000). At times, family members or others who are close to the client (e.g., teachers) provide information to enable the therapist to understand the client, especially in work with children (Mulligan, 2014) but often with clients of all ages (Fisher & Griswold, 2018). During the initial phase of evaluation, occupational therapists strive to understand the client as a person: the context in which they live, work, and play; their perceived strengths and needs related to occupational performance; and their desired goals for occupational engagement (Fisher & Marterella, 2019).

Learning about the client as a person includes identifying their *occupational roles,* which are an individual's playful and productive behaviors that define who the individual is. Roles often indicate what the client values and suggest possible tasks that are important in supporting the identified roles. The therapist then can explore which tasks are easy and which are difficult for the client to perform. Learning the client's perspective about how the environment supports or hinders their roles and tasks further enables the therapist to understand more about the person and their natural contexts (Fisher & Marterella, 2019).

While learning about the client from their perspective, occupational therapists help clients to identify their priorities and goals for occupational therapy—what the client would like to do or do better. The gathered information then guides the occupational therapist to know the focus of the occupational performance analysis, the next phase of evaluation. *Occupational performance analysis* is a method of observation of a person doing an occupation to determine their strengths and weakness. The analysis subsequently leads to intervention planning. Using the identified process helps promote occupation-focused practice. Case Example 5.1 illustrates these points as Jean, the occupational therapist, receives a referral from her team members in a community mental health center.

INTERVENTION PLANNING

Once goals have been collaboratively established, the occupational therapist and client begin to work together to consider options for an intervention plan. The *intervention process* consists of three steps:
1. Planning,
2. Implementation, and
3. Review (AOTA, 2014).

The evaluation process continues throughout intervention, as the therapist monitors the client's responses and modifies the intervention as needed. Thus, the occupational therapist reassesses the client's progress toward goals to determine whether the intervention is effective or whether an intervention plan needs to be modified. Because of the explicit link between evaluation and intervention, it is helpful to consider how evaluation informs each step of the intervention process.

Planning Phase

Evaluation is tied most closely to planning an intervention. An intervention plan draws on the information gathered during the evaluation phase, particularly the client's desired outcomes of therapy and identified goals for therapy. Intervention planning also includes the approach to be used and details of service delivery (AOTA, 2014). As illustrated in the case example of Tonya and Jean (Case Example 5.1), occupational therapists base the intervention plan on the client's desired outcomes and occupational goals to support participation in meaningful life activities (Brown, 2009; Hinojosa et al., 2003, 2017).

Desired outcomes vary in nature and specificity across clients. Examples of desired outcomes for clients at different ages and with various types of disabilities and needs might include:

CASE EXAMPLE 5.1. JEAN AND TONYA: OCCUPATION-FOCUSED PRACTICE

Jean, an occupational therapist, worked in a community outpatient mental health center. **Tonya** sought help through the mental health center because she was feeling "depressed and alone."

During an initial occupational therapy interview, Tonya identified her primary role at this time as a mother of two toddler-age children. She listed the tasks that supported this role as preparing snacks and meals, cleaning, playing with her children, and supporting and fostering their development.

Tonya felt that she was not doing these tasks well; for example, she often started to prepare a meal but then became distracted and changed her plans. She stated that the meals she prepared were not nutritionally complete and that her house was "forever a mess." She stated that she did not feel she really played with the children but rather only watched them.

Tonya had wanted to have children and stay at home with them while they were young, but now she felt isolated. She said that she was not as motivated to keep up with the housework and meal preparation as she would have liked. Tonya acknowledged that she had little enthusiasm to perform the activities she knew were important to her as a mother. She was married, but her husband was out of town 4 days per week for work. She and her family lived on the outskirts of a small town.

Jean learned that Tonya had been in drama clubs during high school and college and enjoyed that period of her life. Further exploration revealed that Tonya liked not only the acting but also the energy level she felt when in contact with large groups of people. Tonya recalled that in college, her grades improved as the pressures of a theater production increased.

Before her children were born, Tonya worked as a kindergarten teacher, where she felt she was able to use her artistic talents in many ways to promote her students' development. Jean listened as Tonya talked about her past, present, and dreams for the future. Tonya said that she would like to be around other people but did not want to be employed while her children were young. She stated she wanted to feel that she was "doing something worthwhile with her life." She also wanted to do a better job caring for her children's daily needs and to "have fun with them."

During the initial evaluation phase, Jean gathered an occupational profile of Tonya. The *occupational profile* is a summary of the client's life constructed by the therapist, including activities, routines, and roles (AOTA, 2014, 2017). Occupational therapists may conduct an informal interview with a client to obtain an occupational profile (as Jean did with Tonya), or they may use assessment protocols to determine how a client spends their time, what they value given their occupational roles and routines, how they engage in interests, and how they obtain feelings of competence.

Two assessment instruments used to gather such data are the Canadian Occupational Performance Measure (COPM; Law et al., 2019) and the Occupational Performance History Interview–II (OPHI–II; Kielhofner et al., 2004). The COPM gathers specific information regarding the occupations the client wants or needs to do and the client's perception of their performance of and satisfaction with these occupations. The OPHI–II provides a more expansive occupational profile.

Jean used her clinical reasoning and decided that she needed to assess Tonya's performance during daily tasks with which Tonya had reported having difficulty (Fisher & Marterella, 2019; Gillen, 2013). Observing occupational performance allows occupational therapists to consider the quality with which the client performs a task and is essential to promote occupation-based evaluation and intervention (Fisher, 2013).

Observing clients engaging in occupations in natural contexts provides the most efficient and valid method of evaluating occupational performance (Gillen, 2013). Jean and Tonya decided that it might be informative for Jean to observe Tonya completing a simple cooking task. Jean could analyze her observations using a nonstandardized analysis or a standardized assessment, such as the Assessment of Motor and Process Skills (AMPS; Fisher & Jones, 2012). *Standardized assessments* are instruments with standard instructions, scoring, and established psychometric properties. *Nonstandardized assessments* are assessments without an examination of psychometric properties or scoring details. Jean chose to do a nonstandardized analysis of Tonya as she prepared lunch for her children with a structured format to inform her assessment and allow here time for other relevant standardized outcome assessments (Fisher & Griswold, 2019).

After interpreting their observation of the client's occupational performance, the therapist then determines whether further evaluation is needed to assess specific client factors or environmental contexts (AOTA, 2014; Fisher & Marterella, 2019). Only the aspects necessary to more thoroughly understand the client's performance need to be assessed. Context of the place of employment might be relevant. For example, visiting a job site would enable the therapist to determine the challenges and supports in that environment. The therapist might consider any physical, social, and cultural aspects of the environment that might be supporting or hindering a client's performance.

In other situations, assessing client factors such as range of motion or strength mi ght help to determine underlying causes of problems in occupational performance (AOTA, 2014). Occupational therapists use their

(Continued)

CASE EXAMPLE 5.1. JEAN AND TONYA: OCCUPATION-FOCUSED PRACTICE *(Cont.)*

clinical judgment to determine whether the assessment of any of these areas will be helpful in better understanding the client and their occupational performance. These areas would be assessed with additional observation or specific assessments or measures as appropriate.

In Tonya's case, Jean determined that she needed more information about how Tonya spent her time each day—the temporal dimension of context. She asked Tonya to keep a log of all activities that she engaged in for a 7-day period, using the Occupational Questionnaire (Smith et al., 1986). This questionnaire asks the client to indicate the importance, sense of competence, and enjoyment for each activity.

When assessing the environment once all the relevant information has been gathered, for some clients, the occupational therapist synthesizes and interprets the results of all evaluation data and identifies the client's strengths and weaknesses (AOTA, 2014). The therapist then shares their interpretation and hypotheses with the client. Further interpretation of the results may occur with the client, and together the therapist and client then establish goals to lead to the client's desired outcomes.

Jean concluded that Tonya was motivated to carry out her role as a mother. On the basis of her performance analysis of her observation of Tonya preparing lunch, Jean reported that Tonya had the motor and process skills to do desired tasks of IADLs that were important for her role as a mother. Motivation and performance skills were Tonya's strengths.

Analyzing Tonya's occupational questionnaire, Jean determined that Tonya engaged in many activities throughout the week that she felt she had to do but did not enjoy doing. Jean noted that Tonya actually engaged in very few activities that were enjoyable to her. She hypothesized that the environment in which Tonya lived was not conducive to social contact with others, particularly adults. Jean also hypothesized that Tonya was frustrated by not using her creative talents.

Jean shared her conclusions with Tonya, who agreed with them and said that she would like to have more contact with other adults and to become involved in drama in some way again. These were Tonya's desired outcomes. Jean and Tonya then identified specific goals and a plan that would enable Tonya to reach her desired outcomes. Setting goals is an important outcome of the evaluation process.

- Living independently at home,
- Engaging in the activities associated with the role of a mother or grandmother,
- Playing with other children on the playground, or
- Feeling emotionally ready to return to work and interact socially with peers.

Often, occupational therapists help the client turn desired outcomes into specific goals that support what the client would like to do. For example, to live independently at home, a client might need to prepare a simple sandwich and pour a cold beverage into a glass. Playing with others on the playground might include collaborating with other children to share playground equipment. The goals are further honed into behavioral objectives on the basis of difficulties that the therapist observed during the occupational performance analysis.

Suppose an occupational therapist observed an older gentleman, who wanted to remain living independently in his home and needed to prepare lunch for himself, to have difficulty choosing the right utensils to make a sandwich and not be able to locate the mustard that he had put into the refrigerator before the assessment began. The therapist can use these observations to write behavioral objectives to support the goal of making a sandwich, contributing to the desired outcome of living independently at home. In this example, adding specific criteria related to locating needed materials for a behavioral objective would indicate improved performance of an observed problem in a desired task.

Similarly, an occupational therapist would use observation results of a child on the playground to refine the goal

of collaborating with others into behavioral objectives. In particular, the therapist might have observed that the child did not ask questions of their peers or respond to peers' questions or comments, which ultimately resulted in failure to take turns during the social interaction intended to support playing together. The therapist could use the observations to write behavioral objectives related to asking a peer a question during play activities and responding to peers' questions and comments.

One can see from these two examples that occupational therapists need to observe the quality of occupational performance to write clear and specific behavioral objectives that emphasize occupation. Because the behavioral objectives are grounded in performance analysis, the intervention plan is client centered and occupation focused. In other words, the intervention plan considers what is important to the client and their current level of occupational performance.

Occupation-focused evaluation includes

- Gathering information from the client's perspective on desired and challenging occupations,
- Observing occupational performance in natural contexts, and
- Using the analysis of an observation of occupational performance to identify behavioral objectives to support the client's desired occupations.

After determining the goals and behavioral objectives with the client, therapists use their clinical reasoning to consider factors that hinder the person from performing at the desired level (Fisher & Marterella, 2019). Options might include client factors (e.g., motivation, internalized routine, body function), environmental demands (e.g., characteristics of people in the environment, space, available assessments and materials), or task demands (e.g., required steps, required actions).

On the basis of the occupational therapist's judgment, they select an intervention approach and theoretical perspective or frame of reference to guide the intervention. The therapist decides whether it is more appropriate to take a *skill acquisition approach* to facilitate learning or relearning of skills, such as manipulating small objects or controlling impulsive behaviors (Kaplan, 2020), or a *restorative approach* to establish or restore underlying abilities, such as muscle strength or skilled movement. Alternatively, the therapist might choose to take a *compensatory approach* and adapt task demands or modify the environment to promote more successful engagement in desired occupations (Fisher & Marterella, 2019).

The occupational therapist should share with the client their knowledge and evidence regarding the different intervention options. In collaboration with the client, the therapist determines the best approach to obtain the identified goals and create a plan for intervention. The therapist uses clinical reasoning, professional experiences, selected theoretical perspective, and evidence-based research to determine reasonable and appropriate methods to reach the desired outcomes.

Implementation Phase of Intervention

As the occupational therapist and the occupational therapy assistant work with a client to implement an intervention plan, they engage in ongoing reassessment to ensure that therapy is meaningful and effectively facilitating progress toward the established goals and objectives. *Reassessment* is the continuous gathering of client performance data at any time other than the initial evaluation and formal reevaluation. As a practitioner implements services, they continually reassess and seek new activities to promote the client's progress.

Activities that are relevant and meaningful to clients have been shown to be more effective in helping them reach the established goals (Hétu & Mercier, 2012; Lough et al., 2012). Monitoring the client's affective response to activities and approaches used during therapy enables occupational therapy practitioners to determine the meaning they hold for the person (Park, 2008; Price, 2009). Such monitoring and ongoing reassessment keep the intervention client centered.

Review: Monitoring Progress

In addition to the ongoing, informal evaluation throughout intervention, the occupational therapist, with the occupational therapy assistant, formally reevaluates a client's performance and progress throughout intervention to modify the intervention plan. A review of ongoing observations and formal assessment data can redirect a practitioner's decision making and services. A practitioner may observe poor performance during a therapy activity, which could lead to a change in the intervention approach or additional formal reevaluation, which, in turn, redirects intervention.

As the review of progress occurs, the therapist moves into the review phase of intervention. The *review phase* is part of reassessment; after a certain period of intervention, progress is determined and the therapist reflects on the need for additional intervention. This may include a formal re-evaluation.

Review time may be built into the intervention plan if allowed by the pragmatic constraints that influence practice. The time frame may be after a certain number of visits or at set intervals (e.g., weekly, monthly), often determined by reimbursement guidelines. *Reimbursement* refers to the payment by insurance agencies to the occupational therapist for the services provided to members as covered by that policy. During these reviews, the desired outcomes, goals, and behavioral objectives of the occupational therapy intervention plan form the basis for determining the effectiveness of the intervention. The initial assessment measures may be repeated to determine change in occupational performance.

It is important for occupational therapists to consider how frequently an assessment can be used for reassessment when choosing the assessments for the initial evaluation. Comparison of assessment data over time enables the therapist and client to objectively measure progress and determine whether therapy should continue or the client should be discharged. Review of the intervention may also facilitate a referral to another professional colleague.

Case Examples 5.2 and 5.3 illustrate very different types of evaluation approaches that address each client's occupational goals. However, in both examples, the occupational therapists gathered information about each client as a person and observed the quality of occupational performance in relevant tasks. The two cases reflect different types of settings in which the occupational therapists worked, which influenced the evaluation process. Finally, the frame of reference the therapists in these examples used further influenced their choice of assessments. Consequently, the evaluation process influenced planning intervention, implementing intervention, and reviewing progress.

Intervention Planning in the Case Examples

In both case examples, the occupational therapists focused on the occupational interests and desires of the clients. Joan (see Case Example 5.2) had preliminary information about her client, so she did not have to spend as much time collecting information for an occupational profile as did Danielle (see Case Example 5.3).

However, Joan did need to do a formal assessment, because the focus of her services was different from that of the occupational therapy services her client had received previously. Joan observed Jose as he engaged in occupations that were important to him in his home so that she could determine his occupational ability and plan appropriate intervention. Joan consciously decided not to further assess Jose abilities around muscle tone, movement, or cognition because information from these types of assessments would not have helped her plan for intervention.

Danielle also began her evaluation by gathering information to construct an occupational profile of Pierre.

CASE EXAMPLE 5.2. JOAN AND JOSE: DESIRED OUTCOMES AND INTERESTS

Joan worked as an occupational therapist for a home-based rehabilitation program. She was allowed four visits to see her client, **Jose,** including time for evaluation and intervention. Jose had experienced a cerebrovascular accident and had already received 2 months of inpatient occupational therapy services.

Joan knew that evaluation was essential to enable her to know what to focus on in intervention; however, she was also very aware that she had limited time to spend with her client and wanted to move into intervention as quickly as possible. She received documentation on Jose from the inpatient rehabilitation setting where he had received services most recently. The documentation Joan received enabled her to quickly establish a therapeutic rapport with Jose. She used the assessment data provided by the previous occupational therapist at the time of discharge and did not need to repeat the same assessments. She also knew Jose's interests, concerns, abilities, and needs from this documentation.

Joan built on her existing knowledge of Jose and directed her attention to how he was doing at home, an area not addressed during inpatient rehabilitation. Thus, Joan focused her evaluation on Jose's current needs, which allowed her to begin intervention almost immediately.

Joan spent the first 10 minutes of her home visit talking with Jose and his wife. She quickly learned through her informal interview that Jose wanted to make his own coffee in the morning, tend to his rose garden, and grill meat for family meals. Although Jose was not independent in all personal ADLs, he and his wife agreed that the routine they had worked out met his needs, and his wife felt comfortable assisting him.

Joan determined that she wanted to assess Jose's occupational performance by observing him performing tasks that were important to him. She decided to use the Assessment of Motor and Process Skills (AMPS; Fisher & Jones, 2012), a standardized assessment instrument, to determine the effort, efficiency, independence, and safety that Jose exhibited during familiar and desired ADLs. For the assessment, she and Jose chose AMPS tasks that directly related to his desired outcomes. Joan observed him potting a rose plant and making a pot of coffee.

From her assessment, including the discussion with Jose and his wife and observing the quality of his occupational performance, Joan gathered a great deal of information about Jose's abilities and needs. She determined that further assessing Jose's specific physical or cognitive skills would not help her plan or implement intervention or review progress. Joan and Jose used his expressed desired outcomes and interests to set goals and plan intervention.

Aware of his abilities and current stage of recovery, Joan decided to use a compensatory approach to support Jose's performance in his desired occupations. At the conclusion of her first visit, Joan began the intervention by making suggestions for modifying Jose's kitchen environment and adapting the task demands in his garden area. Joan efficiently included both evaluation and intervention into the first of her four sessions with Jose.

Joan repeated the AMPS at the end of the intervention period to provide a standardized measure of the progress that Jose had made. Another measure of effectiveness of the occupational therapy intervention was Jose's reported improved participation in the three occupations that he had identified as being important. By using a client-centered and occupation-based approach, Joan was able to help Jose meet his goals of making his own coffee, tending to his roses, and grilling for his family.

She observed Pierre performing desired occupations, but she did so in the clinic setting, not in his work environment. Her observation allowed her to efficiently determine Pierre's motor abilities and skills. Then, consistent with the biomechanical frame of reference, Danielle focused subsequent assessment on the client factors she knew were the underlying cause of Pierre's inability to engage in work tasks; such measurements were required by her facility.

These two case examples illustrate that there is no single right way to complete an evaluation. The process varies on the basis of the client, the information available from other sources, and information gathered during the initial steps of the evaluation process. The pragmatics of service delivery (particularly the number of visits allowed by third-party payers) influence what a therapist can do.

In both cases, Joan and Danielle gathered information about their clients as occupational beings and analyzed their clients' occupational performance. Joan was able to move from her performance analysis to intervention. Her intervention plan came directly from the performance analysis that she had done for evaluation and addressed those occupations of concern in therapy sessions to ensure occupation-based intervention.

Because Danielle further assessed components of body function, as was required by her facility, the focus of her assessment at that time was no longer on occupation, and she ran the risk of switching her intervention focus to that of body function, in particular range of motion (ROM) and strength, rather than occupation. Danielle worked hard to remain occupation focused, particularly as she documented her results.

Documenting Evaluation Results

The evaluation phase concludes with documenting results and reporting recommendations. Most important, occupational therapists need to frame the evaluation results

CASE EXAMPLE 5.3. DANIELLE AND PIERRE: BIOMECHANICAL FRAME OF REFERENCE

Danielle, an occupational therapist in an outpatient clinic that specializes in upper-extremity rehabilitation, took a slightly different approach during evaluation than did Joan in Case Example 5.2. Danielle was working with **Pierre,** a plumber, as a client. Pierre was eager to return to work after sustaining an on-the-job injury to his left hand. He had a tendon repair and was referred for occupational therapy by his orthopedic surgeon. Because of the nature of the injury, Pierre's insurance preapproved eight sessions.

Danielle began her first session by interviewing Pierre to get to know his job requirements and leisure interests. She learned about the types of hand movements that Pierre needed to do at work and looked at the tools and materials he used on the job. She also found out that Pierre bowled regularly with friends and built model trains at home. Pierre said that he could still bowl with

his right hand but was not able to use his left hand to work on his trains.

Pierre was most concerned about returning to work. Danielle observed Pierre using his plumbing tools; she recognized that limited range of motion (ROM) and strength in his left hand were the underlying cause of his difficulty with occupational performance. Danielle knew that her intervention approach would be one of remediation of hand function to support Pierre's job performance and enable him to perform other activities that were important to him.

Danielle selected a biomechanical frame of reference to guide Pierre's evaluation and intervention (Flinn et al., 2008). Further assessment focused on measuring ROM and grip strength in Pierre's left hand, because these factors would be important in monitoring his progress toward his occupational performance goals supporting his roles as plumber and builder of model trains.

using occupation, discussing the client as an occupational being and reporting the observed quality of occupational performance during desired and necessary tasks. Doing so maintains occupation-centered thinking and emphasizes the unique role of occupational therapy (Fisher, 2013). **Documentation** should include information that is relevant and important to address the initial referral for evaluation. The purpose of the referral for evaluation might have been clearly stated or might have been vague in nature. However, remaining focused on occupation helps clients and team members better understand occupational therapy practice.

The referral for Pierre (see Case Example 5.3) read "evaluate and treat ROM and strength: post tendon injury and surgical repair." As an occupational therapist, Danielle documented Pierre's performance in occupations that were meaningful to him. Because of the setting's documentation requirements and the referral, she also documented the underlying body functions of ROM and strength in his hand. To remain occupation focused, Danielle reported on Pierre's occupational performance first, then documented body functions as they related to his occupational performance, as shown in Appendix 5.A, "Sample Occupational Therapy Evaluation Report."

Occupational therapy evaluation results provide valuable information about the client that will be helpful for other professional colleagues, particularly when planning for discharge. Often, the occupational therapist is the professional who is best able to determine how independently and safely a person can perform necessary occupations, information essential in determining discharge readiness and recommendations. Consequently, occupational therapy evaluation reports should be written clearly so that other professionals can easily understand the types of assessment used, the findings, and the interpretation of those findings that relate to occupational performance and subsequent goals and recommendations.

Appendix 5.B, "Occupational Therapy Evaluation Report Template," provides one example of an evaluation report

template based on AOTA's (2018) *Guidelines for Documentation of Occupational Therapy.* The report template leads the occupational therapist through reporting evaluation findings to planning intervention in the Recommendations section. Appendix 5.A illustrates this using the template for Pierre (see Case Example 5.3).

Although facilities often determine the format for evaluation reports, most evaluation reports conclude with recommendations. The recommendations usually include the broad goals for intervention and a suggested approach to use during therapy, and they may include details of services to be provided. To support reimbursement, recommendations often indicate the need for skilled occupational therapy services (AOTA, 2018).

For example, Joan (see Case Example 5.2) might recommend that Jose receive three more occupational therapy visits in which the therapist will use a compensatory approach to modify the demands of tasks and Jose's environment to support his safety and independence in performing desired and necessary IADLs at home. The recommendations should be logically based on the evaluation findings reported.

Even if therapy is not warranted, the report should include recommendations (in the form of suggestions) that address the reason for referral. For example, an elementary-grade student, Eric, was referred to occupational therapy "to determine if sensory processing difficulties are interfering with his ability to attend in the classroom." If the occupational therapist does not find that Eric has sensory processing difficulties and finds no reason for his difficulty in class that warrants occupational therapy services, the therapist still might offer suggestions that the teacher could implement to enhance Eric's ability to engage in schoolwork tasks. The therapist might suggest moving Eric to a location in the classroom with fewer distractions or suggest that the teacher be sure she has Eric's attention before giving instructions or ensure that Eric has all needed supplies before beginning a schoolwork task.

Suggestions for Eric might also include a referral to another professional—for example, to a speech–language pathologist to confirm hearing acuity and processing, which also might influence Eric's schoolwork performance. The recipients of the evaluation report (in this case, Eric's parents and teachers) receive not only a written report of the evaluation findings but also some guidance regarding how to proceed.

All written client information serves as a permanent record of the client's abilities and progress made during intervention. An evaluation report documents the client's performance level at a given time related to their needs and desired outcomes, which can inform others who work with the client in the future.

Such information is especially helpful for clients who are transferred from one facility or type of care to another. In the continuum of health care used in the United States, it is not unusual for a client to receive services in several facilities or different departments within one facility. Information gathered during evaluation often goes into the client's chart for future use by other occupational therapists and professionals in subsequent settings. An occupational therapist at the receiving facility may use and build on previous assessments so that clients do not have to repeat the same assessments and lose valuable intervention time during a limited length of stay.

Occupational therapists should confirm the client's desired outcomes and goals efficiently at the onset of services in a new setting, which helps to establish a therapeutic relationship with the client and keep services client centered. The therapist then can begin intervention almost immediately while continuing to gather more evaluation data throughout intervention. The example of Joan and Jose in Case Example 5.2 illustrates good use of information from another facility.

TYPES OF ASSESSMENTS

Several assessment methods were presented in the three client examples in this chapter. Assessment instruments vary in their specific purpose, procedures for administration and scoring, type of data obtained, and interpretation of results.

It is essential that occupational therapists consider what each assessment measures and how the results are interpreted to ensure a match with the intended use of the evaluation for a given client (Zur et al., 2012). Selecting assessments on the basis of the client's situation and needs allows the occupational therapist to maintain client-centered practice. Furthermore, choosing assessments that focus on occupation emphasizes the unique role of occupational therapy (Fisher, 2013). Therapists should not select assessments just on the basis of their own level of comfort or familiarity; learning new assessments is a professional responsibility.

Knowing the purpose of each assessment being considered for use is essential to enable the occupational therapist to choose the most appropriate assessment for a specific client and the questions to be answered. Some assessments gather information about a client's occupational history, interests, or roles. Other assessments provide guidelines for evaluating occupational performance; still others focus on client factors, context, or activity demands.

Standardized assessments should always be scored in a standardized manner. They provide objective data that can help identify or determine a client's level of function and dysfunction. Results from a standardized test may vary in their usefulness in planning an intervention program, depending on the focus of the assessment and its interpretation. Repeating a standardized assessment can document change over time and provide data for evidence-based research (Mulligan, 2014). Standardized assessments often have specific procedures for administration and scoring that therapists must follow to obtain reliable and valid results. Some standardized assessments require formal training to learn how to administer, score, and interpret, to ensure that the results are reliable.

Many standardized assessments are limited because they measure behaviors in unnatural conditions, unless occupational performance in a natural environment is a condition of testing. Typically, standardized assessments require the client to perform tasks such as stacking 1-inch cubes, sorting cards or objects, squeezing a dynamometer, or determining correct change in a simulated purchasing task in a testing room or clinic and therefore outside a meaningful context.

The results may help the therapist understand a client's abilities, but the therapist then needs to transfer the results to a context and relate the findings to occupational performance. As Gillen (2013) pointed out, the transfer of results from an artificial testing environment does not reflect a client's performance in a natural context. Certainly, standardized assessments in which the occupational therapist observes the client perform activities in a natural context provide the most valid way to measure occupational performance. Such assessments directly support intervention planning because the therapist has observed performance in the real context.

Interpreting the assessment results requires the occupational therapist to first refer back to the stated purpose of the assessment used and then to further consider the focus of interpretation stated in the assessment manual. For example, both the ADL-Focused Occupation-Based Neurobehavioral Evaluation (A–ONE; Árnadóttir, 1990, 2011) and the AMPS (Fisher & Jones, 2012) are based on observation of a person performing ADL tasks in a natural context, so they are both occupation-focused assessments.

Interpretation of these two assessments is different: The A–ONE focuses on underlying neurobehavioral impairments that cause decreased ADL performance, and the AMPS evaluates a person's ability to perform ADLs and IADLs, providing a measure of the quality of a person's motor and process abilities when performing ADL tasks. Assessment manuals provide guidelines for interpreting the results.

Using a variety of methods and tools for assessment provides a range of data to inform an evaluation appropriate to the needs of the client. Occupational therapists draw from different quantitative and qualitative methods, depending on the questions they have about a client.

Case Example 5.4 illustrates an occupational therapist's use of two types of assessments:

CASE EXAMPLE 5.4. LUKE AND CRYSTAL: CRITERION-REFERENCED AND NORM-REFERENCED ASSESSMENTS

Luke, a 10-year-old fifth grader, was referred to occupational therapy by his teacher and the school's special education referral team. Luke had received occupational therapy services as a preschooler for motor skills, particularly for fine motor development. Occupational therapy was discontinued when he entered kindergarten because norm-referenced assessments indicated that his motor development was within age range. At the beginning of second grade, Luke was diagnosed with a language-based learning disability and has received speech–language therapy and help with reading since that time.

Luke's fifth-grade teacher is concerned because Luke is not getting his work done in a timely manner. She reported that he frequently does only half of the required writing, with illegible, sloppy handwriting. She wonders whether his difficulty with written work is because of fine motor and handwriting issues, in addition to his learning disability affecting his spelling. Because of his history of fine motor difficulty in preschool and now handwriting difficulty, the team asked the occupational therapist to assess his fine motor skills as they related to education.

Crystal, the occupational therapist, talked with Luke's teacher and learned that Luke has difficulty with all writing tasks but that his problem is more pronounced when he needs to write several paragraphs at one time. Crystal learned that Luke also does not complete most classroom projects in a timely manner and that the end product is usually incomplete and sloppily done. Crystal found out that Luke finishes his math work, most of which is done in a math workbook. Crystal's focus was not on how well Luke was performing academically but on Luke's performance while doing his schoolwork tasks—his necessary occupation.

During the conversation with Luke's teacher, Crystal arranged to observe Luke during a science activity in which the students would be graphing results from an experiment and writing up the results in paragraph form—both tasks that the teacher indicated would be challenging for Luke to finish in a timely and neat manner. During the observation, Crystal noted that Luke made several trips to gather paper, a ruler, and pencils needed to complete the two tasks. His materials were on top of one another in his workspace, which made it difficult for him to locate materials when he needed them.

Luke paused for long periods during each task. He also played with his ruler and pencils, at one point putting a pencil through a hole in the ruler and spinning the ruler around. Another student sitting near Luke cued him to get back to work. He then worked quickly and wrote without keeping his written work between the lines on the paper.

Crystal noted that Luke held his pencil with a mature grasp and easily manipulated his pencil and other materials in his hands. Crystal concluded that Luke's difficulty in writing was caused not by deficiencies in fine motor skills but by inefficient use of time, space, and materials related to the schoolwork tasks.

Crystal was a calibrated rater for the School Assessment of Motor and Process Skills (AMPS; Fisher et al., 2007) and scored her observations using the criteria in the School AMPS manual. She entered the scores into her School AMPS software program to obtain a school motor performance measure of 2.1 logits and a school process performance measure of 0.03 logits.

The motor performance measure indicated that Luke demonstrated a questionable level of effort in using tools and materials. The process performance measure indicated that he demonstrated a mild to moderate level of inefficiency when organizing time, space, and materials. Transformation of the two performance measures revealed that Luke's motor performance was in the average range when compared with his same-age peers (z score of −1.0), but his process performance was significantly below that of his peers (z score of −2.4). Standardized scores were familiar to other team members and helped them understand Luke's performance in relation to other students of the same age.

Crystal knew that the special education team and Luke's teacher would expect her to assess his fine motor and visual–motor skills, factors that support handwriting. Although her clinical reasoning of the observations when using the School AMPS indicated that these skills were not issues for Luke, she reasoned that specific assessments in these areas would be relatively quick to do and provide information expected by the team. She also saw combining the three assessments as an opportunity to demonstrate to the team the value of a standardized observational assessment over assessments of client factors (Gillen, 2013).

Crystal chose the fine motor control tasks on the Bruininks–Oseretsky Test of Motor Proficiency (BOT2; Bruininks & Bruininks, 2005) and the Beery–Buktenica Developmental Test of Visual–Motor Integration (Beery VMI; Beery & Beery, 2010). Both are standardized assessments of client factors. These two assessments indicated that Luke's fine motor skills and visual–motor integration were in the average range. His performance resulted in a z score of −1.2 as measured by the BOT2 and a standard score of 99, in the 47th percentile, on the Beery VMI. The results from these two standardized assessments confirmed the clinical reasoning of Crystal's observation of Luke in his classroom.

Crystal shared her findings with the team and reported that she had observed Luke having difficulty during the schoolwork tasks. However, she clarified that Luke demonstrated no difficulty with the quality of motor performance when writing during the schoolwork project, and she reported that Luke's scores on the standardized

(Continued)

CASE EXAMPLE 5.4. LUKE AND CRYSTAL: CRITERION-REFERENCED AND NORM-REFERENCED ASSESSMENTS *(Cont.)*

assessments of fine motor and visual–motor skills supported her interpretation. Crystal emphasized that Luke had difficulty completing his schoolwork tasks because of inefficiency in gathering materials and organizing time and space, which caused him to rush to finish his work and compromised the quality of the end product.

Her recommendations to support Luke in the classroom resulted from her observation of his work during schoolwork tasks, in the context in which he typically did these tasks. Crystal used her observations and

problem solved with the teacher ways to support Luke to gather needed tools and materials. Crystal worked with Luke on strategies to keep his desktop more organized as he works. Luke, his teacher, and Crystal developed a plan to help Luke begin working more quickly and sustain work behaviors throughout a task. Because Crystal used a standardized assessment of her observations (i.e., School AMPS), she will be able to document changes in his performance when she observes him later in the school year.

1. A standardized, observational, *criterion-referenced assessment* (i.e., designed to provide a measure of performance that is interpretable in terms of clearly defined and delimited criteria) conducted in the natural environment, and
2. A *norm-referenced assessment* (i.e., designed to provide a measure of performance that is interpretable in terms of clearly defined and delimited criteria) of client factors.

The occupational therapist deliberately chose the assessments she used and carefully considered the information they provided. Each type of assessment provided different information to gain an understanding of the client's abilities and challenges. The occupational therapist used her clinical reasoning to interpret all the findings and to consider intervention.

The example of Luke and Crystal (see Case Example 5.4) demonstrates the use of criterion-referenced assessments and norm-referenced assessments. The School AMPS (Fisher et al., 2007) is a standardized criterion-referenced assessment based on observation in a natural context. This particular assessment allowed Crystal to generate a baseline performance measure (i.e., number) to later compare with Luke's future performance. Crystal's observation of Luke in the classroom provided her with a wealth of information to consider while determining his needs and options for occupational therapy services.

The standardized norm-referenced assessments on fine motor and visual–motor skills ruled out difficulty in these areas but did not add any information to help Crystal plan an intervention for Luke. If Luke had demonstrated difficulty on these two assessments, the results would have informed Crystal of weaknesses in these areas but would not have helped her know what to do for intervention. Furthermore, if Crystal had limited her evaluation to the assessments of client factors that were conducted outside of the natural classroom environment, the results would have led her to logically conclude that Luke did not need occupational therapy services. Fortunately, Crystal observed Luke doing tasks that he needed to do in his classroom, and she saw difficulties that occupational therapy could address. In Luke's case, occupational therapy played an important role to support his schoolwork performance.

EVALUATION IN CONTEXT: PRAGMATIC ISSUES OF EVALUATION

Although the focus of evaluation is on the client, options are often limited by pragmatic constraints on practice. These constraints include reimbursement implications determined by federal, insurance, or facility policies; facility procedures; resources in the community where the client lives; and the occupational therapist's own attributes (Vroman & Stewart, 2014).

Reimbursement

The time many occupational therapists spend on evaluation is constrained by federal, insurance, or facility policies guiding reimbursement (demonstrated in Case Examples 5.2 and 5.3). In some cases, an occupational therapist may have only half an hour for evaluation. In other situations, the facility will be reimbursed only if the therapist engages in intervention during the first visit with a client, which thus limits the amount of formal evaluation time.

Occupational therapists can blend observation of occupational performance and findings from assessments directly into intervention, as Joan did with Jose in Case Example 5.2. Thus, the transition from evaluation to intervention is nearly seamless, leading to time efficiency. For instance, during her interview, Joan discovered that Jose wanted to tend to his rose garden (occupational profile). She observed him pot a plant and scored the observation using the AMPS (Fisher & Jones, 2012). Consequently, at the end of the evaluation, Joan had observed performance in the desired task (i.e., gardening). This observation informed her about how to help Jose participate in his desired occupation. Joan used the entire evaluation process to guide intervention immediately.

When evaluation time is limited, therapists may also rely on screening techniques. Screening is a preliminary assessment process used to determine whether a problem exists. Results of a screening are insufficient for intervention planning but may indicate the need for more extensive evaluation (Vroman & Stewart, 2014). Screening can include observation of the client, review of the client's medical records, or administration of a standardized assessment designed as a screening instrument (Mulligan, 2014).

Because of reimbursement constraints, it is imperative that occupational therapists be clear about the purpose of evaluation and the usefulness of the information gathered for decision making. Therapists need to ensure that they are gathering information that is useful and relevant to the desired purpose. Knowing the potential use of evaluation data and the type of information that is relevant to address a client's needs enables therapists to gather the essential information more efficiently.

In Case Examples 5.2 and 5.3, the therapists began their evaluations by getting to know the clients as people and learning what was important to them, so that further evaluation focused on the clients' goals and supported their occupational interests and performance of desired tasks. In these examples, both therapists quickly determined what other assessment data would enable them to plan and monitor intervention. Both therapists chose assessments with a specific purpose in mind.

Facility Procedures

Each facility has its own way of conducting business. Professionals work together in a variety of ways to gather evaluation information and provide services to clients. The working relationship, or structure of teamwork, to which the facility subscribes influences how occupational therapists work with colleagues who are simultaneously gathering evaluation data. Teams might be multidisciplinary, interdisciplinary, or transdisciplinary in nature.

Coordinating efforts always proves to be efficient, informative, and cost-effective. Clearly identifying each professional's domain of focus and services may help to determine the purpose of their respective evaluations, regardless of the type of team used in a facility. Some evaluation information may be universally desired, and team members can determine who is in the best position to gather that information and share it with the team. Having one professional gather information for the rest of the team reflects client-centered thinking, because the client has to give information or perform similar assessment tasks only once.

The type of setting and the mission and philosophy of the facility, the composition of professionals, and the complexity of clients' needs often determine how professionals coordinate their efforts for evaluation and intervention. In medical settings and frequently in mental health practice, each professional on a multidisciplinary team typically gathers their own assessment data and then shares results with other team members (Falk-Kessler, 2019). This team model may result in an overlap of assessments performed.

In some rehabilitation settings and in many pediatric settings, professionals work as an interdisciplinary team, collaborating in the assessment process. Team members determine the type of assessment data needed and how each member will contribute to the process. They share their respective evaluation results and develop an integrated intervention plan (Falk-Kessler, 2019; Mulligan, 2014).

When a team has worked together in a facility over time, each professional knows the team expectations and focuses on discipline-specific information. Occupational therapists usually gather information to complete an occupational profile and focus on how a disability affects the client's occupational performance; other team members may gather specific client-factor information. When team members coordinate their evaluation efforts, they avoid duplication for the client and reduce costs.

Transdisciplinary teams are commonly seen in early intervention programs for infants and young children (Mulligan, 2014), but they also may be used in other areas of practice. In this model, team members have a stable relationship from working together over time and have shared knowledge and skills, which enables them to observe and record assessment results for one another. With a transdisciplinary team, professional boundaries are blurred, and expertise is shared so that assessment and intervention services are integrated and often done by one person (Mulligan, 2014). Transdisciplinary teams may use an **arena assessment** to conduct an evaluation; one person presents assessment tasks, and each professional gathers their respective information (Mulligan, 2014).

Community Resources

Communities vary greatly in the options and natural supports available to residents. Natural community supports include health care options, religious supports, employment and volunteer opportunities, and leisure and social networks. Communities with senior citizen centers may have a cadre of volunteers who provide supports to older adults to enable them to live longer in their homes.

Knowing the availability of natural supports for all community members helps an occupational therapist ensure that clients are at the right level of independence and, before discharge, have access to supports to help ensure their safety and well-being. Knowing the community options for discharge helps a therapist anticipate goals for clients and make decisions regarding assessment foci. For example, knowing that Meals on Wheels is available for a client might enable the therapist to focus on other aspects of IADLs. When a therapist evaluates a client living in a community that is unfamiliar to the therapist, an environmental assessment might be helpful to identify the broader community resources.

Therapist Attributes

Pragmatically, an occupational therapist's own knowledge and experience naturally limit what they do during an evaluation. Staying abreast of new models of practice and frames of reference, as well as the implications of new perspectives for evaluation and intervention, enables therapists to reflect current professional thinking. Reviewing and critiquing evidence related to how best to evaluate or enhance occupational performance informs therapists of the best practices known to date (Baker & Tickle-Degnen, 2019). In addition, knowing a range of assessment instruments enables a therapist to practice in a client-centered manner; learning new assessment instruments should be part of a therapist's ongoing professional competence objectives.

LEARNING A NEW ASSESSMENT

Learning is a process that requires time and practice, and learning a new assessment procedure or instrument is no exception. Some assessments require specific education and certification processes. For example, the Sensory Integration and Praxis Tests (Ayres, 1989) and the AMPS (Fisher & Jones, 2012) both require that occupational therapists take a course, practice using the assessment, and then demonstrate standardized use or calibration of scoring. Other assessments, such as the Sensory Profile (Dunn, 2014), the Occupational Performance History Interview–II (Kielhofner et al., 2004), and the Canadian Occupational Performance Measure (Law et al., 2019), require the therapist to study the administration manual and practice the assessment according to described procedures to competently administer, score, and interpret the results.

In all cases, an occupational therapist learning a new assessment instrument should know the purpose of the assessment and the type of information it will provide. The therapist should have read the manual and know, before using the assessment with a client, how to administer, score, and interpret the results. Practice administering the assessment is essential to acquiring competence in its use.

Some assessments require standardized administration, which means that the occupational therapist must use very specific directions and responses during administration. Giving too much or too little information or doing the assessment tasks incorrectly, including not giving instructions as described in the assessment manual, can influence the client's response and invalidate the results. Some assessments do not require specific wording in directions given to the client; the manual provides parameters for client instructions.

When one is learning a new assessment, a single reading of a manual is never sufficient, even for experienced occupational therapists. Tests that have standardized administration may require the therapist to create note cards or other prompts as reminders of what to do next or what to observe while assessing. The therapist needs to imagine using the assessment instrument, then practice using it, possibly without another person present, before giving the assessment to another person who is not a client. Some instruments have objects to present to a client, such as blocks, small toys, or pegs and a pegboard. Therapists may need to know which side of the client to sit on, because it may affect test administration.

Once the occupational therapist is comfortable with the assessment instrument's items, their order of presentation, and the scoring of a person's performance, they should practice giving the instrument to another person with the same characteristics as the population for whom the assessment was intended. This practice person may be a friend or colleague, but therapists learning a new assessment must anticipate a response from someone who might be less able.

Occupational therapists should be prepared to provide certain types of support as appropriate. For example, the assessment manual may have specific guidelines to follow when a person makes an error; therapists need to know in advance what constitutes an error as well as how to respond. Some assessments end after a person has made a certain number of errors, so therapists should know when to end the assessment.

Learning a new instrument can be daunting. However, the rewards of learning and using a new assessment protocol are worth every minute of preparation. Furthermore, preparation increases the accuracy of the assessment findings and ensures that the therapist is competent in administering and interpreting the assessment. The final result is a valid, ethical, fair evaluation process leading to increased confidence when reporting the results and using them to plan intervention.

New assessments will continue to be developed as the profession evolves. The influence of the *OTPF* (AOTA, 2014) and the focus on observing occupational performance will generate new protocols that highlight what occupational therapists do best—evaluate and promote occupational performance and engagement in occupation. Occupational therapists will have many opportunities to learn new assessments throughout their careers, to stay current in practice, and to provide the quality of services that they want to offer to clients.

THERAPEUTIC USE OF SELF DURING EVALUATION

Regardless of the type of assessment used or the constraints on evaluation and practice, occupational therapists should always consider how they are influencing the evaluation process. The value of establishing a positive working relationship with clients has been important to occupational therapists throughout the profession's history (Peloquin, 2003). Use of one's own personal and professional attributes, termed *therapeutic use of self*, promotes collaboration with a client.

Therapeutic use of self continually used by occupational therapists throughout the evaluation process helps the therapist and the client determine what occupation is of greatest concern and what tasks the therapist might observe the client perform. If the task is difficult for the client to perform successfully, the experience will likely trigger frustration, sadness, anger, or despair. The therapist must be ready to support the client as appropriate. Poor performance may lead to a goal and motivation for therapy; it also may be the point at which the therapist needs to help the client consider other options in their life and find meaning in new activities. Using one's self in this way, as a medium of therapy, is considered the "art of therapy" and is just as important as the theoretical and technical knowledge and skills that therapists possess (Peloquin, 2003).

SUMMARY

Evaluation provides the foundational information upon which occupational therapy services are built. The process begins with getting to know the client as a person and understanding the occupations that are important to them. The occupational therapist examines the client's occupational performance in tasks that are relevant, important, and challenging to the client. The therapist may determine that further assessment of client factors, context, or task demands would provide greater understanding of a client's strengths and limitations. The evaluation process is as long or short as necessary to enable the therapist to plan and implement appropriate occupational therapy services, although context may limit the time for the formal evaluation.

Many methods can provide information that might be interesting; however, a longer evaluation is not necessarily a better one. The occupational therapist must determine the salient information to answer the questions posed by the referral and support the client's desire and need to participate in meaningful life experiences. A sound evaluation process leads to informed planning and intervention services.

QUESTIONS

1. The author describes how evaluation leads to intervention planning in Case Example 5.1. What other assessments might you have used with Tonya?
2. Can you think of some additional types of interventions that Jean might have developed for Tonya on the basis of the information provided? Are there other areas on which you would have focused?
3. Reflect on a case with which you are familiar. When reviewing interventions to consider making changes, what kind of information would have made you consider changing the intervention plan? Identify specific data that you would want to gather before changing the plan with the client in the case you chose.
4. In Case Example 5.2, how might the evaluation (and possibly the intervention) have been different if the number of visits had not been limited?
5. Think about a case with which you are familiar. What were the critical elements that needed to be included in the documentation to justify occupational therapy intervention in that setting?
6. In Case Example 5.1, what strategies might Jean have used to develop a therapeutic rapport with Tonya that supported occupational therapy intervention?
7. Consider a case of your own. What other type of evaluation questions might you ask to enhance the focus of evaluation and intervention on occupation? What assessments or methods would help you glean the desired information?
8. Look at each case example. Different therapists often approach cases in a different manner; how would you approach each of these cases in a way that is different from the way the case is handled here?

REFERENCES

American Occupational Therapy Association. (2014). Occupational therapy practice framework: Domain and process (3rd ed.). *American Journal of Occupational Therapy, 68*(Suppl. 1), S1–S48. https://doi.org/10.5014/ajot.2014.682006

American Occupational Therapy Association. (2017). AOTA occupational profile template. *American Journal of Occupational Therapy, 71*(Suppl. 2), 7112420030. https://doi.org/10.5014/ajot.2017.716S12

American Occupational Therapy Association. (2018). Guidelines for documentation of occupational therapy. *American Journal of Occupational Therapy, 72*(Suppl. 2), 7212410010. https://doi.org/10.5014/ajot.2018.72S203

Árnadóttir, G. (1990). *The brain and behavior: Assessing cortical dysfunction through activities of daily living.* St. Louis: Mosby.

Árnadóttir, G. (2011). Impact of neurobehavioral deficits on activities of daily living. In G. Gillen (Ed.), *Stroke rehabilitation: A function-based approach* (3rd ed., pp. 456–500). St. Louis: Mosby.

Ayres, A. J. (1989). *Sensory Integration and Praxis Tests.* Los Angeles: Western Psychological Services.

Baker, N., & Tickle-Degnen, L. (2019). Evidence-based practice. In B. A. B. Schell & G. Gillen (Eds.), *Willard and Spackman's occupational therapy* (13th ed., pp. 498–512). Philadelphia: Wolters Kluwer.

Beery, K. E., & Beery, N. A. (2010). *The Beery–Buktenica Developmental Test of Visual–Motor Integration* (6th ed.). Bloomington, MN: Pearson.

Brown, C. (2009). Functional assessment and intervention in occupational therapy. *Psychiatric Rehabilitation Journal, 32,* 162–170. https://doi.org/10.2975/32.3.2009.162-170

Bruininks, R. H., & Bruininks, B. D. (2005). *Bruininks–Oseretsky Test of Motor Proficiency* (2nd ed.). Bloomington, MN: Pearson.

Dunn, W. (2014). *Sensory Profile 2.* Bloomington, MN: Pearson.

Falk-Kessler, J. (2019). Professionalism, communication, and teamwork. In B. A. B. Schell & G. Gillen (Eds.), *Willard and Spackman's occupational therapy* (13th ed., pp. 556–571). Philadelphia: Wolters Kluwer.

Fisher, A. G. (2013). Occupation-centred, occupation-based, occupation-focused: Same, same or different? *Scandinavian Journal of Occupational Therapy, 20,* 162–173. https://doi.org/10.3109/11038128.2012.754492

Fisher, A. G., Bryze, K., Hume, V., & Griswold, L. A. (2007). *School Assessment of Motor and Process Skills.* Fort Collins, CO: Three Star Press.

Fisher, A. G., & Griswold, L. A. (2018). *Evaluation of social interaction* (4th ed.). Fort Collins, CO: Three Star Press.

Fisher, A. G., & Griswold, L. A. (2019). Performance skills: Implementing performance analyses to evaluate the quality of occupational performance. In B. A. B. Schell & G. Gillen (Eds.), *Willard and Spackman's occupational therapy* (13th ed., pp. 335–350). Philadelphia: Wolters Kluwer.

Fisher, A. G., & Jones, K. B. (2012). *Assessment of Motor and Process Skills* (7th ed., rev.). Fort Collins, CO: Three Star Press.

Fisher, A. G., & Marterella, A. (2019). *Powerful practice: A model for authentic occupational therapy.* Fort Collins, CO: Center for Innovative OT Solutions.

Flinn, N. A., Jackson, J., McLaughlin Gray, J., & Zemke, R. (2008). Optimizing abilities and capacities: Range of motion, strength, and endurance. In M. V. Radomski & C. A. Trombly (Eds.), *Occupational therapy for physical dysfunction* (6th ed., pp. 573–597). Philadelphia: Lippincott Williams & Wilkins.

Gillen, G. (2013). A fork in the road: An occupational hazard? *American Journal of Occupational Therapy, 67,* 641–652. https://doi.org/10.5014/ajot.2013.676002

Hétu, S., & Mercier, C. (2012). Using purposeful tasks to improve motor performance: Does object affordance matter? *British Journal of Occupational Therapy, 75,* 367–376. https://doi.org/10.4276/030802212X13433105374314

Hinojosa, J., Kramer, P., Royeen, C. B., & Luebben, A. (2003). Core concept of occupation. In P. Kramer, J. Hinojosa, & C. B. Royeen (Eds.), *Perspective on human occupation: Participation in life* (pp. 1–17). Philadelphia: Lippincott Williams & Wilkins.

Hinojosa, J., Kramer, P., & Royeen, C. B. (2017). Core concept of occupation. In J. Hinojosa, P. Kramer, & C. B. Royeen (Eds.), *Perspective on human occupation: Theories underlying practice* (2nd ed., pp. 23–38). Philadelphia: Lippincott Williams & Wilkins.

Hocking, C. (2001). Implementing occupation-based assessment. *American Journal of Occupational Therapy, 55,* 463–469. https://doi.org/10.5014/ajot.55.4.463

Ideishi, R. I. (2003). Influence of occupation on assessment and treatment. In P. Kramer, J. Hinojosa, & C. B. Royeen (Eds.), *Perspectives in human occupation: Participation in life* (pp. 278–296). Philadelphia: Lippincott Williams & Wilkins.

Kaplan, M. (2020). Frame of reference for motor acquisition. In P. Kramer, J. Hinojosa, & T. H. Howe (Eds.), *Frames of reference for pediatric occupational therapy* (4th ed., pp. 391–424). Philadelphia: Wolters Kluwer.

Kielhofner, G., Mallinson, T., Crawford, C., Nowak, M., Rigby, M., Henry, A., . . . Walens, D. (2004). *A user's guide to the Occupational Performance History Interview–II* (Version 2.1). Chicago: Model of Human Occupation Clearinghouse, Department of Occupational Therapy, University of Illinois.

Law, M., Baptiste, S., Carswell, A., McColl, M. A., Polatajko, H., & Pollock, N. (2019). *Canadian Occupational Performance Measure* (5th ed., rev.). Altona, MB: COPM, Inc.

Lough, C. L., Rice, M. S., & Lough, L. G. (2012). Choice as a strategy to enhance engagement in a colouring task in children with autism spectrum disorders. *Occupational Therapy International, 19,* 204–211. https://doi.org/10.1002/oti.1337

Mulligan, S. (2014). *Occupational therapy evaluation for children: A pocket guide* (2nd ed.). Philadelphia: Lippincott Williams & Wilkins.

Park, M. (2008). Making scenes: Imaginative practices of a child with autism in a sensory integration–based therapy session. *Medical Anthropology Quarterly, 22,* 234–256. https://doi.org/10.1111/j.1548-1387.2008.00024.x

Peloquin, S. M. (2003). The therapeutic relationship: Manifestations and challenges in occupational therapy. In E. B. Crepeau, E. S. Cohn, & B. A. B. Schell (Eds.), *Willard and Spackman's occupational therapy* (10th ed., pp. 157–170). Philadelphia: Lippincott Williams & Wilkins.

Price, P. (2009). The therapeutic relationship. In E. B. Crepeau, E. S. Cohn, & B. A. B. Schell (Eds.), *Willard and Spackman's occupational therapy* (11th ed., pp. 328–341). Philadelphia: Lippincott Williams & Wilkins.

Simmons, D. C., Crepeau, E. B., & White, B. P. (2000). The predictive power of narrative data in occupational therapy evaluation. *American Journal of Occupational Therapy, 54,* 471–476. https://doi.org/10.5014/ajot.54.5.471

Smith, N. R., Kielhofner, G., & Watts, J. H. (1986). The relationships between volition, activity pattern, and life satisfaction in the elderly. *American Journal of Occupational Therapy, 40,* 278–283. https://doi.org/10.5014/ajot.40.4.278

Vroman, K., & Stewart, E. (2014). *Occupational therapy evaluation for adults: A pocket guide* (2nd ed.). Philadelphia: Lippincott Williams & Wilkins.

Weinstock-Zlotnick, G., & Hinojosa, J. (2004). Bottom-up or top-down evaluation: Is one better than the other? *American Journal of Occupational Therapy, 58,* 594–599. https://doi.org/10.5014/ajot.58.5.594

Zur, B., Johnson, A., Roy, E., Rudman, D. L., & Wells, J. (2012). Beyond traditional notions of validity: Selecting appropriate measures for occupational therapy practice. *Australian Occupational Therapy Journal, 59,* 243–246. https://doi.org/10.1111/j.1440-1630.2012.01007.x

APPENDIX 5.A. SAMPLE OCCUPATIONAL THERAPY EVALUATION REPORT

Facility/Agency Name
Occupational Therapy Evaluation Report
Name: Pierre Sample
Date of Birth: November 25, 1996
ID #: 77007
Date of Evaluation: January 31, 2020
Age: 23 years
Primary Diagnosis: Limited function postinjury and postsurgery of flexor pollicis longus

Referral Information

Pierre was referred by A-1 Hand Surgery, Inc., 5 weeks post-surgical repair of flexor pollicis longus in his left hand, surgical restrictions removed. Referral was for evaluation and intervention to restore hand function to return to work.

Client Information

Pierre sustained his injury while working as a plumber, when equipment crushed his hand. No prior relevant medical history. Presenting problems include an inability to use his left hand for work-related tasks as well as leisure activities and some IADLs.

Occupational Profile

Pierre reported that he lives with his girlfriend, who does most of the meal preparation and is willing to do household chores that he typically does until his hand function returns. He said he has adapted self-care tasks so that he is independent. Pierre reported working for a local plumbing company, where he primarily installs pipes and heating systems in new home construction. He described his primary job tasks to include drilling holes, cutting and fitting pipes, and soldering. He usually works with one other plumber when he goes out to a job site. Pierre said he enjoys his job and is working toward advancing his status. He stated that his boss is holding his job for him.

In addition to work, Pierre reported that he is an avid bowler and bowls 2–3 times a week for a social outlet. Pierre stated that he can continue bowling because he bowls with his uninjured right hand. He also builds model trains, which he began doing with his father when he was a young boy. Building model trains has become a large part of Pierre's identity; his trains have been shown in many public events, particularly around the holidays. Pierre expressed concern regarding his inability to pinch the tiny train parts with his left hand. He reported that after experiences recovering from past sports injuries in high school, he knows he needs to do his exercises and is eager to begin therapy. His goals are to return to work and to building model trains.

Assessments Used

Evaluation included gathering information from Pierre regarding difficulties in task performance, observation of his performance during tasks he reported he needed for his job, and goniometric measurements, as well as evaluation of grip strength.

Analysis of Occupational Performance

When Pierre cut and soldered pipes of 2-inch diameter, he demonstrated decreased force when holding the pipe with his left hand, resulting in the pipe slipping from his grip. He hesitated to initiate cutting and soldering and paused several times to reposition the pipe as he cut it. He had difficulty aligning a fitting onto the pipe due to the lack of stability to hold the pipe and keep it from tipping.

Other Evaluation Results

Evaluation of left thumb range of motion (ROM) indicated moderate limitation. Active ROM (AROM for thumb MP was 30° and thumb interphalangeal 55°. Secondary to prolonged immobility, lumbrical strength for Digits 2–4 was manual muscle testing (MMT) score of 3, limiting grasp and pinch. Evaluation of strength for flexor pollicis longus was MMT score of 2. Dynamometer results found a left grasp of 70 pounds. Secondary to AROM limitation, pinch strength was not evaluated. Sensory evaluation noted no deficits in sensory functioning.

Summary and Analysis

At the time of the initial evaluation, Pierre demonstrated limited left-hand function that is hindering his return to work as a plumber because he needs his left hand to grasp and support copper pipe of 1-inch diameter. When observed cutting and soldering pipes, Pierre was unable to grip and stabilize the pipes and fittings with his left hand, resulting in his inability to do routinely performed work tasks. Pierre had limited ROM and strength in left-hand flexors and thumb adduction and opposition. He was unable to oppose and achieve forceful thumb flexion to pinch and pick up objects less than 3 inches in diameter, resulting in a nonfunctional grasp. An important leisure activity of building trains is also compromised. He is able to perform personal ADLs with adaptation, and he is independent with necessary IADLs. Pierre's goals of returning to work and engaging in all leisure activities are realistic. He is motivated to participate in occupational therapy to achieve his goals.

Recommendations

Outpatient occupational therapy services are recommended to address left-hand function, postsurgical repair of flexor pollicis longus, and intrinsic muscle weakness, to meet the goal of grasping and manipulating tools and materials, as required to return to work. Services include eight sessions over a 4-week period of time and a home exercise program. Adapted handles on work tools will enable return to work before obtaining full ROM and strength.

Danielle Exemplar, MS, OTR/L
Occupational Therapist

APPENDIX 5.B. OCCUPATIONAL THERAPY EVALUATION REPORT TEMPLATE

Facility/Agency Name
Occupational Therapy Evaluation Report
Name: (Client's Full Name)
Date of Birth:
ID #: (given by facility/agency)
Date of Evaluation:
Age:
Primary Diagnosis: (if known)
Reason for Referral
Include the referral source, reason for referral, and the presenting primary concerns.
Client Information
Describe the client's present performance level relative to the referral and related past and current medical information, including precautions.
Occupational Profile
Include information about the client's current living situation, employment status, and leisure activities. For each relevant occupation (e.g., work, education, leisure, ADLs), discuss the tasks necessary, context (social and physical environment), and satisfaction level. Discuss the client's occupational history if it provides information about the client's ability to adapt to the presenting situation. Identify the client's self-identified strengths, limitations, desired outcomes or goals, and priorities.
Assessments Used
Results may be organized in a variety of formats. Often the information in this section is organized by the evaluation procedure used, by areas of occupation, or by the assessment.
Analysis of Occupational Performance
Provide a synthesis of the observation of performance. Information in this section highlights the focus of occupational therapy.
Other Evaluation Results
Report other assessment data gathered. This format of reporting will be determined by the facility, and specific findings may be included in an appendix.
Summary and Analysis
Synthesize and interpret all findings, relating them to problems in occupational performance. Summarize the data as they relate to the concerns stated in the referral. Include expected outcomes and prognosis.
Recommendations
Recommendations for occupational therapy services, if warranted, should include the focus of planned intervention, intervention approach, and service delivery model, with suggested frequency and duration of services. The recommendations should address the reason for referral and reflect the client's occupational goals and priorities noted earlier in the report.

Note. Based on "Guidelines for Documentation of Occupational Therapy," by American Occupational Therapy Association, 2018, *American Journal of Occupational Therapy*, Vol. 72, Suppl. 2.

Administration of Evaluation and Assessments

6

Rebecca L. Simon, EdD, OTR, FAOTA, and Paula Kramer, PhD, OTR, FAOTA

CHAPTER HIGHLIGHTS

- Assessment categories
- Considerations for assessment administration
- Developing competence in use of assessments
- Preparing the assessment environment
- Types of error in assessment
- Implications for intervention

KEY TERMS AND CONCEPTS

- Assessment environment
- Capability
- Capacity
- Classical test theory
- Criterion-referenced assessments
- Interview technique
- Interviews
- Ipsative assessments
- Item bias
- Item response theory
- Nonstandardized assessments
- Normative assessments
- Observation
- Occupational profile
- Open-ended interviews
- Performance assessments
- Psychometrics
- Questionnaires
- Rater bias
- Reliability
- Semistructured interviews
- Simulated situation
- Standardized assessments
- Structured interviews
- Test-taker variables
- Therapeutic relationship
- Therapeutic use of self
- Validity

INTRODUCTION

The process of occupational therapy always begins with the evaluation of the client (American Occupational Therapy Association [AOTA], 2014). The formal or informal assessment tools chosen by occupational therapists may vary on the basis of client and context, but when administering and interpreting an assessment tool, therapists must carefully consider the facts known about the client, which are drawn largely from the screening and occupational profile (Asher, 2014) in addition to the specific assessment tools themselves.

This chapter details general principles regarding categories of assessments and includes a detailed discussion of factors that guide the administration of each type of assessment. It is essential that occupational therapy practitioners understand how to use both standardized and nonstandardized assessments and have a general understanding of contextual factors, including environmental and cultural components. Sources of errors in testing are also reviewed. The chapter concludes with a brief description of how the findings from assessments influence the development of an intervention plan and determine the effectiveness of the intervention.

ASSESSMENT CATEGORIES

Occupational therapists generally use a combination of standardized and nonstandardized assessments (e.g., observation, checklist, interviewing, screening) to identify a client's overall strengths and limitations. Reports from both standardized and nonstandardized instruments, as well as clinical observations, can help therapists gain a comprehensive picture of the client's occupational performance.

The purpose of an evaluation is to obtain useful information about the client and the client's life situation. Occupational therapists use data from assessments to identify the client's strengths and limitations and obtain useful information about the client's life. This information assists the therapist in developing an appropriate and meaningful intervention plan. The evaluation process is "focused on finding out what a client wants and needs to do; determining what a client can do and has done; and identifying supports and barriers to health, well-being, and participation" (AOTA, 2014, p. S13). Occupational therapists use clinical reasoning in the evaluation process. After screening, the first major step in the evaluation process is selecting the most appropriate assessment, which is influenced by "client

---

needs, practice settings, and therapists' frames of reference or practice models" (AOTA, 2014, p. S13).

Standardized

Best practice requires therapists to use standardized assessments whenever possible, although they should be combined with some nonstandardized assessments to get a complete picture of the client. Piernik-Yoder and Beck (2012) found that 90% of occupational therapists use standardized assessments several times per year. They noted that the most frequent reasons for choosing a specific assessment tool were to meet the needs of a client and the availability of that tool in the work environment. Choosing a tool based on its availability contradicts best practice for careful selection and use of outcome measures.

Standardized assessments are structured with standard administration procedures; their measurement properties are studied with normative data. When standardized assessments are administered in the recommended manner they provide reliable and valid data. If modifications are made when the assessment is administered, the standardization of the tool is affected, and the results are compromised. In many situations, laws governing practice and reimbursement, including the Individuals With Disabilities Education Improvement Act of 2004 (IDEA; P. L. 108-446) and the Improving Medicare Post-Acute Care Transformation Act of 2014 (IMPACT Act; P. L. 113-185), require the use of standardized assessments to ensure those receiving services truly qualify for them. Many standardized assessments are also appropriate for reevaluation because therapists can compare the retest scores, performance measures, or behavioral indicators to identify changes in a client's performance.

When determining which standardized assessment to use, occupational therapists should read the specific literature on testing tools to increase their knowledge of available assessment options, including their advantages and limitations. This knowledge also assists therapists in determining whether the assessment can be used as part of a reevaluation. In situations in which a standardized assessment is not designed for reevaluation, therapists should look for another standardized assessment that addresses the same domain or area of concern to obtain comparison data.

Standardized assessments are accompanied by specific set procedures or protocols. It is essential that evaluators follow these guidelines to ensure that the testing environment and procedures are the same for all clients who undergo evaluation using that assessment. Following standardized procedures when administering the assessments is necessary to obtain reportable, valid results. Many standardized assessments also have specific processes for data analysis.

There are three types of standardized assessments:

1. *Normative assessments* compare data obtained with a normed sample.
2. *Criterion-referenced assessments* determine a set score for mastery and compare data obtained with the set score.
3. *Ipsative assessments* have standardized procedures but no normed sample and are individualized to the client so that the same domain can be compared over time.

Normative assessments

The test developer designs a normative assessment from data using research conducted on a specific sample of people (i.e., the normative group). Often, the normative group is the "normal" population, or normed sample. Data from a normed sample forms a probability distribution shaped like a bell curve, with the scores of a majority of the people clustered in the center.

When occupational therapists obtain data about a client from a normative assessment, they can compare the client's scores, behaviors, or performance with those of the normed sample. At times, test developers may design an assessment for a group with a specific disability that becomes another sample for comparison with clients in that specific population. This standardization often describes how the person with a specific disability performs relative to both the normed sample and other people with the specific disability. It is critical that therapists understand to whom the client is being compared and explicitly state this information in the evaluation summary report.

For example, in the case of a manual dexterity evaluation, there may be a normed sample for those with use of both upper extremities and a sample for those who have use of only one extremity. If therapists are assessing a person with only one extremity, they need to be sure to compare the results with the latter sample because comparing them with the former sample will not necessarily provide valid results. It is essential that evaluating therapists consider this when reflecting on the evaluation process and report it clearly.

Occupational therapists must consider the psychometric integrity and potential limitations of the normative assessment tool when interpreting data from it. *Psychometrics* includes the reliability and validity evidence, responsiveness of the scale, the sample size and demographics of the normed sample, and the standard error of measurement. These factors are important in judging the value of the data from the assessment and to understanding the client's abilities and limitations.

Reliability refers to the consistency of the results provided by the scores on an assessment, whereas *validity* refers to how true the scores are to the underlying theory and concepts that the assessment claims to measure. Reliability is necessary, but not sufficient, to determine psychometric integrity. A measure's scores can be reliable but not valid, but valid scores on a measure may provide reliable information. For example, a set of items with simple hand movements may be a reliable test, but it may not be valid as a hand function test if functional activities are not within the types of items designed in the test. A measure with evidence of reliability is relatively free of measurement error. Reliability estimates can range from 0 to 1.00 in the traditional test theory approach (i.e., classical test theory methods where correlations are mainly employed). Generally, a reliability of 0.75 or higher indicates that a measure has strong evidence of reliability in a certain context, such as on repeated administration or between raters (Andresen, 2000).

There is no single score or system to determine an assessment's validity evidence; rather, there are many different types. Therefore, therapists do not have one score they can use to determine validity. In reality, many of the assessments occupational therapists use do not meet the standards of having multiple pieces of validity evidence. However, the assessment selected may be the only available instrument or the best instrument available for the purpose. Please refer to Chapter 9, "Psychometric Properties Related to Standardized Assessments," for a complete discussion of psychometric concepts related to testing.

It is also important to understand how to read the literature related to assessment and understand what constitutes a high-quality tool. Occupational therapists should always seek assessments with the most psychometric integrity. If an assessment's psychometric integrity is relatively low, therapists need to consider whether other assessments are available for the population of interest. If there is a better assessment, it is the therapist's ethical responsibility to obtain and use it.

There are times when occupational therapists may decide to use a particular assessment with lower psychometric integrity for a specific reason; the assessment may be the only assessment that exists to measure the construct of interest or the only assessment standardized for a particular age range. When this decision is made, therapists should be clear about why they have made this choice. Greater familiarity with an assessment is not sufficient justification for choosing an assessment with less psychometric integrity. Sometimes the only assessment available for testing a specific construct or trait has weak psychometric integrity; in such cases, therapists should report the limitations of the assessment in the evaluation report and summary.

Some normative assessments frequently used by occupational therapists are the

- Sensory Integration and Praxis Tests (Ayres, 1989),
- Lowenstein Occupational Therapy Cognitive Assessment (Itzkovich et al., 2000),
- Assessment of Motor and Process Skills (AMPS; Fisher & Jones, 2012),
- School Version of the Assessment of Motor and Process Skills (School AMPS; Fisher et al., 2007), and
- Test of Visual–Perceptual Skills (Martin, 2017).

This is not intended to be an exhaustive list, and readers are directed to the resources listed in Chapter 3, "Assessment Identification and Selection," to familiarize themselves with databases and guidelines that can assist with assessment selection.

Criterion-referenced assessments

Criterion-referenced assessments measure how well a person performs against a set of criteria rather than against another person or normative data. The developer of a criterion-referenced assessment selects items that reflect mastery of the area of concern or content. This type of assessment is distinguished from the more established, norm-referenced assessment in that the criterion-referenced assessment will examine performance in relation to a specific task that is a part of a larger domain (Ricketts, 2009).

Developing an assessment on the basis of a particular criterion begins with the construction of a table of specifications that lists the indicators associated with each component specification. These indicators may be considered competencies in other areas of practice, such as medicine (Ricketts, 2009). For example, in occupational therapy, if assessment developers wanted to assess the ability to dress oneself, they would begin by identifying the component aspects of dressing (e.g., selecting clothes, putting on a shirt, putting on pants or a skirt, putting on socks, putting on shoes) and measuring those specific tasks.

Criterion-referenced assessments generally provide an established score that reflects mastery. A person's score on a criterion-referenced assessment reflects how well the person performs against the set score for mastery. A criterion-based assessment does not compare scores, behaviors, or performances with a norm; instead, the focus is on the mastery of the area of interest.

Sometimes a test developer selects criteria for a criterion-referenced assessment for which normative information is available. When using a criterion-referenced assessment, occupational therapists cannot use information about the normal range of the criteria as a basis for comparing the client's performance against the known norm. Comparing criterion-referenced data with normative-referenced data is like comparing apples and oranges.

It is important for evaluators to recognize the difference between the two types of tests and how to interpret both sets of data. Criterion-referenced data are based on mastery; normative-referenced data are based on performance as it relates to a normative sample, as described earlier. A criterion-referenced assessment cannot become a normative assessment just because normative data are available. Driving tests, course exams, and the National Board for Certification in Occupational Therapy® examination are all criterion-referenced assessments.

Some criterion-referenced assessments that occupational therapists might use with a client are the

- School Function Assessment (Coster et al., 1998),
- Performance Assessment of Self-Care Skills (Rogers et al., 2016), and
- Kohlman Evaluation of Living Skills (Thomson & Robnett, 2016).

Another popular tool, the Miller Function and Participation Scales (Miller, 2006), is both norm- and criterion-referenced. The performance component of the tool is norm-referenced, and the participation component is criterion-referenced. Again, this is just a sample of such assessments and is not meant to be an exhaustive list.

Just as with normative assessments, the psychometric integrity of criterion-referenced assessments and other limitations identified in the test manual must be examined. Again, occupational therapists must determine which assessment is most appropriate to use on the basis of several factors, not just comfort, familiarity, and availability.

Ipsative assessments

Ipsative assessments have standardized procedures and are individualized so that people compare themselves in the same domain across time. Frequently, present performance is contrasted with previous performance in a specific domain. Two common forms—interview-based and observation-based assessments—do not have specific expected outcomes. Ipsative assessments use a standardized method of collecting data so that therapists can obtain information from different clients under consistent conditions.

Developers of ipsative assessments outline the specific procedures, the order in which they are to be followed, and sometimes the conditions that are most appropriate for administering the assessment. The purpose is to ask a standardized set of questions to elicit a clear understanding of the client's life, then compare those answers over time to note improvement or decline (Cynkin & Robinson, 1990; Law et al., 2005; Mosey, 1986). This type of assessment can be extremely beneficial for therapists working with clients for a length of time or therapists seeing a client later in treatment (or after discharge) in a different setting.

A common ipsative assessment used by occupational therapists is the Canadian Occupational Performance Measure (Law et al., 2019). This assessment can be used to identify areas of need for the client over time and in different settings. Other ipsative assessments include the Pediatric Volitional Questionnaire (Geist et al., 2002), the Pediatric Interest Profiles (Henry, 2000), and the Meaningful Activity Participation Assessment (Eakman et al., 2010). Again, this is not meant to be an exhaustive list of ipsative assessments used by occupational therapists.

Nonstandardized

Nonstandardized assessments have no standard administration procedures or study of measurement properties against a normative sample, One method of grouping nonstandardized assessments is by the techniques used for gathering information. These categories can be labeled *watching* (i.e., observation), *measuring* (i.e., observation using instruments for performance measures), *listening* (i.e., interviews), and *asking* (i.e., written questionnaires). The most basic techniques are observation and interviewing.

Observation-based assessments

Observation involves occupational therapists directly perceiving the actions of a client and then recording what they see. Observation can be aided by the use of an assessment or unaided. Many assessments of ADLs and IADLs originated with unaided observation of activities and behaviors that led to the development of standardized observational assessments. The AMPS (Fisher & Jones, 2012) is an example of a standardized observational assessment.

Observation has advantages over interviews and questionnaires. First, observation allows occupational therapists to witness how a client performs in a specific situation directly, without the rationalization or explanation therapists might interject during an interview and without the bias inherent in a self-report or proxy-report questionnaire. Second, observational assessment does not rely on the client's interpretation of questions or memory of events or activities.

To ensure an observational assessment is accurate and consistent, therapists must be unbiased and experienced in delivering the assessment. This can be a disadvantage for some therapists who lack training in the specific area being assessed. Observational assessments usually require extensive time to gather accurate information. Some can take an hour or more to perform or may require multiple sessions.

These disadvantages must be weighed in each practice setting to determine whether observation is appropriate.

Performance-based assessments

Occupational therapists often select **performance assessments** to measure functional limitations. For example, therapists can assess reaching and standing balance with the Berg Balance Scale (Berg et al., 1989); walking speed with the Timed Get-Up-and-Go Test (Wall et al., 2000), and specific developmental motor skills with tools such as the Bruininks–Oseretsky Test of Motor Proficiency, Second Edition (Bruininks & Bruininks, 2005). Therapists also use dynamometers to test hand strength, which is independent of context (i.e., grip strength simply tells the evaluator that the client has a certain strength that is above, below, or average).

Unlike ADL and IADL observations, performance assessments often focus on a specific body function, client factors, and performance skills, and any associated impairments. Performance assessments often rely on calibrated instruments for measurement. Therefore, they are independent of individual judgment and not as susceptible to influence from the client or rater bias as are observations, interviews, and questionnaires. However, because performance assessments focus on the function of a specific body part, they usually ignore the environment and the person as a whole. This often means that another assessment will be needed to understand the person in context. Performance assessments may also assess cognitive functioning. These assessments require the client to perform a cognitive task, such as telling time on an analog clock or spelling or reading given words.

Interviews

Interviews are another common means of gathering information. The **interview technique** involves a conversation between the occupational therapist and the client or a proxy. Optimally, an interview should involve direct interaction with the client. When direct interaction is not possible, a therapist, with the client's permission, can conduct an interview with a proxy, or someone who has sufficient knowledge of the client's situation to act on his or her behalf (e.g., spouse, parent, significant other, or caregiver). A proxy may also be used if the client is a minor or is legally incapable of being interviewed. Whenever possible, therapists should conduct interviews in person to observe the respondent's reactions and behaviors. When an in-person interview is impossible, therapists can interview the client by telephone or through virtual means.

Interviews range from structured to open ended. **Structured interviews** contain specific questions that occupational therapists ask in a specific order. The Collaborative Occupational Measure of Performance and Change over Time™ (Stube & Hanson, 2016) is an example of a tool that requires questions be asked of clients in a specific order and has detailed administration procedures. When an interview is highly structured, the information obtained is more likely to be consistent across interviewees. **Semistructured interviews,** including the Occupational Performance History Interview–II (Kielhofner et al., 2004), are also used. In a semistructured interview, some questions are structured, and some obtain both a detailed understanding of the client's life and a broad look at the impact of the client's illness or disability.

Open-ended interviews allow interviewees to tell their story in the manner that is most comfortable, sharing their lived experience. For example, the occupational profile is meant to be an open interview guide that allows evaluating occupational therapists to ask questions about various areas of occupational performance but leaves much room for interpretation. The *occupational profile* is a "summary of a client's occupational history and experiences, patterns of daily living, interests, values, and needs" (AOTA, 2014, p. S13). The information is obtained from the client's perspective through both formal interview techniques and casual conversation and leads to an individualized, client-centered approach to intervention (AOTA, 2014).

An advantage of these less structured and open-ended interviews is that they provide occupational therapists with an opportunity to obtain more or clarifying information. Probing is more likely to be used in these types of interviews. When the occupational therapist asks clarifying questions, the client can explain answers to difficult-to-comprehend questions, and a much more vivid and rich picture of the client's occupational performance may be achieved that includes culture and context that may be overlooked in a structured interview.

Interview information can be recorded using written notes, audiotaping, or videotaping for later review. Audiotaped interviews allow independent raters to score the data and ensure verification of interpretation. Audiotaping is often done in qualitative research but not in practice. Whenever a person is audio- or videotaped, occupational therapists must obtain written consent from that person. This written consent should identify who will have access to the data and what the therapist will do with the audio- or videotapes after the evaluation is completed.

When interpreting data from an interview, occupational therapists must consider the method of data collection (e.g., face-to-face vs. remote contact, structured vs. open ended) because it can affect the credibility of the information obtained. One challenge for therapists during an interview is to establish rapport with the client or proxy so that he or she shares information truthfully. Therapists conducting open-ended interviews need advanced training on how to engage the client in a guided conversation to solicit appropriate information and identify confabulation (a symptom of various memory disorders in which made-up stories fill in any gaps in memory). It is important that therapists realize that an open-ended interview is not a give-and-take conversation with the interviewee but a guided exchange designed to elicit specific information.

The occupational profile, for example, is a template that can be completed after or during a client interview. Because this document can be used as a interview method or to guide the interview process, it includes information about the client's needs, problems, and concerns about performance of occupations. It is in the analysis that occupational therapists can specifically identify supports and barriers related to occupational performance and identify targeted outcomes (AOTA, 2014).

In some settings, interviews will not constitute effective evaluations on their own. Certain settings, such as schools, require the use of a standardized tool by law. Although the interview can provide valuable information, it cannot stand alone and is not an acceptable tool to determine the need for services. In settings in which laws (e.g., IDEA, IMPACT Act) require standardized assessments, it is prudent to combine the interview process with standardized assessments to obtain a complete picture of the client and ensure reimbursement and appropriate development of meaningful and acceptable interventions.

Questionnaires

Questionnaires are sets of questions that occupational therapists may ask clients to gather more information, or they can include a choice of responses designed for surveying a particular trait, behavior, or concept. The two major advantages of questionnaires are the (1) ease of administration and (2) low cost. The client or proxy can complete the questionnaire, as with an interview, with or without the therapist being present. A highly structured questionnaire in which the client answers multiple-choice or true–false questions (called *forced-choice responses*) provides highly reliable information. Clients can complete a self-report questionnaire at their convenience and can easily be interrupted or stopped. Although questionnaires are easy for therapists to administer, they have many disadvantages. Questionnaires with highly structured and clearly worded questions provide valid and reliable information, but those with vague or difficult-to-interpret questions provide questionable information. Moreover, the information obtained using questionnaires may be less accurate than information obtained from direct observations or interviews.

For example, when completing a questionnaire, a client can easily misinterpret a question. If clients misunderstand a question asked during an interview, occupational therapists have a chance to probe for clarification or additional information. Clients can be less accurate when reporting their own behavior than when a therapist is directly observing it. In addition, clients may be unable to judge their own abilities accurately or may answer a question with personal bias. Again, unlike during an interview or observation, therapists do not have an opportunity to seek clarification or probe for more in-depth understanding. However, a well-designed questionnaire provides therapists with ways to detect untruths and biases through questions designed to test the veracity of the client's answers.

Finally, clients' ability to complete a questionnaire depends on their understanding of the language as well as their reading and cognitive abilities. In cases in which therapists are unsure of the client's ability to complete the questionnaire independently, they should read the questionnaire to the client and help the client complete it. Examples of questionnaires with quality psychometric components include the recently updated Role Checklist (Scott et al., 2019), which has better reliability and validity than the original Role Checklist (Oakley et al., 1986); the Sensory Profile (Dunn, 2014); and the Sensory Processing Measure (Parham et al., 2010).

CONSIDERATIONS FOR ASSESSMENT ADMINISTRATION

To address client needs, occupational therapists select assessments on the basis of the purpose of the evaluation, therapists' skills, the amount of time available for administration, and the assessment's requirements (e.g., equipment, space, expertise). Typically, therapists begin by conducting an initial screening to obtain general information about the client. Screening often includes a review of referral information; general observations; or other information provided by documentation on file, the client, significant others, or other professionals.

On the basis of screening data, occupational therapists may decide to proceed with a full evaluation. They must then decide which assessments to administer and develop a plan to conduct the evaluation. The evaluation plan must be realistic and created in such a manner that therapists can appropriately carry it out under real circumstances, in a natural environment if possible, and be sensitive to the client's situation. Sometimes space, equipment, resources, or expertise limits the choice of available assessments tools.

Because professionals in many disciplines use the same assessments, occupational therapists may revise the evaluation plan on the basis of which assessments others in the practice setting are using. If an assessment administered by another professional provides information needed to complete the occupational therapy evaluation, occupational therapists should obtain and use that information in preparing their final evaluation summary. When using information from another professional's report, therapists should always reference the other professional's report and the specific assessments the professional used.

Once occupational therapists have developed an evaluation plan, they inform the client about the process of the evaluation and what the client will be expected to do during each step in the process. It is important to tell the client how long the evaluation will take and what exactly it will involve. Clients have the right to be informed about the purpose of each assessment and how the results will be used.

Moreover, clients have the absolute right to refuse an evaluation or a specific assessment without consequences, and occupational therapists need to accept their refusal without repercussion. When the client is a child, the family or legal guardian should be involved in the explanation process and has the right to refuse an evaluation. If the client is an adult but not capable of understanding the rationale for an assessment, therapists should inform the designated health proxy about the focus and purpose of the selected assessments.

In the past, it was customary to discuss such issues with family members and significant others. However, since passage of the Health Insurance Portability and Accountability Act of 1996 (P. L. 104-191), only persons who have been formally designated by the client or hold a health proxy for the client can be involved in this process. In the case of the evaluation of a minor, information must be provided to the parent or legal guardian. In the case of a client who is unable to give consent, the legal guardian or health proxy must be included in discussions regarding the evaluation. A client's refusal to participate in portions of the evaluation should be reported as a part of the evaluation, but their refusal should not affect the outcome or plan for service. Occupational therapists are responsible for explaining the evaluation process in a manner that is appropriate for the client and should choose wording that is easily understood by all involved.

DEVELOPING COMPETENCE IN USE OF ASSESSMENTS

Standardized assessments are generally multifaceted; often, they are not easy for occupational therapists to master until they have practiced with them repeatedly. Therapists should first study and rehearse an unfamiliar assessment before administering it to a client. Therapists must always read the assessment manual carefully. This thorough reading provides an understanding of the scope and purpose of the assessment. Most manuals discuss the administration procedures for the assessment, identify its limitations, and present facts about its psychometric integrity. The manual also explains what therapists will learn about the client from the assessment. For example, the manual might explain that therapists will learn about a client's strengths, limitations, performance skills, personal characteristics, roles, and values. Some manuals are more extensive than others. Some assessments require extensive training and certification, as discussed in Chapter 5, "Evaluation in the Intervention Planning Process." This can be both a cost and a time factor for therapists, but it is critical for appropriate use.

It is helpful for occupational therapists to examine the published literature on any assessment they are considering using. Research and clinical narratives provide important information about an assessment and its efficacy in a practice situation. An assessment should not be used simply because of its availability and commonality to the setting. It should be chosen because it suits the needs of the client, at that particular time and in that particular setting. The following sources provide up-to-date and relevant information about standardized assessments:

- Buros Center for Testing website (https://buros.org)
- Educational Testing Service website (http://ets.org/tests)
- Health and Psychosocial Instruments (HaPI) database (published by Behavioral Measurement Database Services; https://www.bmdshapi.com)
- Rehabilitation Measures Database (https://www.sralab.org/rehabilitation-measures).

These sources can provide occupational therapists with a broader understanding of an assessment and its appropriate use.

If there is little published information on an assessment, it would be wise for the occupational therapist to seek out someone with more experience evaluating people like the therapist's client to identify whether more appropriate assessments are available.

Once occupational therapists decide that a standardized assessment is appropriate and will provide useful data, they must develop competence in administering it efficiently (Exhibit 6.1). Therapists should practice administering the assessment until they are competent in the mechanics of giving directions and manipulating materials. Therapists should also practice administering the assessment to several age-appropriate people without disabilities.

EXHIBIT 6.1.	Developing Competence in Administering an Evaluation

- Read the assessment manual thoroughly.
- Review published literature about the assessment.
- Become competent in administration of the assessment.
- Get feedback on your administration of the assessment from an experienced therapist.
- Have an experienced therapist review your interpretation of the assessment.
- Use a combination of standardized and nonstandardized assessments to get a complete picture of the client.
- Write an accurate report, including strengths and areas of concern.

Source. Developed by J. Hinojosa and P. Kramer. Used with permission.

Once occupational therapists have obtained basic competence in administering an assessment, they should have someone with experience observe them administering that assessment and provide feedback to help them refine skills and confirm that the data collected are reliable and accurate. Therapists must develop competence in appropriately interpreting the data by practicing scoring and interpreting them. At times it is helpful to ask a more experienced therapist to review the raw data and interpretation to determine whether that therapist would come to the same conclusion.

As with standardized assessments, occupational therapists must establish competence in administering and interpreting nonstandardized assessments. Therapists can practice administering nonstandardized assessments by observing and interviewing people without disabilities and then interpreting the data to enhance skill development and competence.

After mastering administration of an assessment, occupational therapists need to become competent in writing up the results in a clear, concise summary. In this written summary, therapists present evidence and provide clear baseline data to either support the need for occupational therapy or illustrate that the client has adequate occupational performance. The written summary should give an overall perspective on the client's ability to function and participate in occupations, highlighting strengths as well as limitations. Therapists must keep the report as objective as possible, even when interpreting results. All written reports must be accurate and portray data honestly. Therapists should state actual scores and resulting interpretations. Therapists should not make conclusions that are not supported by the data.

PREPARING THE ASSESSMENT ENVIRONMENT

Occupational therapists need to consider the *assessment environment*—both the physical environment and the psychological environment—when administering an assessment. Therapists are part of the environment, and they play an important role in ensuring that the environment is optimal for obtaining the appropriate data. The assessment environment should be conducive to eliciting true performance skills and abilities from the client. The environments needed for standardized and nonstandardized assessments, as discussed in the following sections, can be distinctly different. The type of assessment and the occupational performance components being assessed will determine the appropriate environmental setting for the assessment. The realities of the setting and the reimbursement system in which therapists work may also influence the assessment environment.

Appropriate Environments for Standardized Assessments

Because standardized assessments compare a person's performance with normative or criterion-referenced data, some standardized assessments specifically prescribe the type of testing environment the occupational therapist must create. If such a description exists, therapists must follow it exactly to achieve valid results. This may include chair-to-table height, specific measurements of distance, client positioning, and other calibrated efforts to ensure consistency. If the assessment manual provides no description of the assessment environment, therapists should create an environment that they believe will foster the client's optimal performance. In most situations, the natural environment may not be the best setting for a standardized assessment, because it tends to have distractions that may impede optimal performance. The optimal assessment environment should be comfortable, private, well lit, distraction free, and quiet.

When choosing the environment, occupational therapists must consider the requirements of the assessment. Some assessments require specific equipment; others require a large amount of space. Occupational therapists should make sure that the environment and equipment for a particular assessment are available before administering the assessment so that the results are not compromised. When therapists administer a standardized assessment in a controlled clinical setting, it is assumed that the client will demonstrate optimal performance. If therapists administer a standardized assessment in a noisy room with distractions, the results would not be valid, and the client may not demonstrate optimal performance.

Appropriate Environments for Nonstandardized Assessments

Most nonstandardized assessments do not specify the characteristics of the testing environment. The most trustworthy information is generally obtained when the assessment is conducted in the most natural environment. For example, occupational therapists can tell more about a child's attention skills in the school setting if they observe the child's performance in the classroom rather than in a clinical environment. Similarly, therapists can gather more information about the home maintenance skills of a woman recovering from a cerebrovascular accident by observing her as she navigates her kitchen at home than by observing her performance in the adapted kitchen in the hospital.

Occupational therapists obtain more accurate and realistic information about the client's true occupational performance skills when they use the natural environment for a nonstandardized assessment. Similarly, clients are more likely to provide more information during an interview when they are in a comfortable, familiar setting. When therapists collect data in a more natural, comfortable environment, the data tend to be more trustworthy.

However, it is often not possible or realistic for occupational therapists to administer an assessment in the natural environment. In these situations, therapists must be creative and develop an appropriate *simulated situation* to obtain valid information about clients' skills and abilities. An effective simulated environment should have characteristics similar to those of the natural environment. For example, to assess cooking skills, therapists would use an appropriate setting that has a stove, pots, and pans. To evaluate bathroom transfer skills, therapists should choose a setting as close as possible to that in the client's home.

In addition, simulated environments may be helpful in increasing the client's comfort with the assessment process. A newer trend is the use of simulated assessments that involve virtual reality. Zhang et al. (2003) effectively used a virtual reality environment for assessment of clients with brain injury. Others have since gone on to use virtual reality tools to assess function in clients after stroke (Adams et al., 2019) and a child's ability to self-feed (Persky et al., 2018). Several simulated driving experiences and assessments are available, including the DriverLab at the Toronto Rehabilitation Institute's iDAPT Centre for Rehabilitation Research (https://kite-uhn.com/labs), Carnetsoft driving simulator (https://cs-driving-simulator.com/), and other standardized tools. As always, it is important that therapists confirm the validity of simulation tools. Wynne et al. (2019) found that although driving simulators were highly used, only half of those on the market provide a valid assessment of skill.

Sometimes occupational therapists cannot create a simulated environment to match the natural environment. In this situation, they might strive to create a simulated environment that is ergonomically correct for both them and the client to increase the comfort of both. Therapists should provide the client with a proper setting, appropriate table height, and a footrest for the client's feet and adhere to safety precautions. Proper ergonomics will increase the potential for optimal performance during the assessment.

Psychological Environment for Assessment

From a psychological perspective, occupational therapists should try to help the client become an active participant in the assessment process. Establishing rapport with the client increases the client's comfort level, which is critical because people tend to perform better when they are comfortable than when they are anxious. Therapists should start an evaluation by introducing themselves. At this point, it is important to find out how the client likes to be addressed. Many older clients prefer to be addressed by their surnames and are offended when they are addressed by their first names, especially by someone who is younger. It is essential to build rapport and not offend the client before the start of the evaluation.

Occupational therapists should explain the assessment to the client and answer any questions the client may have. If the client is a child accompanied by a caregiver, it is important to acknowledge and speak to all parties and not ignore either the child or the guardian. If an interpreter is present, it is important to make eye contact with the client and speak directly to the client as if he or she could understand. This direct, rapport-building communication relieves anxiety and creates a more client-centered atmosphere. In addition, when the client knows the rationale for the assessment and what is expected of him or her while completing the assessment, the client is likely to be a more active participant in the process.

Occupational therapists should also consider the client's personality and timetable when scheduling the assessment. Whenever possible, therapists should administer the assessment when the client is most alert and responsive. Therapists will obtain the best results when the client is alert and calm; however, they have to work within the constraints of the system and should recognize that a client's mood and frame of mind will affect the quality of information obtained from the assessment. If this occurs, it should be reflected in the evaluation report.

Therapeutic Relationship

The *therapeutic relationship* often begins when occupational therapists first meet the client. Often this is at the initial evaluation. In most situations, building rapport with the client assists the evaluation process. In the developing relationship between the therapist and the client, the client is in a vulnerable position. The client depends on the therapist to explain the nature of the evaluation and the intervention process. This relationship is bidirectional, but in most cases, the client relates to this information from a position of trust rather than a position of knowledge.

Occupational therapy practitioners bring their knowledge about the impact of occupation on engagement and participation and "use this information, coupled with theoretical perspectives and clinical reasoning, to critically observe, analyze, describe, and interpret human performance" (AOTA, 2014, p. S12) during the evaluation process. Practitioners and clients, together with caregivers, family members, and other relevant participants, work together in the evaluation process to develop the most comprehensive understanding of the client possible. The therapist is trusted to provide honest and meaningful information that will assist the client in improving function. The client also needs to trust that the therapist has the required expertise to carry out the evaluation and intervention plan. Typically, people are more comfortable with those whom they feel they know. Building rapport between therapist and client helps to build comfort, trust, and a basis for open communication. The interpersonal aspects of the occupational therapy process help therapists to provide assistance more effectively (Canton & Taylor, 2012; Taylor, 2008). Once a relationship of trust has been established, therapists must fulfill the ethical responsibility not to abuse this trust and to provide expert care to the best of their abilities (AOTA, 2015).

Once clients develop trust in the occupational therapist, they may feel more able to reveal important aspects of their life, fears, and concerns. As clients reveal information that is more personal, they become more aware of their own thoughts and feelings, which enables them to come to terms with personal reactions to illness, injury, or disability. Strong rapport between the client and therapist also can empower clients to feel comfortable enough to ask awkward or difficult questions that they otherwise might not have asked. Strong rapport also allows clients to reveal strengths and abilities. The information gained from this relationship helps the therapist to choose assessments that will meet clients' needs.

Ultimately, this information helps the occupational therapist construct a client-centered evaluation and then a client-centered intervention. Throughout this process, the best interests of the client must be the therapist's primary concern. Thus, the therapist must be careful that the nature of the evaluation does not impede the establishment of rapport.

Evaluator and Situational Issues

Every occupational therapist has specific strengths and limitations that influence the choice and use of assessments. A wide variety of factors may influence therapists' selection of tools, including their background knowledge, ability to handle test pieces, and analytic reasoning. Therapists most commonly gravitate toward assessments that they are more comfortable with, or that are readily available, rather than researching the best assessment to use. Therefore, self-reflection can be useful for therapists to become aware of what factors influence their choice of assessments. Using evidence to choose assessment tools will lead to a willingness to explore new or alternative assessments rather than repeatedly using one assessment. Therapists should choose assessments that are most appropriate for the client and the client's needs rather than those they like and feel comfortable administering.

Occupational therapists' mindset or attitude at the time of the assessment may also influence its administration. For example, a therapist who is not feeling well or who is having a bad day may have difficulty attending to the tasks at hand. Therapists must maintain heightened awareness to prevent personal situations from influencing the evaluation. Thus, when administering and interpreting evaluation data, therapists must consider themselves as a possible intervening variable. It is always important for therapists to consider therapeutic use of self during the process. *Therapeutic use of self* refers to the therapist's "planned use of his or her personality, insights, perceptions and judgments as part of the therapeutic process" (Punwar & Peloquin, 2000, p. 285). Although this therapeutic use of self is extremely effective during intervention, therapists must be careful not to let any preconceived notions influence the evaluation process.

Occupational therapists must consider the entire evaluation experience. During an evaluation, the therapist and client form an exclusive relationship within a shared lived experience. Although the primary focus is on the client, the therapist is responsible for analyzing the data to develop an appropriate intervention plan for the client. The knowledge that the therapist gains about the client during the evaluation; the rapport that is established; and the feelings, both emotional and intuitive, of the therapist toward the client make the evaluation experience richer. When interpreting data, therapists should consider other factors about themselves as evaluator and how these factors may have influenced any portion of the assessment. Any recommendations for the intervention plan must reflect both what

has been learned from the total evaluation and the shared experience.

It is critical that occupational therapists realize that the results of the evaluation can have a long-term effect on the client's life. For example, when a child is evaluated in a school system, the results of the data may lead to a classification (e.g., class placement) that may follow that child for many years. The results of the evaluation are also read by family members, teachers, and other team members who will form an opinion of the child's strengths and needs on the basis of the assessment. For older adult clients, assessment data and the subsequent evaluation summary may determine whether a client is capable of living alone or must be in a supervised placement—again, an impact that goes beyond clients themselves. Therapists must be certain of the integrity of the assessments and the accuracy of their data when writing evaluation summaries that may result in high-stakes decision making (Plake & Spies, 2005).

TYPES OF ERROR IN ASSESSMENT

Assessment is the first step in the occupational therapy process (AOTA, 2014), and occupational therapists make important decisions, such as intervention planning and implementation, on the basis of assessment data. Therefore, it is critical that evaluators try to minimize errors in the assessment process. Errors occur as a result of the assessment itself in the form of item bias, or they can be made by raters who score the test or the client's behavior or performance. Therapists should control for error when assessing a client for areas of strength and weakness to ensure that the data are an accurate reflection of the client's abilities. Choosing the best assessment available for the purpose, ensuring that therapists are competent in the administration of the assessment, and adequately preparing the client for the tasks the client needs to perform can keep errors to a minimum.

Item Bias

Item bias occurs when people of similar abilities perform differently on a given assessment or test item because of age, gender, ethnic, cultural, socioeconomic, or other group differences. Items can be biased when they contain content or language that is unfamiliar to, or interpreted differently by, different groups (see Chapter 13, "Accommodating Diversity in Assessment and Evaluation").

When choosing an assessment, occupational therapists should know the group of people for whom the instrument was originally designed and whether it was validated on other specific groups of interest. For example, the 36-item Short-Form Health Survey (SF-36®; Ware & Sherbourne, 1992), one of the most widely used measures of quality-of-life health status, was originally designed to measure the same eight health domains for adults ages 18 years or older. The SF-36 provides psychometrically based Physical Component Summary (PCS) and Mental Component Summary (MCS) scores. The tool was initially designed as a generic health status measure and validated with large groups of people with various health problems. Because none of these groups contained people whose primary means of mobility was a wheelchair, the developers wrote questions about mobility for people who could walk. To make this instrument unbiased for people who use wheelchairs, the word *walk* was replaced with the word *go*. Item bias may introduce errors into an assessment; people with equal abilities should be able to attain the same score. Therapists should research the populations used for standardization in the assessment manual or other literature about the assessment.

Occupational therapists should always consider the psychometric properties of an instrument. ***Classical test theory*** relies on the psychometric concepts of reliability, validity, and responsiveness. This theory divides total scores into two components: (1) the true score and (2) a margin for error. This approach cannot separate individual ability from item difficulty.

Item response theory (IRT), frequently associated with educational and psychological assessments, has become more important to occupational therapy. IRT is sometimes referred to as *latent* (or *underlying*) *trait theory*. This theory, developed in the 1960s as a means of separating item difficulty from underlying individual abilities (respondent traits), involves a series of statistical procedures. IRT views the problem in terms of probability that a person's response will be in a certain category (Embretson & Reise, 2000). A variant of IRT, Rasch analysis, was used extensively in evaluating the underlying response format of the FIM® (Uniform Data System for Medical Rehabilitation, 1997). These analyses have shown that the FIM has three underlying scales: (1) Self-Care, (2) Motor, and (3) Cognitive Functions (Cohen & Marino, 2000).

Although further discussion of psychometrics is beyond the scope of this chapter, the differences between classical test theory and IRT and their implications for health care are discussed in detail in several publications (Chang & Reeve, 2005; DeMars, 2018; Hays et al., 2000; Schwartz & Rapkin, 2004). IRT analyses can also be used to determine whether raters are using the same standards of measurement and can assess whether physical functioning, as assessed by a particular measure, is based on the person's response, the properties of the questions asked, or the severity of a rater's observation.

Evaluator Variables

Rater bias, also known as *observer bias,* is another source of error in assessments. It occurs when different evaluators disagree in their assessment of the same person (i.e., no *interrater reliability*) or when the same evaluator scores the same person differently on repeated testing (i.e., no *intrarater reliability*). If different therapists assessing the same person use different standards of measurement (i.e., if some are more lenient than others), results are not comparable across therapists. Therapists need special training and testing against a standard to eliminate this possibility. For this reason, some assessments, such as the AMPS (Fisher & Jones, 2012), require therapists being trained in its use be calibrated to ensure reliability of ratings.

A more subtle rater bias takes the form of coaching a client (Victor & Abeles, 2004). An occupational therapist may coach, or "push," a client to perform beyond the client's normal capacity. Sometimes this situation occurs because the therapist believes that the client has more skills than are being shown during the evaluation. At other times, it occurs because the therapist and client have developed a rapport, so the therapist views that particular client with a subtle bias. Other therapist factors also contribute to the validity of assessment results. The therapeutic relationship, for example, contributes to the quality of a client's performance. A therapist facilitates the client's optimal performance when the client trusts the therapist and feels that the therapist is concerned about them. In addition, the amount of experience that a therapist has in administering and interpreting a specific assessment can influence the results. As therapists gain more experience in administering an assessment, they become more comfortable and skilled. When therapists first learn to administer an assessment, they usually focus on the mechanics of administration, giving less attention to the client's behaviors and performance. Practice and experience allow therapists to become skilled in the mechanics involved in administering an assessment and increase focus on the client.

Likewise, multiple experiences provide occupational therapists with pragmatic knowledge about when to give breaks; they allow them to be more sensitive to clients' moods and manipulate the environment to ensure best performance within the standardized procedures. Schell and Schell (2008) described the pragmatic reasoning developed by skilled therapists that considers everyday realities that affect service delivery. Skilled therapists use the evaluation process to establish a solid therapeutic relationship with the client and the client's significant others.

Test-Taker Variables

Many ***test-taker variables*** can affect an assessment. Tolerance for pain or discomfort and fatigue can influence clients' scores on an assessment. In addition, the process of being evaluated may stress clients. Clients realize that the occupational therapist will make decisions about them using the data collected. Clients are also conscious of the fact that information gathered using an assessment may determine the services they receive or the level of independence with which they will live. Even very young children seem to realize that they are being observed and judged during an evaluation. Children from certain cultures, particularly boys from American Indian and African American subcultures, are very reluctant to engage in the evaluation process (Astone et al., 2015). Some individuals may want to obtain a certain outcome from the assessment (e.g., return to work, funding from a certain payer) and will attempt to manipulate the test. Therapists with more experience may be able to more easily identify malingerers or people who have used the Internet to identify how to answer questions and present themselves in such a way that will ensure their desired result (Suhr & Gunstad, 2007).

Anxiety and stress are always important concerns. A moderate amount of anxiety can enhance performance in a testing situation; however, too little or too much anxiety can result in poor performance. Therefore, occupational therapists should try to make clients at ease in the testing situation. Therapists should inform clients about what the assessment involves and what they will be asked to do. Moreover, therapists should outline the procedures the assessment will entail; knowledge of the process can reduce client anxiety. Questioning clients about prior experiences with testing and their views on testing can provide information that will promote rapport and provide therapists with some insights into clients.

Anxiety, stress, depression, or paranoia may also be concerns during the evaluation process. If anxiety, stress, depression, or paranoia appear to interfere with clients' ability to complete the assessment, therapists may have to adjust the evaluation plan and perhaps refer the client appropriately to another professional. Therapists must continually reaffirm the purpose and goal of the occupational therapy evaluation, but they must also be responsive to clients.

Sometimes clients' beliefs and views about testing influence their behavior or performance. Clients who do not care about the results or who do not understand the purpose of the assessment may put little effort into the process of evaluation. Clients may not be motivated to perform well on an assessment when they believe that assessment scores will not reflect real abilities. When a client's beliefs or views about testing appear to be interfering with the collection of valid assessment data, the therapist needs to adjust the evaluation plan. The therapist may decide to report the limited data collected or may decide to explore other options with the client.

Clients' physical status can interfere with their ability to complete an assessment. During the administration of an assessment, the occupational therapist might observe that a client has limited energy, activity tolerance, or physical stamina. The therapist should modify the evaluation plan to match the client's physical capacity to complete the assessment. Sometimes the therapist will need to postpone the assessment until the client has sufficient physical capacity.

Influence of Previous Testing Activities

A comprehensive evaluation usually involves several assessments, and the order in which they are administered needs to be planned. The activities involved in one assessment may influence performance on another assessment. Some testing demands may lead to fatigue or inability to attend to a task. Some assessments involve tasks that may excite a specific client, and others contain questions that may upset a client, so it is critical that therapists consider the order in which the specific assessments are administered. Occupational therapists must consider what they have learned about the client from the screening. The evaluation plan considers the demands that each assessment will put on the client.

At times, facility policies and third-party payers determine which evaluations are used and how they are administered. Therapists may have to adhere to these policies. However, in either situation, therapists should make the experience as comfortable as possible for the client and should indicate any demands that the evaluation is placing on the client in the ensuing report. Therapists have a dual responsibility to both the client and the facility.

Performance Versus Capacity

Three components of a comprehensive evaluation are the client's (1) capacity, (2) capability, and (3) performance.
1. *Capacity* is a person's ability to execute a task in a controlled, hypothetical, or optimal situation.
2. *Capability* is what a person can do in the daily environment.

3. *Performance* is what a person actually does in the real world (Nasreddine et al., 2005).

The World Health Organization's (2001) *International Classification of Functioning, Disability and Health* indicates that a standardized environment is needed to assess a person's capacity. Because *capacity* depends on such an environment, occupational therapists should attempt to standardize across different environments. *Capability* is the ability to conduct tasks in the person's own environment—not the standardized environment. The capability of an individual does not reflect what they do in real life but what they are capable of doing in their own environment. *Performance*—what a person actually does in a given situation—provides a true picture of the person's functional status. It better reflects the assistance a person may need to function in the home environment, whereas capacity may be a better measure for determining the course and type of therapeutic intervention (Holsbeeke et al., 2009).

Personal factors (e.g., motivation, personality) can influence performance; coaching may influence capacity. During the administration of an assessment and when writing the report, occupational therapists need to consider what they have learned about the client's performance, capacity, and capability as they relate to the intervention planning process.

IMPLICATIONS FOR INTERVENTION

The evaluation process necessitates that occupational therapists obtain trustworthy data. To do so requires the accurate administration of assessments and candid observations of the client's performance and behaviors. Therapists derive a complete picture of the client through data from reliable and valid assessments, including observations and interviews with the client. The data are tempered by therapists' judgment and clinical reasoning skills, often gained through experience. A thorough evaluation, combined with consultation with the client whenever possible, is a complex process, providing the foundation for the development of a sound intervention plan. An intervention plan developed from inadequate data or data that were not gathered in an organized and standardized manner is like a house built on an inadequate foundation. Just as a house may not stand without the proper infrastructure, an intervention plan may not be adequate or successful without a basis in strong evaluative data.

Identifying clear outcomes for the client requires the administration of a comprehensive and sound evaluation that provides clear baseline data. If clear baseline data do not exist, it is difficult to determine the extent of the client's progress. Occupational therapists are often able to identify tasks that clients are able to do after a course of intervention, but without clear baseline data, it is often hard to determine exactly what has changed to account for the improved performance.

SUMMARY

Administering and interpreting assessments require competence and skills. The role of evaluator is one of the more daunting roles undertaken by occupational therapists. Evaluation serves as the basis for understanding the client, determining the client's needs, and developing a plan for intervention. Therapists must become familiar and competent in administering various assessments while at the same time being able to gather nonstandardized data that are critical to understanding occupational performance. They need to understand the psychometric data and protocols used in standardized tests and the nature of the various assessments. Moreover, therapists must consider the complexities of the assessments, the environment, and the potential variables that might affect the outcome of the assessments.

Organizing and understanding all the information that is necessary to perform a comprehensive evaluation is like managing a three-ring circus—one must be aware of many factors at the same time to ensure a comprehensive and accurate evaluation.

QUESTIONS

1. Describe the process that an occupational therapist would use to develop skills in administering a standardized assessment. Why is such an extensive process necessary?
2. Select a criterion-referenced assessment and review the manual. What elements are used to determine mastery?
3. Select a norm-referenced assessment and review the manual. What specific components are used for the normative data?
4. Select an ipsative assessment and review the manual. What specific components are used to develop the test?
5. How would the environment influence the administration of a developmental assessment for a young child?
6. Consider your own life and self-observations. Can you identify any factors that would influence your ability to administer a standardized assessment? How?
7. Do you think it would be easier for you to administer a standardized assessment to a child or an adult? Why?
8. If a language barrier exists when evaluating, even with an interpreter, what steps might you take to develop rapport? What do you think are potential pitfalls, and how might these be overcome?

REFERENCES

Adams, R. J., Ellington, A. L., Armstead, K., Sheffield, K., Patrie, J. T., & Diamond, P. T. (2019). Upper-extremity function assessment using a glove orthosis and virtual reality system. *OTJR: Occupation, Participation and Health, 39*, 81–89. https://doi.org/10.1177/1539449219829862

American Occupational Therapy Association. (2014). Occupational therapy practice framework: Domain and process (3rd ed.). *American Journal of Occupational Therapy, 68*(Suppl. 1), S1–S48. https://doi.org/10.5014/ajot.2014.682006

American Occupational Therapy Association. (2015). Occupational therapy code of ethics (2015). *American Journal of Occupational Therapy, 69*, 6913410030. https://doi.org/10.5014/ajot.2015.696S03

Andresen, E. M. (2000) Criteria for assessing the tools of disability outcomes research. *Archives of Physical Medicine and Rehabilitation, 81*(Suppl. 2), S15–S20. https://doi.org/10.1053/apmr.2000.20619

Asher, I. E. (Ed.). (2014). *Asher's occupational therapy assessment tools: An annotated index.* Bethesda, MD: AOTA Press.

Astone, N. M., Popkin, S. J., Sandstron, H., & Dubay, L. (2015). *Promoting healthy families and communities for boys and young men of color: Race, ethnicity, and gender.* Washington DC: Urban Institute.

Ayres, A. (1989). *Sensory Integration and Praxis Tests (SIPT): Manual* (Updated ed.). Los Angeles: Western Psychological Services.

Berg, K., Wood-Dauphinee, S., William, J. I., & Gayton, W. D. (1989). Measuring balance in the elderly: Preliminary development of an instrument. *Physiotherapy Canada, 41*, 304–311. https://doi.org/10.3138/ptc.41.6.304

Bruininks, B., & Bruininks, R. (2005). *Bruininks–Oseretsky Test of Motor Proficiency, Second Edition: BOT-2.* Minneapolis: NCS Pearson/AGS.

Canton, P., & Taylor, E. W. (2012). *The handbook of transformative learning: Theory, research, and practice.* San Francisco: Jossey-Bass.

Chang, C., & Reeve, B. (2005). Item response theory and its applications to patient-reported outcomes measurement. *Evaluation and the Health Professions, 28*, 264–282. https://doi.org/10.1177/0163278705278275

Cohen, M., & Marino, R. (2000). The tools of disability outcomes research functional status measures. *Archives of Physical Medicine and Rehabilitation, 81*(Suppl. 2), S21–S29. https://doi.org/10.1053/apmr.2000.20620

Coster, W., Deeney, T., Haltiwanger, J., & Haley, S. (1998). *School Function Assessment.* San Antonio: Psychological Corporation.

Cynkin, S., & Robinson, A. (1990). *Occupational therapy and activities health: Toward health through activities.* Boston: Little, Brown.

DeMars, C. E. (2018). Classical test theory and item response theory. In P. Irwing, T. Booth, & D. J. Hughes (Eds.), *The Wiley handbook of psychometric testing: A multidisciplinary reference on survey, scale and test development* (pp. 49–73). Hoboken, NJ: Wiley Blackwell.

Dunn, W. (2014). *Sensory Profile 2.* New York: Pearson.

Eakman, A., Carlson, M., & Clark, F. (2010). The Meaningful Activity Participation Assessment: A measure of engagement in personally valued activities. *International Journal of Aging and Human Development, 70*, 299–317. https://doi.org/10.2190/AG.70.4.b

Embretson, S. E., & Reise, S. P. (2000). *Item response theory for psychologists.* Mahwah, NJ: Erlbaum.

Fisher, A. G., & Jones, K. B. (2012). *Assessment of Motor and Process Skills* (7th ed., rev.). Fort Collins, CO: Three Star Press.

Fisher, A. G., Bryze, K., Hume, V., & Griswold, L. A. (2007). *School Assessment of Motor and Process Skills.* Fort Collins, CO: Three Star Press.

Geist, R., Kielhofner, G., Basu, S., & Kafkes, A. (2002). *The Pediatric Volitional Questionnaire (PVQ), Version 2.0.* Chicago: University of Illinois at Chicago, Department of Occupational Therapy, Model of Human Occupation Clearinghouse.

Hays, R. D., Morales, I. S., & Reise, S. P. (2000). Item response theory and health outcomes measurement in the 21st century. *Medical Care, 38,* 1128–1142. https://doi.org/10.1097/00005650-200009002-00007

Health Insurance Portability and Accountability Act of 1996 (HIPAA), Pub. L. 104–191, 42 U.S.C. § 300gg, 29 U.S.C §§ 1181–1183, and 42 U.S.C. §§ 1320d–1320d9. Retrieved from http://www.hhs.gov/ocr/hipaa

Henry, A. D. (2000). *The Pediatric Interest Profiles: Surveys of play for children and adolescents.* San Antonio: Therapy Skill Builders.

Holsbeeke, L., Ketelaar, M., Schoemaker, M. M., & Gorter, J. W. (2009). Capacity, capability, and performance: Different constructs or three of a kind? *Archives of Physical Medicine and Rehabilitation, 90,* 849–855. https://doi.org/10.1016/j.apmr.2008.11.015

Improving Medicare Post-Acute Care Transformation Act of 2014, Pub. L. 113–185, 42 U.S.C. § 1305.

Individuals With Disabilities Education Improvement Act of 2004, Pub. L. 108–446, 20 U.S.C. §§ 1400–1482.

Itzkovich, M., Elazar, B., Averbuch, S., & Katz, N. (2000). *Lowenstein Occupational Therapy Cognitive Assessment (LOTCA) battery manual* (2nd ed.). Pequannock, NJ: Maddak.

Kielhofner, G., Mallinson, T., Crawford, C., Nowak, M., Rigby, M., Henry, A., & Walens, D. (2004). *The Occupational Performance History Interview II.* Chicago: University of Illinois.

Law, M., Baptiste, S., Carswell, A., McColl, M. A., Polatajko, H., & Pollack, N. (2019). *Canadian Occupational Performance Measure* (5th ed., rev.). Altona, MB: COPM, Inc.

Martin, N. A. (2017). *Test of Visual Perceptual Skills* (4th ed.). Novato, CA: Academic Therapy Publications.

Miller, L. J. (2006). *Miller Function and Participation Scales.* San Antonio: Harcourt Assessment.

Mosey, A. C. (1986). *Psychosocial components of occupational therapy.* New York: Raven Press.

Nasreddine, Z. S., Phillips, N. A., Bédirian, V., Charbonneau, S., Whitehead, V., Collin, I., . . . Chertkow, H. (2005). The Montreal Cognitive Assessment, MoCA: A brief screening tool for mild cognitive impairment. *Journal of the American Geriatrics Society, 53,* 695–699. https://doi.org/10.1111/j.1532-5415.2005.53221.x

Oakley, F., Kielhofner, G., Barris, R., & Reichler, R. K. (1986). The Role Checklist: Development and empirical assessment of reliability. *OTJR: Occupation, Participation and Health, 6,* 157–170. https://doi.org/10.1177/153944928600600303

Parham, L. D., Ecker, C., Miller Kuhaneck, H., Henry, D. A., & Glennon, T. J. (2010). *Sensory Processing Measure.* Torrance, CA: Western Psychological Services.

Persky, S., Goldring, M. R., Turner, S. A., Cohen, R. W., & Kistler, W. D. (2018). Validity of assessing child feeding with virtual reality. *Appetite, 123,* 201–207. https://doi.org/10.1016/j.appet.2017.12.007

Piernik-Yoder, B., & Beck, A. (2012). The use of standardized assessments in occupational therapy in the United States. *Occupational Therapy in Health Care, 26,* 97–108. https://doi.org/10.3109/07380577.2012.695103

Plake, B. S., & Spies, R. A. (2005). *The sixteenth mental measurements yearbook.* Lincoln, NE: Buros Institute of Mental Measurements.

Punwar, A. J., & Peloquin, S. M. (2000). *Occupational therapy: Principles and practice.* Philadelphia: Lippincott Williams & Wilkins.

Ricketts, C. (2009). A plea for the proper use of criterion-referenced tests in medical assessment. *Medical Education, 43,* 1141–1146. https://doi.org/10.1111/j.1365-2923.2009.03541.x

Rogers, J., Holm, M., & Chisholm, D. (2016). *Performance Assessment of Self-Care Skills, version 4.1.* Pittsburgh: University of Pittsburgh.

Schell, B., & Schell, J. (2008). *Clinical and professional reasoning in occupational therapy.* Baltimore: Lippincott Williams & Wilkins.

Schwartz, C. E., & Rapkin, B. D. (2004). Reconsidering the psychometrics of quality of life assessment in light of response shift and appraisal. *Health and Quality of Life Outcomes 2,* 16. https://doi.org/10.1186/1477-7525-2-16

Scott, P. J., McKinney, K. G., Perron, J. M., Ruff, E. G., & Smiley, J. L. (2019). The Revised Role Checklist: Improved utility, feasibility, and reliability. *OTJR: Occupation, Participation and Health, 39,* 56–63. https://doi.org/10.1177/1539449218780618

Stube, J., & Hanson, D. (2016). *COMPACT™ orientation and procedure manual.* Retrieved from https://med.und.edu/occupational-therapy/_files/docs/compact-administration-manual.pdf

Suhr, J. A., & Gunstad, J. (2007). Coaching and malingering: A review. In G. J. Larrabee (Ed.), *Assessment of malingered neuropsychological deficits* (pp. 287–311). New York: Oxford University Press.

Taylor, R. R. (2008). *The intentional relationship: Occupational therapy and use of self.* Philadelphia: F. A. Davis.

Thomson, L., & Robnett, R. (2016). *KELS: Kohlman Evaluation of Living Skills* (4th ed.). Bethesda, MD: AOTA Press.

Uniform Data System for Medical Rehabilitation. (1997). *Guide for the Uniform Data Set for Medical Rehabilitation (including the FIM® instrument), version 5.1.* Buffalo, NY: Author.

Victor, T. L., & Abeles, N. (2004). Coaching clients to take psychological and neuropsychological tests: A clash of ethical obligations. *Professional Psychology: Research and Practice, 35,* 373–379. https://doi.org/10.1037/0735-7028.35.4.373

Wall, J. C., Bell, C., Campbell, S., & Davis, J. (2000). The Timed Get-Up-and-Go test revisited: Measurement of the component tasks. *Journal of Rehabilitation Research and Development, 37,* 109–113.

Ware, J. E., & Sherbourne, C. D. (1992). The MOS 36-item Short-Form Health Survey (SF-36): I. Conceptual framework and item selection. *Medical Care, 30,* 473–483. Retrieved from https://www.jstor.org/stable/3765916?origin=JSTOR-pdf&seq=1

World Health Organization. (2001). *International classification of functioning, disability and health.* Geneva: Author.

Wynne, R. A., Beanland, V., & Salmon, P. M. (2019). Systematic review of driving simulator validation studies. *Safety Science, 117,* 138–151. https://doi.org/10.1016/j.ssci.2019.04.004

Zhang, L., Abreu, B. C., Seale, G. S., Masel, B., Christiansen, C. H., & Ottenbacher, K. J. (2003). A virtual reality environment for evaluation of a daily living skill in brain injury rehabilitation: Reliability and validity. *Archives of Physical Medicine and Rehabilitation, 84,* 1118–1124. https://doi.org/10.1016/S0003-9993(03)00203-X

Contextual Evaluation to Support Participation

Kristie K. Patten, PhD, OT/L, FAOTA, and Yu-Lun Chen, MS, OT

7

CHAPTER HIGHLIGHTS

- Influence of context on evaluation
- Evaluating a client's context
- Supporting participation through evaluation
- Contextual evaluation to support participation
- Client-centered, occupation-based evaluation
- Contextual evaluation to support inclusion

KEY TERMS AND CONCEPTS

- Activity Card Sort
- Bottom-up approach
- Client-centered evaluation
- Community Integration Questionnaire
- Context
- Craig Handicap Assessment and Reporting Technique
- Culture
- Environment
- Function
- Goal-directed activities
- Inclusion
- In-Home Occupational Performance Evaluation for Providing Assistance
- Natural context
- Nonstandardized assessment of context
- Occupational profile
- Participation
- Personal context
- Poles of function
- Social context
- Social model of disability
- Standardized assessment of context
- Strength-based assessment
- Temporal context
- Top-down approach
- Virtual environment
- Work Environment Impact Scale

INTRODUCTION

Occupational therapists' assessment provides an understanding of people as occupational beings and identifies their participation in life roles. A unique skill of the occupational therapist is to evaluate the whole client within their context. During an assessment, therapists learn about the client's ability to engage and participate in home, school, workplace, and community life, in part by looking at the client's functioning in occupations.

Evaluation must consider factors that empower and make possible clients' engagement and participation in positive health-promoting occupations (Wilcock & Townsend, 2008). According to the American Occupational Therapy Association's (AOTA, 2014) *Occupational Therapy Practice Framework: Domain and Process (OTPF)*, the context includes a person's cultural, personal, temporal, virtual, physical, and social aspects. When considering these factors, therapists examine the variety of interrelated conditions within and surrounding the client that influences their occupational performance. AOTA's (2015) *Standards of Practice for Occupational Therapy* highlight that, in addition

to the client's ability to participate in activities and occupations, the occupational therapist evaluates the environments and context in which these activities and occupations occur.

Doucet and Gutman (2013) wrote about two **poles of function.** In the **top-down approach, function** should be "defined and measured by the client's performance of life roles and meaningful activities that are a part of that role" (p. 7). The other pole is a **bottom-up approach** to evaluation and looks at "specific discrete body impairments that affect larger daily life activities" (p. 7). The authors argued that *function* is defined by both poles. An evaluation that examines a client's context must use information from both poles to understand the influence of context and the environment on the client's participation.

INFLUENCE OF CONTEXT ON EVALUATION

When occupational therapists are conducting evaluations, context matters. **Context** refers to a variety of interrelated conditions that are within and surrounding the client and includes the client's external physical and social environments. Within these surrounding environments, a client's daily life occupations occur (AOTA, 2014). *Contexts* are broadly and comprehensively defined in the *OTPF* as cultural, personal, temporal, virtual, physical, and social. Table 7.1 defines these areas and, because the client is not limited to the individual level, outlines examples of context for the person, groups, and populations.

Some contexts are external to clients (e.g., virtual), some are internal to clients (e.g., personal), and some may have both external features and internalized beliefs and values (e.g., cultural). A client who has difficulty performing effectively in one context may be successful when the context is changed. The context within which clients engage in their occupations is unique for each client. Occupational therapists can only assess a client's actual occupational performance when they examine the influence of the physical, cultural, personal, temporal, and social contexts and the influence of personal and social environments. Furthermore, the extent, amount, and quality of a client's participation may be influenced by the context in which the occupational therapist administers the assessment (AOTA, 2014).

TABLE 7.1. Types of Contexts and Environments

CATEGORY	DEFINITION	EXAMPLES
Contexts		
Cultural	Customs, beliefs, activity patterns, behavioral standards, and expectations accepted by the society of which a client is a member. The cultural context influences the client's identity and activity choices.	▪ *Person:* A person delivering Thanksgiving meals to home-bound individuals ▪ *Group:* Employees marking the end of the work week with casual dress on Friday ▪ *Population:* People engaging in an afternoon siesta or high tea
Personal	"Features of the individual that are not part of a health condition or health status" (WHO, 2001, p. 17). The personal context includes age, gender, socioeconomic status, and educational status and can also include group membership (e.g., volunteers, employees) and population membership (e.g., members of society).	▪ *Person:* A 25-year-old unemployed man with a high school diploma ▪ *Group:* Volunteers working in a homeless shelter ▪ *Population:* Older drivers learning about community mobility options
Temporal	The experience of time as shaped by engagement in occupations; the temporal aspects of occupation that "contribute to the patterns of daily occupations" include "rhythm . . . tempo . . . synchronization . . . duration . . . and sequence" (Larson & Zemke, 2003, p. 82; Zemke, 2004, p. 610). The temporal context includes stage of life, time of day or year, duration and rhythm of activity, and history.	▪ *Person:* A person retired from work for 10 years ▪ *Group:* A community organization's annual fundraising campaign ▪ *Population:* People celebrating Independence Day on July 4
Virtual	Environment in which communication occurs by means of airwaves or computers and in the absence of physical contact. The virtual context includes simulated, real-time, and near-time environments, such as chat rooms, email, video conferencing, and radio transmissions; remote monitoring through wireless sensors; and computer-based data collection.	▪ *Person:* Friends who text message each other ▪ *Group:* Members who participate in a video conference, telephone conference call, instant message, or interactive white board use ▪ *Population:* Virtual community of gamers
Environments		
Physical	Natural and built nonhuman surroundings and the objects in them. The natural environment includes geographic terrain, plants, and animals as well as the sensory qualities of the surroundings. The built environment includes buildings, furniture, tools, and devices.	▪ *Person:* Individual's house or apartment ▪ *Group:* Office building or factory ▪ *Population:* Transportation system
Social	Presence of, relationships with, and expectations of persons, groups, or populations with whom clients have contact. The social environment includes availability and expectations of significant individuals, such as spouse, friends, and caregivers; relationships with individuals, groups, or populations; and relationships with systems (e.g., political, legal, economic, institutional) that influence norms, role expectations, and social routines.	▪ *Person:* Friends, colleagues ▪ *Group:* Occupational therapy students conducting a class get-together ▪ *Population:* People influenced by a city government

Note. WHO = World Health Organization.

EVALUATING A CLIENT'S CONTEXT

Frequently, assessing context involves both standardized and nonstandardized assessments. Using both types of assessments provides a broad perspective of the client's lived world and is useful in understanding the client's strengths and the challenges the client may be facing. When deciding which assessments to use, the occupational therapist must consider what kind of information would be most helpful in planning an occupation-based intervention.

Standardized assessments, when administered according to established procedures, provide valid and reliable results. When occupational therapists use a *standardized assessment of context,* it is critically important that they select an assessment that was standardized on an appropriate population with the same demographics and disabilities as the client being assessed. In occupational therapy, only a few standardized assessments exist that specifically address the context of a client. These assessments address personal context, temporal context, and the environment and are discussed in the next section.

Standardized Assessments of the Personal Context

Personal context refers to demographic features of the person, such as age, gender, socioeconomic status, and educational level, that are not part of a health condition (World Health Organization [WHO], 2001). The personal context has a direct influence on assessment results. For example, age, educational status, and gender can affect performance, which interacts with the health condition.

This is illustrated in a study by Klaas et al. (2010), who assessed participation of 194 children and adolescents with spinal cord injuries (SCI). The study showed that young people with physical disabilities participated more often and reported higher levels of enjoyment in informal activities than formal activities. However, their participation in formal activities was more socially engaged and community based. Personal contexts, including the child's age, sex, and injury level, affected aspects of informal participation. Formal participation was related to the child's age and caregiver education.

For standardized assessments, validity studies are often associated with the personal context to establish discriminative validity. One example is the study by Rosenberg et al. (2010) that compared children with and without disabilities on the Children Participation Questionnaire (CPQ). Scores on the CPQ differed between groups; children with disabilities participated in fewer activities, in lower frequencies, and with less independence.

Known groups also differ on adult measures. The *Activity Card Sort* (ACS; Baum & Edwards, 2008) is a standardized assessment that evaluates an adult's amount and level of involvement in various activities, including instrumental activities, low-demand leisure activities, high-demand leisure activities, and social activities.

Another validity study conducted in Jordan with healthy young and older adults and adults with multiple sclerosis (MS; Hamed & Holm, 2013). The study found that the Arab Heritage Activity Card Sort differentiated these groups in current and retained participation levels, whereas the healthy adults (combining young and older adults) reported significantly greater current participation and retained participation, but not previous participation, than adults with MS. When comparing adults with MS with healthy young and older adults, adults with MS had significantly lower retained participation than the healthy young adults, which was not significantly different from healthy older adults. These are all powerful examples of how context affects assessment.

According to the *OTPF,* the personal context includes gender (AOTA, 2014). Gender differences are seen in the *Community Integration Questionnaire* (CIQ; Willer et al., 1994), which was developed as an outcome measure for persons with brain injury. Using the CIQ, researchers have found some interesting relationships among client factors, context, occupations, and community integration among clients with head injury (Ritchie et al., 2014). Client contexts, including gender and age, also affect community integration in clients with SCIs (Kratz et al., 2015). Women with SCI tend to have greater home integration postrehabilitation, and men tend to have higher productivity. Young clients with SCI tend to be more integrated in terms of home and productivity dimensions, whereas older clients have more limited community integration.

Standardized Assessment of the Temporal Context

Temporal context includes stage of life, time of day or year, duration, rhythm of activity, and history. Depending on the stage of life one is in, results of assessments will vary, and assessments may even measure different constructs. A factor analysis study of the first edition of the ACS (Sachs & Josman, 2003) confirmed the original factors with slight variation for older adults and young adults (i.e., students). The ACS items for the older adults clustered into four categories: (1) IADLs, (2) leisure, (3) demanding leisure, and (4) maintenance activities. For the young adults, the items clustered into five categories: (1) IADLs, (2) leisure, (3) demanding leisure, (4) maintenance, and (5) social recreational activities. This analysis of construct validity suggests that the ACS measures slightly different constructs on the basis of personal characteristics of the individual.

The *Craig Handicap Assessment and Reporting Technique* (CHART; Whiteneck et al., 1992) was developed to assess community participation among people with SCI. It has been demonstrated that CHART scores are affected by contextual factors, such as race or ethnicity, marital status, change of locomotion methods, education, and employment, at the time after discharge (Hiremath et al., 2017). Contextual factors that continuously predict better community participation at 1, 5, and 10 years after discharge include being employed and educated. Conversely, being widowed, being African American, and having locomotion methods of wheelchair or transitioned from ambulation to wheelchair predicted significantly lower CHART scores at all time points. Although the CHART's scores are based on normative data and it only measures objective aspects of participation, the CHART is a well-established measure of community integration for people with disabilities.

Context clearly affects clients' performance on an assessment. The environment where occupations occur and how the client interacts with the personal and social environments also have a substantial effect on the evaluation process and individual assessments.

Standardized Assessment of the Environment

Assessments of the environment relevant to occupational therapists are examinations of the interaction between person and environment that enables accomplishment of occupations. The goal of most environmental measures is to determine whether the environment constrains or supports a person's occupational performance and what can be adapted or changed to enhance that person's performance. These assessments give occupational therapists information about what environmental elements enable or interfere with a person's participation in life activities as the therapist determines what services the client may need. For example, a parental report of environmental barriers to participation may highlight the importance of home-based occupational therapy intervention to optimize participation (Law et al., 2013). By modifying or adapting the environment, occupational therapists can improve clients' participation and decrease levels of caregiver assistance.

Contextual assessments for children often emphasize the role of the physical and social environments in promoting skill development. The goal of many assessments of children's contexts is to determine the transactions between the environment and child. These assessments emphasize the elements of the context known to promote development (e.g., parent support and responsiveness, availability of toys and learning materials). For example, research has shown that high-quality home environments predict positive well-being of preschool children who entered the child welfare system as infants (Harden & Whittaker, 2011). Specifically, cognitive stimulation and emotional support in the home predicted higher cognitive and language scores, decreased behavioral problems, and increased social skill.

In contrast, adult assessments emphasize the safety and accessibility of the physical environment, workplace supports, or social supports in a community context. In much of occupational therapy practice, contexts are informally assessed, with a focus on understanding the supports and constraints available in the environment. Few assessments of the environment have been developed, perhaps because environments are dynamic and complex and change rapidly over time and space. It often is difficult to determine how a person will move through environments and how contexts will change over time.

The environmental assessments that have been developed tend to focus on one environment (e.g., home or work) and tend to focus on a single problem (e.g., physical access, fall prevention, social participation). Assessments of the home environment have focused on barriers to function, particularly for persons using wheelchairs or mobility devices, and safety for older adults who are at risk for falling or other injuries. These assessments often identify barriers and problems that need to be modified to promote optimal function and safety (Pighills et al., 2011).

As the environment is evaluated more thoroughly, it is becoming more relevant to look at the caregivers in the environment in innovative assessments. For example,

the *In-Home Occupational Performance Evaluation for Providing Assistance* (Keglovits et al., 2015) looks at the environmental barriers that may affect performance of daily caregiving activities and caregivers' confidence in and satisfaction with their ability to perform their caregiving occupations.

Measures of a person's work environment have been developed to identify potential environmental modifications that can increase safety, access, and optimal function. They assess the worker's perception of the social environment, including peer and supervisor support. Research has shown that a supportive work environment is predictive of employee productivity and well-being (Dorman, 2009). The social environment is highlighted in this research, which shows how important it is to consider both physical and social environments.

For example, the *Work Environment Impact Scale* (Corner et al., 1997) assesses the experience of persons with disabilities in their workplace. Both physical and social factors are considered, including transportation, safety, lighting, time, equipment, tools, sound, and architecture. In addition, the social environment is assessed, including attitudes, social climate, social support, communication, and expectations. Table 7.2 presents examples of contextual assessments that consider both the physical and the social environments.

Nonstandardized Assessment of a Client's Context

To develop a client's comprehensive occupational profile, the occupational therapist uses nonstandardized assessment strategies to learn about the client's personal lived experience and the context of their life. Using observations, interviews, photographs, and engagement in an art activity to conduct a *nonstandardized assessment of context* can provide the therapist with rich, insightful information about the client's life. Observations offer the opportunity to see the client interact with others in context. Interviews allow the client to express their perceptions and feelings about life. Viewing photographs offers a glimpse into the client's current and past life. Finally, drawing or painting a picture can facilitate the client's expression of their context. For example, a child's picture of their family or home can provide the therapist with useful information that the child is unable to express verbally.

Although the *occupational profile* typically is used to identify occupations that are meaningful to the person, it can also be used to explore context. The occupational therapist can ask the client how the physical context of their life supports or hinders those occupations. Furthermore, the therapist can explore the client's social context and obtain the client's view about the role it plays in their life. It is up to the therapist to creatively ask questions in a nonthreatening manner to determine the role of context in the client's life and learn how it may support active participation.

Nonstandardized Assessment of the Client's Personal Context

In the *OTPF*, personal context includes qualities that are not part of the client's health condition or health status (AOTA, 2014). During an interview or from the chart, the therapist

TABLE 7.2. Sample Assessments of Context

ASSESSMENT	PURPOSE	CONTEXT
Children		
Home Observation for Measurement of the Environment (Bradley et al., 2003; Caldwell & Bradley, 1984)	Four versions that assess home context of infants, young children, school-age children, and adolescents	*Physical:* Lighting, safety, equipment, and toys *Social:* Interpersonal relationships, social support, family organization, community life, and use of services
Test of Environmental Supportiveness (Bundy, 1999; Skard & Bundy, 2008)	Assesses supportiveness of the environment for play for children 18 months to 15 years	*Physical:* Safety, objects, accessible space *Social:* Caregiver support, availability and competence of peers
Adults		
Housing Enabler (Iwarsson & Slaug, 2001)	Measures physical and architectural barriers, with a primary focus on home accessibility of older persons	*Physical:* Indoor and outdoor housing barriers that are a safety concern *Social:* Not assessed
In-Home Occupational Performance Evaluation (Stark et al., 2010)	Measures performance and satisfaction of home activities, and calculates ratings of the influence of environmental barriers for each of the prioritized activities	*Physical:* Environmental barriers that influence performance of client-prioritized activities *Social:* Not assessed
In-Home Occupational Performance Evaluation for Providing Assistance (Keglovits et al., 2015)	Measures person–environment fit in the home to assist caregivers	*Physical:* Environmental barriers to performance of daily caregiving activities *Social:* Subjective confidence in and satisfaction with ability of caregiver to assist with activities
Safety Assessment of Function and the Environment for Rehabilitation–Health Outcome Measurement and Evaluation (Chiu et al., 2001)	Assessment of a person's ability to function safely in the home, with 14 safety domains	*Physical:* Safety hazards, mobility, ADLs, and IADLs *Social:* Living situation, communication, family support
Westmead Home Safety Assessment (Clemson, 1997)	Identifies fall hazards in the home environment of older adults	*Physical:* Fall hazards *Social:* Not assessed
Work Environment Impact Scale (Corner et al., 1997)	Measures the fit between the client and aspects of the environment	*Physical:* Accessibility, arrangement, design, comfort, and sensory qualities *Social:* Time and productivity demands, work schedules, coworker interactions, supervisor communication, and client and customer interactions
Work Environment Scale (Moos, 1994)	Measures workers' perceptions of a workplace's social environment and its impact on morale	*Physical:* Not assessed *Social:* Interpersonal interaction, social communication exchanges, cohesion among workers, friendship and support provided by coworkers and management

can get information about the client's age and socioeconomic status. Information about the client's gender is more difficult to obtain. Although observation may be a beginning point, information about gender identification is best obtained through a guided conversation with the client.

Although some questions can be answered straightforwardly, others may require the occupational therapist to probe gently into the client's self-identity. Occupational therapists must be open to ideas, practices, and preferences that are different from their own. Therapists must conduct the interview in a sensitive and nonjudgmental manner to get accurate information.

Nonstandardized Assessment of the Environment

Obviously, the best way to understand a client's environment is to observe the physical environment and the objects in it. If this is not possible, the occupational therapist can obtain this information by having the client describe their nonhuman world. When the therapist is interviewing clients, it is critical to ask them to describe their world, including the geographic terrain, plants, and animals (AOTA, 2014). The therapist can also ask clients to share photographs of their lives. With clients' permission, the therapist can also ask significant others in the clients' lives to share photographs.

Nonstandardized Assessment of the Client's Social Context and Culture

A client's **culture** is unique to that person and how they practice the customs, beliefs, standards, and expectations of the culture with which they identify. Although clients may describe themselves as a member of a specific culture, their practices may be unique to their situation. Again, observation is a good beginning point, but occupational therapists need to be careful not to make generalizations based on observation alone. As with the personal context, the most effective method of obtaining information is directly from the client. During the interview, therapists should let clients describe their cultural practices. Therapists can sensitively ask these questions and must be open to ideas, practices, and preferences that are different from their own.

Nonstandardized Assessment of the Social Aspects of the Client's Context

A client's **social context** consists of people with whom they interact. The social context is constructed around the significant others and important activities in the client's life. If possible, observing the client's interactions with significant others (e.g., spouse, friends, caregivers) provides insightful information about the client's social life. It is also helpful to ask about important occupations that may be done in a social context of groups or clubs.

Nonstandardized Assessment of the Virtual Environment

The **virtual environment** is becoming increasingly important in people's lives; it includes communication by means of airwaves or computers with no physical contact with another person (AOTA, 2014). Some examples of these interactions are emails, social networking sites, chat rooms, and videoconferencing. When interviewing the client, the occupational therapist can obtain useful information about the client's participation. Furthermore, the therapist can explore how important participation in the virtual environment is to the client.

SUPPORTING PARTICIPATION THROUGH EVALUATION

There is an adage in most testing that what one evaluates or assesses is what one will treat or, in education, what one will study. If the occupational therapy evaluation does not address participation in life through engagement in occupations but only focuses on the bottom-up pole at the impairment level, chances are that impairment is what the occupational therapy intervention will address. Participation must be central to the evaluation process to successfully fulfill occupational therapy's charge to facilitate engagement and participation in occupations in context. **Participation** means sharing with others, taking part in an activity, or being involved in a life situation. Participation in life's activities is an important aspect of health

and quality of life. Law (2002) described its importance: "Through participation, we acquire skills and competencies, connect with others and our communities, and find purpose and meaning in life" (p. 640). Participation in occupations is a central concept to occupational therapists and defines an essential goal of intervention.

WHO (2001) defined *participation* as involvement in a life situation and considered it to be a key indicator of health. WHO (2001) recognized the complexity of participation by stressing the interrelationships between body function and structure, activity, personal factors, and environment characteristics. A person's participation does not occur in isolation and must be considered in relationship to their abilities and the environment in which they live. Occupational therapists can assess participation only by considering the contexts in which people live, work, and play. The concept implies engagement in a life situation or life activity but does not always mean performing the activity.

For example, a person can meaningfully participate in an activity by observing that activity, partially performing it, performing it in an adapted way, or directing others to perform it. All of these types of performing imply engaged involvement, which is the essence of participation. Key aspects of participation that relate to health are that the person can make decisions about participating, finds the activity to be meaningful, and participates in opportunities that are consistent with their life goals.

By definition, assessments of participation consider the contexts of a person's activities, recognizing that the physical, social, temporal, and cultural context can support or constrain participation. In the measurement of participation, the concept of *environment* is dynamic—that is, it varies across time and space, because contexts change with activities and roles. The environment has an essential role in determining the quality, frequency, and level of a person's participation in life activities.

Because the environment can contribute to disability, comprehensive evaluation to understand the basis for disability and to plan intervention includes assessment of the environment. In the *International Classification of Functioning, Disability and Health* (*ICF*; WHO, 2001), **environment** is broadly defined to include physical, social, cultural, economic, and organizational components. In the *OTPF* (AOTA, 2014), environment and its various components are recognized under the broad term of *context*.

The majority of occupational therapy measures assess the client's occupational performance (i.e., how a person completes an activity or task). Measures of participation are challenging to conceptualize, given the dynamic and evolving nature of participation. Scholars (e.g., Law, 2002; Law et al., 2005) have discussed the difficulty of measuring participation. It is not only a broad concept but also a multidimensional and complex one. Participation measures need to consider not only the person, environment, and occupation but also the interactions of these variables. Rather than defining specific attributes of the person, their occupations, and relevant environments, participation assessments have to examine the transaction of these variables.

It can be argued that measures of participation have certain characteristics. Scholars have attempted to define the characteristics of this broad, multidimensional concept and have made assumptions about how to measure it. The field has yet to reach consensus on how to measure participation (Coster & Khetani, 2008; Law, 2002; Law et al., 2005); nevertheless, in recent years, a number of participation measures have been published, and sample measures are presented in Table 7.3. Some defining characteristics of existing participation measures include that they

- Use self-report or caregiver report,
- Focus on a person's everyday occupations or common occupations,
- Consider a person's natural environment or multiple environments,
- Focus on activities that are goal directed, and
- Assess the perceived importance of participation and associated feelings of well-being or satisfaction.

Self- or Caregiver Report

Measures of participation are most often self-reported scales that define participation across environments and time.

Coster and Khetani (2008) discussed the temporal and spatial aspects of participation that are inherent in the meaning of the term. Through self-report or caregiver report, participation is assessed as a personal and individualized experience. By using self-report, the evaluator gains a perspective on the opportunities and environmental supports available to the client and how they participate in those opportunities.

Various methods have been developed to elicit self-report. Many instruments, such as the Life Habits Assessment (Fougeyrollas et al., 1998) and the Late Life Function and Disability Instrument (Haley et al., 2002; Jette et al., 2002), use a questionnaire that can be administered as an interview or in paper-and-pencil format. Other measures (e.g., ACS; Baum & Edwards, 2001, 2008) use a card-sort activity in which the client identifies the amount and level of involvement in activities as depicted on the cards. Measures tend to be organized by activities, occupations, or roles and rate the frequency of participation, the supports necessary to participate, how well a person performs in that role or occupation, satisfaction with participation, and restrictions or limitations.

TABLE 7.3. Sample Measures of Participation

ASSESSMENT	PURPOSE	HOW DOES IT MEASURE PARTICIPATION?
Children		
Children's Assessment of Participation and Enjoyment (CAPE; King et al., 2004) and Preferences for Activities of Children (PAC; King et al., 2004)	Measures how a child (with or without disabilities) participates in everyday activities outside of schoolwork or home chores in the context of the natural environment (CAPE) and their preference for doing activities (PAC)	Examines how a child participates, including diversity (number of activities done), intensity (frequency of participation), and enjoyment of activities. The CAPE reflects participation in the following areas: ■ Formal and informal activities ■ Recreation ■ Active physical ■ Social ■ Skill based ■ Self-improvement
School Function Assessment (Coster et al., 1998)	Measures a child's participation in academic and social school-related activities	Assesses participation; assistance and adaptations to perform tasks; and school-related performance in physical, cognitive, and behavioral tasks. Includes sections on level of participation in 6 school activity settings: ■ General or special education classroom ■ Playground ■ Transportation to and from school ■ Bathroom ■ Transition to and from class ■ Mealtimes
Participation and Environment Measure in Children and Youth (Coster et al., 2010)	Examines environmental impact on children's participation in home, school, and community settings for 5–17-year-olds with and without disabilities	Identifies numbers of activities done, frequency, level of involvement, number of activities in which change is desired, and 2 summary scores of environmental barriers to and supports for participation in 3 settings: ■ Home ■ School ■ Community
Young Children's Participation and Environment Measure (Khetani et al., 2015)	Examines caregiver perception of their children's participation within home, school and community settings for 0- to 5-year-olds with and without disabilities	Identifies numbers of activities done, frequency, level of involvement, number of activities in which change is desired, and 2 summary scores of environmental barriers and supports for participation in 3 settings: ■ Home ■ School ■ Community

(Continued)

TABLE 7.3.   Sample Measures of Participation (Cont.)

Adults		
Activity Card Sort (Baum & Edwards, 2001, 2008)	Identifies levels of occupation and activity participation to develop intervention goals and measure outcome of intervention	Evaluates an adult's amount and level of involvement in various activities, including: ▪ Instrumental activities ▪ Low-demand leisure activities ▪ High-demand leisure activities ▪ Social activities
Craig Handicap Assessment and Reporting Technique (Whiteneck et al., 1992)	Designed to assess community participation among people with spinal cord injury, then expanded with a cognitive section to use with people with cognitive impairments, including persons with traumatic brain injury, stroke, and multiple sclerosis	Asks the client to indicate time spent performing each task in five domains or roles: ▪ Physical independence ▪ Mobility ▪ Occupation ▪ Social integration ▪ Economic self-sufficiency
Late-Life Function and Disability Instrument (Haley et al., 2002; Jette et al., 2002)	Assessment of physical function and disability of community-dwelling older adults. Measures functional limitations (inability to perform activities encountered in daily routines) and disability (inability to participate in major life tasks and social roles).	Function Scale assesses participation in 32 physical activities, and Disability Scale evaluates self-reported limitations in and frequency of performing 16 major life tasks. The client reports how limited they feel in doing a particular task and how often they do that task.
Life Habits Assessment (Fougeyrollas et al., 1998)	Measure of social participation, life habits, and daily activities of people with disabilities	Appraises the quality of social participation by judging the difficulty clients have carrying out life habits in the following areas: ▪ Daily activities ▪ Nutrition ▪ Fitness ▪ Personal care ▪ Communication ▪ Housing ▪ Mobility ▪ Social roles ▪ Responsibility ▪ Interpersonal relationships ▪ Community life ▪ Education ▪ Employment ▪ Recreation
London Handicap Scale (Jenkinson et al., 2000)	Measures global function and disability among adults with chronic, multiple, or progressive diseases	Rates a person's perception of independence from no disadvantage to extreme disadvantage in the areas of: ▪ Physical independence ▪ Social integration ▪ Economic self-sufficiency
Community Integration Questionnaire (Willer et al., 1994)	Outcome measure for persons with brain injury that rates home, work, and community activities that require both physical and cognitive performance	Examines frequency of the activities performed and whether they are done jointly in the following areas: ▪ Home integration ▪ Social integration ▪ Productivity in work, school, and volunteer activities

Everyday Occupations and Roles

Occupational therapy has traditionally categorized occupations as ADLs, IADLs, rest and sleep, education, work, play, leisure, and social participation (AOTA, 2014). As noted by Coster and Khetani (2008), measures of child participation are often organized by role or life situations. Examples of life situations defined in the *ICF* (WHO, 2001) include recreation and leisure, engagement in play, education, self-care, and work. Occupational therapists also recognize the importance of assessing the subjective experience embedded in these occupations and roles.

The meaning that a person gives to an occupation is essential to determining how it matches their life roles. For example, cooking may be leisure to one person, work to another, and an IADL to a third. In evaluations of participation, perception of the experience can be as important as actual performance. For example, a family may rate a child's performance as independent when it is actually supported by equipment, adapted methods, and physical assistance. When these adapted methods are integrated into a family's everyday life, the family often considers them as natural and routine and would not consider the child's dependence on supports to be a lack of independence.

Natural Contexts and Multiple Environments

Context is of particular interest when occupational therapists are evaluating participation because different environments can support, enhance, or restrict participation. When an assessment does not specify the context, the occupational therapist should consider multiple environments to rate assessment items, because performance can change in different environments.

Child measures of participation often include home, school, and community sections, with the realization that occupational performance and participation may differ by setting. A client who has difficulty performing effectively in one context may be very successful when the context is changed (AOTA, 2014).

Occupational therapists assess adult participation by examining how a person functions in their natural context, with emphasis on essential daily living activities, including ADLs, social participation, and mobility. A *natural context* is a typical environment that the individual experiences on a day-to-day basis, such as school, work, home, or play settings, as opposed to a contrived environment such as a hospital or therapeutic setting. Attempting to assess in the natural context makes an accurate indication of participation more likely. Simulated task performance in a clinic kitchen or hospital bathroom may not be indicative of performance in the natural context.

Goal-Directed Activities

Goal-directed activities are sets of tasks that have an expected outcome or achievement, such as cleaning a room or learning to write. Because participation in life activities is goal directed and purposeful, participation measures consider the purpose of activity to the person. A person's goal in a specific activity (e.g., swimming, work) determines both the meaning of participation and the intervention plan. For example, if the goal of going to the movies is to be with friends, then independent mobility in the theater or understanding the movie's plot may not be important aspects of participating in this activity. Activities such as housekeeping are perceived to be work to some people and leisure to those who derive great pleasure from maintaining a clean home. A child's learning in school can be work and lead to a career, but it is also a social activity that enables learning about society and culture unrelated to work as an adult.

The meaning a person assigns to an activity may determine whether that activity is a desired or appropriate focus for a rehabilitation program. For example, when a mother with multiple sclerosis finds that baking cookies with her 10-year-old daughter has become difficult, it is important to know whether she values baking as a leisure pursuit or as a time for the mother–daughter relationship. If baking is an important and desired activity, the occupational therapist can adapt the techniques to bake; if mother–daughter interaction is most important, the therapist can recommend a substitute joint activity.

Well-Being and Satisfaction

Participation in meaningful occupations has a direct and substantial effect on health and quality of life (Coster & Khetani, 2008; Law, 2002; Wilcox, 1998). Most measures of participation include personal satisfaction, similar to measures of quality of life. The key difference between measures of quality of life and of participation is that most scales that rate quality of life do not specify certain occupations or human functions. In contrast, participation measures link satisfaction and well-being to a client's involvement in specific activities.

CONTEXTUAL EVALUATION TO SUPPORT PARTICIPATION

Occupational performance was defined by Forsyth et al. (2014) as doing a task related to participation, so how can contextual evaluation be used to assess participation? How do occupational therapists evaluate the varied contexts and understand the effects of these on occupations? More important, how can a contextual evaluation support participation by revealing what the barriers and supports are in the environment?

By adopting a client-centered, strength-based, and occupation-based approach to evaluation and choosing assessments that consider the contextual factors that support or hinder participation, occupational therapists can develop a more informed understanding of the conditions that are necessary for the client to "achieve health, well-being, and participation in life through engagement in occupation" (AOTA, 2014, p. S2). This stance cannot be an afterthought to the evaluation process. Including participation in baseline measures during the evaluation process can help therapists focus on this unique area of practice (Kessler & Egan, 2012).

CLIENT-CENTERED, OCCUPATION-BASED EVALUATION

Client-centered evaluation is a defining principle of occupational therapy practice; it guides how occupational therapists evaluate performance strengths and concerns, select goals, plan interventions, and assesses the effects of an intervention program. This principle has been a defining construct of occupational therapy over time (Yerxa, 1967), across international borders (AOTA, 2014; Barrett et al., 2020; Canadian Association of Occupational Therapists [CAOT], 2013; Wilcock, 1998), and across areas of practice (Law & Mills, 1998). Elements of a client-centered approach include demonstrating respect for clients, involving clients in decision making, advocating with and for clients in meeting their needs, and recognizing clients' experience and knowledge (CAOT, 2013).

In a client-centered evaluation, the occupational therapist assesses the client's ability to engage in meaningful occupations and the interplay among performance, activity demands, and context (Rogers & Holm, 2009). A primary goal of evaluation is to understand the person as an occupational being. Through evaluation of a client's participation in work, school, leisure, and play in natural physical, social, and cultural contexts, the therapist develops an occupational profile to use in establishing goals and in framing and interpreting further analysis of performance. On the basis of data from the occupational profile and other assessments, the therapist develops intervention goals and strategies that enhance the client's participation in the occupations most important to them (Law, 2002).

Occupation-based intervention is a highly individualized process because it incorporates the unique perspective of the client, the client's occupational performance problems, and the performance context (Rogers & Holm, 2009). These principles—the use of a client-centered approach, the understanding of a person as an occupational being, and the focus on the client's participation in life roles—have important implications for the evaluation process, the types of assessments selected, the methods used to assess clients, and the interpretation of evaluation results.

A client-centered approach recognizes that the client's perspective is the most important one in the evaluation and intervention process. Client-centered evaluations may be more accurate than nonindividualized assessments. Fleischer et al. (2019) found that using a client-centered evaluation, such as the Canadian Occupational Performance Measure (Law et al., 2019), detected greater perceived impairment among breast cancer survivors than the Disabilities of the Arm, Shoulder, and Hand (Gummesson et al., 2003), a standardized but nonindividualized assessment. Accuracy of assessment information is critical in establishing client-centered interventions.

Almost always, the client and their caregivers have the most accurate understanding of the client's strengths, limitations, and priorities. Client-centered evaluation includes the client's perceptions of and concerns about performance, roles, interests, goals, and priorities.

A client-centered approach counters the traditional medical model, in which an expert determines a diagnosis and prescribes a treatment based on that diagnosis. In a traditional medical model, the client is the recipient of the treatment but is not actively involved in making treatment decisions. On the basis of the client's diagnosis and performance deficits, professionals determine the treatment approach. In such an approach, it becomes unlikely that treatment goals meet the client's interests and concerns. Because the traditional medical approach promotes passivity and dependency, it contradicts the goal of the occupational therapist that clients actively engage and fully participate in work, daily living, and leisure roles.

In a client-centered evaluation, the occupational therapist helps the client identify and prioritize the occupations and activities that become the focus of intervention. By determining with the client what occupations are most relevant to them, the therapist can design meaningful interventions. When the therapist facilitates the client's self-direction and values the client's self-identified goals,

the client becomes invested in the intervention program and is motivated to achieve the outcomes. As a result, outcomes are likely to be more satisfying and important to the client. In addition, the probability that outcomes are successfully achieved increases (Law, 1998).

A client-centered approach supports the client's perception that they can make decisions about intervention and can problem solve how to adapt activities to enhance participation. This approach encourages the client's sense of self-determinism and promotes their confidence in making decisions and directing therapy services toward their own goals. Three core psychological needs that are at the heart of self-determination theory—autonomy, competence, and relatedness (Ryan & Deci, 2000)—can be fostered in a client-centered, strength-based approach to evaluation. Many clients who receive occupational therapy have disabilities that endure throughout their lifetimes; therefore, promoting and respecting clients' self-determinism encourages them to independently manage services and direct the personal assistance they need.

Strength-Based Approach to Evaluation

An evaluation of a client's context must examine the client's strengths, motives, habits, and skills. These assessments are by nature strength based, but a *strength-based assessment* goes a step further and looks at what about the disability experience can help shape occupations. As Dunn et al. (2013) stated,

> It is even more important to consider a strengths approach when people have obvious challenges. Complexities are just another feature of a person's overall characteristics; for example, having severe spasticity likely means a person moves slowly and without precision; it might also mean that the person can sit quietly and pay attention to what is going on in the room. When we point out what is helpful about a person's characteristics, we acknowledge that the disabilities do not define them as human beings. We might describe a person as "intellectually disabled" or as "working best with structure and routines in place." By stating what the person can do, we set the stage for fostering participation on that person's terms. (p. 1)

A person's spasticity is irrelevant when they are sitting quietly to watch television but may become a challenge when the person tries to change the channel. The context and how it can support participation is the crux of a strength-based approach. Evaluation and interventions can focus on adaptations to support this preferred activity. Knowing how the person's spasticity affects their performance can provide the basis for designing an adaptation for channel changing. Therefore, in a strength-based approach, spasticity is a feature to understand and focus on the client's abilities, rather than the "deficit." This innovative approach requires a more intensive look at how context can support participation.

A contextual evaluation must take into account the strengths of the person, and often this is neglected in favor of focusing on the barriers to participation. During the assessment, the occupational therapist must actively listen to the priorities and goals of the client. Many therapists acquired their professional skills at a time when the focus of assessment and, consequently, intervention was identifying what was wrong with a person and then attempting to fix it (Dunn et al., 2013). The traditional medical model led to people with disabilities being acted on by professional experts who defined them in terms of their impairments and then sought to remediate those impairments.

For example, autobiographical narratives and interviews with self-advocates with autism spectrum disorder (ASD) suggest that although remediation may be needed at times, these individuals have not built their lives on remediated weaknesses; rather, they seek assistance in modifying and adapting their environments and building on their strengths and unique interests to engage in meaningful occupations that foster participation (Kotler & Koenig, 2012). As one self-advocate noted, "The autism spectrum is inclusive of more than a series of impairments; many of the traits we possess can be, in the proper contexts, strengths or at least neutral attributes" (Ne'eman, 2010).

Occupational therapists are in a unique position to offer innovative services that embrace a client-centered, occupation-based, and strength-based practice for adolescents and adults with autism. By being a central agent of change in this paradigm shift, occupational therapists can be at the forefront of using restricted interests as meaningful occupation rather than impairments with people who have ASD (Patten Koenig, 2019). This shift has to take place at the evaluation stage or it will not be incorporated into intervention in a meaningful way. Table 7.4 provides sample assessments that occupational therapists can use to foster a strength-based practice.

In particular, much of the current literature on autism has negatively referred to the interests of persons diagnosed with ASD as perseverative, restrictive, and obsessive. Historically, the focus of intervention has been on the need to extinguish these interests to "normalize" the person. An innovative strength-based practice emphasizes the need to recognize these interests as part of the individual. This innovation has to start with the contextual evaluation. The

occupational profile must answer two questions for a contextual evaluation:

1. What aspects of the environments or contexts does the client see as supporting engagement in desired occupations?
2. What aspects of the environments or contexts does the client see as inhibiting?

CONTEXTUAL EVALUATION TO PROMOTE INCLUSION

Because disability is often associated with the medical model and with individual deficit and pathology that require remediation, this association drives the deficit-based approach to evaluation that focuses on individual factors and contextual factors that relate specifically to that individual. However, individual factors are not the only barrier to successful participation; the context itself can be an important barrier to participation and inclusion and needs to be considered. ***Inclusion*** provides opportunities for people with disabilities to learn, work, play, and participate alongside their peers without disabilities. Contextual barriers, such as physical inaccessibility, lack of social support, and negative attitudes, often hinder one's participation and inclusion in society.

For example, Beukelman and Mirenda (2013) identified a participation model for individuals with complex communication needs. In this model, the two components of participation are (1) access and (2) opportunity. Both are required for full participation and inclusion with use of augmentative and alternative communication. Opportunity may be as simple as belief in the individual's skill and competence by the professionals around them, even before evaluation of individual abilities.

In line with the ***social model of disability*** (Goering, 2015), which interprets disability within a social context and as a result of societal barriers, true contextual evaluation provides a more holistic and complementary perspective on a client's challenges to full participation. A contextual evaluation goes well beyond individual factors

TABLE 7.4. Sample Measures That Assess Strengths	
ASSESSMENT	**HOW DOES IT MEASURE STRENGTHS?**
Child Occupational Self-Assessment (Kramer et al., 2014)	▪ Identifies interests of the child ▪ Self-assesses competence and value of everyday activities ▪ Self-identifies goals
Canadian Occupational Performance Measure (Law et al., 2019)	▪ Self-determines goals that indicate autonomy and individual goal priorities
Behavioral and Emotional Rating Scale (Epstein, 2004)	▪ Self-evaluates of strengths for children ages 11–18 years ▪ Measures parent evaluation of strengths for children ages 5–18 years ▪ Identifies strengths, including interpersonal, intrapersonal, career, and affective strengths ▪ Assesses family involvement and school functioning
Survey of Favorite Interests and Activities (Smerbeck, 2017)	▪ Identifies interests, including potential benefits of interests in competence development ▪ Includes adaptive Coping subscale that looks at how interests foster happiness, emotional coping, and skill development

and may have a more significant impact in identifying factors that influence actual participation. Shifting the focus from individual deficits to contextual barriers, contextual evaluation can address restraining environments and promote a more inclusive society for individuals with various needs.

Occupational therapists can facilitate social inclusion by evaluating contextual and environmental barriers and advocating for changes. For example, an occupational therapist working with a student with ASD can evaluate peer and teacher attitudes toward the student and their knowledge about autism. If negative peer attitudes are identified, the therapist can promote the use of class or schoolwide peer intervention, which has shown positive effects on peer attitudes and acceptance (Armstrong et al., 2017; Gillespie-Lynch et al., 2015).

This contextual evaluation of the students' social environment complements the client-centered evaluation of social participation, but it adds an outward focus that looks at determinants of participation that are not under the client's control but do have a significant impact on participation. Furthermore, it enables a change toward a more inclusive environment that supports individuals with divergent needs.

SUMMARY

Context is an important part of a client's life, yet ways of exploring context have been limited. It is important to determine whether context serves as a support or deterrence to participation in occupations. There are standardized and nonstandardized ways to evaluate context.

An important nonstandardized way for assessing context is through the occupational profile, which provides the basis for the occupational therapist and client to identify priority goals and essential outcomes that become the focus of intervention. By evaluating the client's participation in life roles, the occupational therapist can construct an occupational profile that explores the client's natural contexts. Participation assessments often use self-report or interview with the client, consider the client's everyday occupations and natural environments, and evaluate goal-directed activities. Participation assessments also may assess the client's satisfaction with participation and their perception of barriers. This chapter includes discussions of participation assessments that give insight into the client and their contextual life.

Assessment of the client's environment is included in holistic evaluation of their occupations and participation. Assessments of a child's environments often focus on contextual factors that promote development of specific skills, such as play. Assessments of an adult's environments tend to measure safety, accessibility, comfort, and social supports. The strength-based assessment can ensure the performance of a contextual evaluation that supports participation. The measures described in this chapter are part of the occupational therapist's evaluation toolbox and enable a comprehensive understanding of a client's occupations, the constraints and supports in the client's environment, and the ability of the client to participate in different environments.

QUESTIONS

1. What role does context play in a client's life?
2. How can the occupational profile be used to explore context?
3. How can a participation assessment tell the therapist about the client's context?
4. Identify three standardized assessments that can be used to explore context. What aspect of context can be identified through each?
5. Why is an occupation-based evaluation important to a therapist's evaluation process? How does it complement observational assessments of performance?
6. What is a strength-based approach? How does it change the focus of evaluation?
7. How can the evaluation of context affect inclusion and belonging?

REFERENCES

American Occupational Therapy Association. (2014). Occupational therapy practice framework: Domain and process (3rd ed.). *American Journal of Occupational Therapy, 68*(Suppl. 1), S1–S48. https://doi.org/10.5014/ajot.2014.682006

American Occupational Therapy Association. (2015). Standards of practice for occupational therapy. *American Journal of Occupational Therapy, 69*(Suppl. 3), 6913410057. https://doi.org/10.5014/ajot.2015.696S06

Armstrong, M., Morris, C., Abraham, C., & Tarrant, M. (2017). Interventions utilising contact with people with disabilities to improve children's attitudes towards disability: A systematic review and meta-analysis. *Disability and Health Journal, 10,* 11–22. https://doi.org/10.1016/j.dhjo.2016.10.003

Barrett, K., Coppola, S., & Alvarez, L. (Eds.). (2020). *International occupational therapy: Strategies for working and learning abroad.* North Bethesda, MD: AOTA Press.

Baum, C. M., & Edwards, D. (2001) *Activity Card Sort.* St. Louis, MO: Washington University School of Medicine.

Baum, C. M., & Edwards, D. (2008). *Activity Card Sort* (2nd ed.). Bethesda, MD: AOTA Press.

Beukelman, D. R., & Mirenda, P. (2013). *Augmentative and alternative communication: Supporting children and adults with complex communication needs.* Baltimore: Brookes.

Bradley, R. H., Corwyn, R. F., McAdoo, H. P., & Coll, C. G. (2003). The home environments of children in the United States Part I: Variations by age, ethnicity, and poverty status. *Child Development, 72,* 1844–1867. https://doi.org/10.1111/1467-8624.t01-1-00382

Bundy, A. (1999). *Test of Environmental Supportiveness.* Fort Collins: Colorado State University.

Caldwell, B., & Bradley, R. (1984). *Home Observation for Measurement of the Environment.* Little Rock: University of Arkansas at Little Rock.

Canadian Association of Occupational Therapists. (2013). *Enabling occupation II: Advancing an Occupational Therapy Vision for Health, Well-being, & Justice through Occupation (2nd ed.).* Ottawa: CAOT Publications.

Chiu, T., Oliver, R., Marshall, L., & Letts, L. (2001). *Safety Assessment of Function and the Environment for Rehabilitation (SAFER) tool manual.* Toronto: COTA Comprehensive Rehabilitation and Mental Health Services.

Clemson, L. (1997). *Home fall hazards: A guide to identifying fall hazards in the homes of elderly people and an accompaniment to the assessment tool, the Westmead Home Safety Assessment (WeHSA).* West Brunswick, Australia: Coordinates Publications.

Corner, R. A., Kielhofner, G., & Lin, F.-L. (1997). Construct validity of a work environment impact scale. *Work, 9,* 21–24. https://doi.org/10.3233/WOR-1997-9104

Coster, W., & Khetani, M. A. (2008). Measuring participation of children with disabilities: Issues and challenges. *Disability and Rehabilitation, 30,* 639–648. https://doi.org/10.1080/09638280701400375

Coster, W., Deeney, T., Haltiwqanger, J., & Haley, S. M. (1998). *School Function Assessment.* San Antonio, TX: Pearson Education.

Coster, W., Law, M., & Bedell, G. (2010). *The Participation and Environment Measure in Children and Youth (PEM–CY).* Boston: Boston University.

Dorman, J. P. (2009). Statistical tests conducted with school environment data: The effect of teachers being clustered in schools. *Learning Environments Research, 12,* 85–99. https://doi.org/10.1007/s10984-009-9054-y

Doucet, B. M., & Gutman, S. A. (2013). Quantifying function: The rest of the measurement story. *American Journal of Occupational Therapy, 67,* 7–9. https://doi.org/10.5014/ajot.2013.007096

Dunn, W., Koenig, K. P., Cox, J., Sabata, D., Pope, E., Foster, L., & Blackwell, A. (2013). Harnessing strengths: Daring to celebrate everyone's unique contributions, Part 2. *Developmental Disabilities Special Interest Section Quarterly Newsletter, 36,* 1–4.

Epstein, M. H. (2004). *BERS–2: Behavioral and Emotional Rating Scale—second edition.* Austin: Pro-Ed.

Fleischer, A., Fisher, M., & Bunger, L. (2019). Support for client-centered evaluations for detecting functional impairments among breast cancer survivors one to five years after treatment. *American Journal of Occupational Therapy, 73,* 7311500018. https://doi.org/10.5014/ajot.2019.73S1-RP203A

Forsyth, K., Taylor, R. R., Kramer, J. H., Prior, S., Richie, L., Whitehead, J., . . . Melton, J. (2014). The Model of Human Occupation. In B. A. B. Schell & M. E. Scaffa (Eds.), *Willard and Spackman's occupational therapy* (12th ed., pp. 505–526). Baltimore: Lippincott, Williams & Wilkins.

Fougeyrollas, P., Noreau, L., Bergeron, H., Cloutier, R., Dion, S. A., & St-Michel, G. (1998). Social consequences of long term impairments and disabilities: Conceptual approach and assessment of handicap. *International Journal of Rehabilitation Research, 21,* 127–141. https://doi.org/10.1097/00004356-199806000-00002

Gillespie-Lynch, K., Brooks, P. J., Someki, F., Obeid, R., Shane-Simpson, C., Kapp, S. K., . . . Smith, D. S. (2015). Changing college students' conceptions of autism: An online training to increase knowledge and decrease stigma. *Journal of Autism and Developmental Disorders, 45,* 2553–2566. https://doi.org/10.1007/s10803-015-2422-9

Goering, S. (2015). Rethinking disability: The social model of disability and chronic disease. *Current Reviews in Musculoskeletal Medicine, 8,* 134–138. https://doi.org/10.1007/s12178-015-9273-z

Gummesson, C., Atroshi, I., & Ekdahl, C. (2003). The Disabilities of the Arm, Shoulder, and Hand (DASH) outcome questionnaire: Longitudinal construct validity and measuring self-rated health change after surgery. *BMC Musculoskeletal Disorders, 4*(1), 11. https://doi.org/10.1186/1471-2474-4-11

Haley, S. M., Jette, A. M., Coster, W. J., Kooyoomjian, J. T., Levenson, S., Heeren, T., & Ashba, J. (2002). Late Life Function and Disability Instrument: II. Development and evaluation of the function component. *Journals of Gerontology, Series A: Biological Sciences and Medical Sciences, 57,* M217–M222. https://doi.org/10.1093/gerona/57.4.m217

Hamed, R., & Holm, M. B. (2013). Psychometric properties of the Arab Heritage Activity Card Sort. *Occupational Therapy International, 20*(1), 23–34. https://doi.org/10.1002/oti.1335

Harden, B. J., & Whittaker, J. V. (2011). The early home environment and developmental outcomes for young children in the child welfare system. *Children and Youth Services Review, 33*(8), 1392–1403. https://doi.org/10.1016/j.childyouth.2011.04.009

Iwarsson, S., & Slaug, B. (2001). *The Housing Enabler—an instrument for assessing and analysing accessibility problems in housing.* Nävlinge, Sweden: Veten & Skapen HB & Slaug Data Management.

Jenkinson, C., Mant, J., Carter, J., Wade, D., & Winner, S. (2000). The London Handicap Scale: A re-evaluation of its validity using standard scoring and simple summation. *Journal of Neurology, Neurosurgery, and Psychiatry, 68,* 365–367. https://doi.org/10.1136/jnnp.68.3.365

Jette, A. M., Haley, S. M., Coster, W. J., Kooyoomjian, J. T., Levenson, S., Heeren, T., & Ashba, J. (2002). Late Life Function and Disability Instrument: I. Development and evaluation of the disability component. *Journals of Gerontology, Series A: Biological Sciences and Medical Sciences, 57,* M209–M216. https://doi.org/10.1093/gerona/57.4.M209

Kratz, A. L., Chadd, E., Jensen, M. P., Kehn, M., & Kroll, T. (2015). An examination of the psychometric properties of the Community Integration Questionnaire (CIQ) in spinal cord injury. *Journal of Spinal Cord Medicine, 38*(4), 446–455. https://doi.org/10.1179/2045772313Y.0000000182

Keglovits, M., Somerville, E., & Stark, S. (2015). In-Home Occupational Performance Evaluation for Providing Assistance (I–HOPE Assist): An assessment for informal caregivers. *American Journal of Occupational Therapy, 69,* 6905290010. https://doi.org/10.5014/ajot.2015.015248

Kessler, D., & Egan, M. (2012). A review of measures to evaluate participation outcomes poststroke. *British Journal of Occupational Therapy, 75,* 403–411. https://doi.org/10.4276/030802212X13470263980757

Khetani, M. A., Graham, J. E., Davies, P. L., Law, M. C., & Simeonsson, R. J. (2015). Psychometric properties of the Young Children's Participation and Environment Measure. *Archives of Physical Medicine and Rehabilitation, 96,* 307–316. https://doi.org/10.1016/j.apmr.2014.09.031

King, G., Law, M., King, S., Hurley, P., Hanna, S., Kertoy, M., & Young, N. (2004). *Children's Assessment of Participation and Enjoyment (CAPE) and Preferences for Activities of Children (PAC).* San Antonio: Harcourt Assessment.

Klaas, S. J., Kelly, E. H., Gorzkowski, J., Homko, E., & Vogel, L. C. (2010). Assessing patterns of participation and enjoyment in children with spinal cord injury. *Developmental Medicine and Child Neurology, 52*(5), 468–474. https://doi.org/10.1111/j.1469-8749.2009.03552.x

Kotler, P. D., & Koenig, K. P. (2012). Authentic partnerships with adults with autism: Shifting the focus to strengths. *OT Practice, 17,* 6–9.

Kramer, J., ten Velden, M., Kafkes, A., Basu, S., Federico, J., & Kielhofner, G. (2014). *The Child Occupational Self-Assessment (COSA) Version 2.2.* Chicago: Model of Human Occupation Clearinghouse, Department of Occupational Therapy, College of Applied Health Sciences, University of Illinois at Chicago.

Larson, E., & Zemke, R. (2003). Shaping the temporal patterns of our lives: The social coordination of occupation. *Journal of Occupational Science, 10,* 80–89. https://doi.org/10.1080/14427591.2003.9686514

Law, M. (1998). Does client-centered practice make a difference? In M. Law (Ed.), *Client-centered occupational therapy* (pp. 19–29). Thorofare, NJ: Slack.

Law, M. (2002). Participation in the occupations of everyday life. *American Journal of Occupational Therapy, 56,* 640–649. https://doi.org/10.5014/ajot.56.6.640

Law, M., Anaby, D., Teplicky, R., Khetani, M. A., Coster, W., & Bedell, G. (2013). Participation in the home environment among children and youth with and without disabilities. *British Journal of Occupational Therapy, 76,* 58–66. https://doi.org/10.4276/030802213X13603244419112

Law, M., Baptiste, S., Carswell, A., McColl, M., Polatajko, H., & Pollock, N. (2019). *Canadian Occupational Performance Measure* (5th ed., rev.). Altona, MB: COPM, Inc.

Law, M., Dunn, W., & Baum, C. (2005). Measuring participation. In M. Law, C. Baum, & W. Dunn (Eds.), *Measuring occupational performance: Supporting best practice in occupational therapy* (2nd ed., pp. 107–128). Thorofare, NJ: Slack.

Law, M., & Mills, J. (1998). Client-centered occupational therapy. In M. Law (Ed.), *Client-centered occupational therapy* (pp. 1–18). Thorofare, NJ: Slack.

Moos, R. (1994). *Work Environment Scale manual* (3rd ed.). Palo Alto, CA: Consulting Psychologists Press.

Ne'eman, A. (2010). The future (and the past) of autism advocacy, or why the ASA's magazine, *The Advocate,* wouldn't publish this piece. *Disability Studies Quarterly, 30*(1). Retrieved from http://dsq-sds.org/article/view/1059/1244

Patten Koenig, K. (2019). A strength based frame of reference for autistic individuals. In P. Kramer, J. Hinojosa, & T. Howe (Eds.), *Frames of reference for pediatric occupational therapy* (4th ed., pp. 496–522). Baltimore: Lippincott Williams & Wilkins.

Pighills, A. C., Torgerson, D. J., Sheldon, T. A., Drummond, A. E., & Bland, J. M. (2011). Environmental assessment and modification to prevent falls in older people. *Journal of the American Geriatrics Society, 59*(1), 26–33. https://doi.org/10.1111/j.1532-5415.2010.03221.x

Ritchie, L., Wright-St. Clair, V. A., Keogh, J., & Gray, M. (2014). Community integration after traumatic brain injury: A systematic review of the clinical implications of measurement and service provision for older adults. *Archives of Physical Medicine and Rehabilitation, 95,* 163–174. https://doi.org/10.1016/j.apmr.2013.08.237

Rosenberg, L., Jarus, T., & Bart, O. (2010). Development and initial validation of the Children Participation Questionnaire (CPQ). *Disability and Rehabilitation, 30,* 1633–1644. https://doi.org/10.3109/09638281003611086

Rogers, J., & Holm, M. (2009). The occupational therapy process. In E. B. Crepeau, E. S. Cohn, & B. A. B. Schell (Eds.), *Willard and Spackman's occupational therapy* (11th ed., pp. 428–434). Philadelphia: Lippincott Williams & Wilkins.

Ryan, R. M., & Deci, E. L. (2000). Self-determination theory and the facilitation of intrinsic motivation, social development, and well-being. *American Psychologist, 55,* 68–78. https://doi.org/10.1037/0003-066X.55.1.68

Sachs, D., & Josman, N. (2003). The Activity Card Sort: A factor analysis. *OTJR: Occupation, Participation and Health, 23,* 165–176. https://doi.org/10.1177/153944920302300404

Skard, G., & Bundy, A. C. (2008). Test of Playfulness. In L. D. Parham & L. S. Fazio (Eds.), *Play in occupational therapy for children* (2nd ed., pp. 71–94). St. Louis: Mosby/Elsevier.

Smerbeck, A. (2017). The Survey of Favorite Interests and Activities: Assessing and understanding restricted interests in children with autism spectrum disorder. *Autism, 23,* 247–259. https://doi.org/10.1177/1362361317742140

Stark, S., Somerville, E., & Morris, J. (2010). In-Home Occupational Performance Evaluation (I–Hope). *American Journal of Occupational Therapy, 64,* 580–589. https://doi.org/10.5014/ajot.2010.08065

Wahl, H.-W., Fänge, A., Oswald, F., Gitlin, L. N., & Iwarsson, S. (2009). The home environment and disability-related outcomes in aging individuals: What is the empirical evidence? *The Gerontologist, 49,* 355–367. https://doi.org/10.1093/geront/gnp056

Whiteneck, G. G., Charlifue, S. W., Gerhart, K. A., Overholser, J. D., & Richardson, G. N. (1992). Quantifying Handicap: A new measure of long-term rehabilitation outcomes. *Archives of Physical Medicine and Rehabilitation, 73,* 519–526.

Wilcock, A. A. (1998). Reflections on doing, being, and becoming. *Canadian Journal of Occupational Therapy, 65,* 248–256. https://doi.org/10.1177/000841749806500501

Wilcock, A. A., & Townsend, E. A. (2008). Occupational justice. In E. B. Crepeau, E. S. Cohn, & B. B. Schell (Eds.), *Willard and Spackman's occupational therapy* (11th ed., pp. 192–199). Philadelphia: Lippincott Williams & Wilkins.

Willer, B., Ottenbacher, K. J., & Coad, M. L. (1994). The Community Integration Questionnaire: A comparative examination. *American Journal of Physical Medicine & Rehabilitation, 73,* 103–111. https://doi.org/10.1097/00002060-199404000-00006

World Health Organization. (2001). *International classification of functioning, disability and health.* Geneva: Author.

Yerxa, E. J. (1967). Authentic occupational therapy [Eleanor Clarke Slagle Lecture]. *American Journal of Occupational Therapy, 21,* 1–9.

Zemke, R. (2004). Time, space, and the kaleidoscopes of occupation [Eleanor Clarke Slagle Lecture]. *American Journal of Occupational Therapy, 58,* 608–620. https://doi.org/10.5014/ajot.58.6.608

Nonstandardized Assessments

Aimee J. Luebben, EdD, OTR, FAOTA; Charlotte Brasic Royeen, PhD, OTR/L, FAOTA, ASAHP, FNAP; and Keli Mu, PhD, OTR/L

8

CHAPTER HIGHLIGHTS

- Standardized versus nonstandardized testing
- Why use nonstandardized testing?
- When to use nonstandardized assessments
- AOTA Occupational Profile Template as a guide to choosing additional assessments
- Using nonstandardized assessments

KEY TERMS AND CONCEPTS

- Bottom-up assessments
- Central tendency
- Class evidence
- Duration recording
- Elements of nonstandardized assessment
- Environment bias
- Event recording
- Halo effect
- Interactive reasoning
- Interview
- Ipsative-referenced assessments
- Item bias

- Occupational profile
- Occupation-based therapy
- Observation
- Operations of nonstandardized assessments
- Outcomes of nonstandardized assessments
- Person-related bias
- Questionnaires
- Rate recording
- Research Pyramid
- Screening
- Semistructured interviews

- Severity or leniency
- Standardization
- Structured assessments
- Structured interviews
- Testing bias
- Time sampling
- Top-down assessment
- Triple Aim
- Unstructured assessments
- Unstructured interviews
- Visual sampling

INTRODUCTION

During this era of the **Triple Aim,** which consists of improving patients' experience of care, increasing the use of evidence-based care, and reducing the cost of health care per person (Wilkinson et al., 2017), it is imperative for occupational therapists to be rigorous and reliable in how they use standardized and nonstandardized testing. Both standardized and nonstandardized assessments are critical in providing a valid view into the occupational needs of a person or population.

This chapter begins with an introduction to nonstandardized assessments as a method of information gathering, including a discussion of how nonstandardized assessments relate to standardized assessments. It then presents why and when occupational therapists use nonstandardized assessments. The remainder of the chapter reviews four major categories of nonstandardized assessment methods: (1) observation, (2) interview, (3) questionnaire, and (4) performance.

STANDARDIZED VERSUS NONSTANDARDIZED TESTING

What makes an assessment standardized? **Standardization** "implies uniformity of procedure in administering and scoring the test" (Anastasi & Urbina, 1997, p. 6). **Standardization** means that each time an occupational therapist administers a standardized assessment, the therapist administers and scores it in the same manner. It also means that the environmental conditions under which the assessment is administered are prescribed. Standardized assessments have psychometric data regarding their reliability and validity.

In addition, most standardized assessments are categorized as either criterion referenced or norm referenced. A *criterion-referenced assessment* allows comparison of clients' results with a defined criterion. A *norm-referenced assessment* allows comparison of the results of an individual with those of a group of people, often people with similar characteristics or conditions. When occupational therapists administer a standardized assessment and do not follow the procedures prescribed in the manual, the assessment is no longer considered standardized and is therefore not valid in terms of scoring. In such a case, the compromised standardized assessment may only be used as a clinical observation without standardized scoring because the psychometric properties of the assessment established previously—that is, its reliability and validity—are no longer maintained. Romli et al. (2019) provided an excellent overview of the standardized tests that occupational therapists use in practice, and the reader is referred to their article for further information on the use of standardized assessments in occupational therapy.

Table 8.1 compares the characteristics of standardized and nonstandardized assessments and shows that different types of data are pertinent to each. One is highly personalized; the other is highly related to the performance of others. The nature of the assessment settings differs, as does the type of data generated. Each assessment approach requires the utmost professional skill and commitment of the occupational therapist to gathering "true" or internally valid patient data and patient-reported information during the assessment process.

Nonstandardized assessments may not be uniform in administration or scoring. In addition, full and complete psychometric data about the assessment may not exist. Because nonstandardized testing is not built on prescribed processes of administration and scoring, it allows for flexibility and individualization. Standardized assessments are norm referenced or criterion referenced; nonstandardized tests are individualized. Individualized assessments are also called *ipsative-referenced assessments* (*ipsitive* is an alternative spelling); the word *ipsative* is derived from the Latin *ipse*, "of the self." Anastasi and Urbina (1997) acknowledged that although "the ipsative frame of reference may be the most suitable for intraindividual comparisons, such as

those needed in the assessment of interests and other preferences, normative reference data are necessary for individual comparisons" (p. 370). This refers to the need for normative data when comparing one person against other people with similar age and gender, as opposed to just comparing the person against themselves.

Nonstandardized assessments using an ipsative reference provide a unique opportunity for occupational therapists to delve deeply into the person or a group in the natural environment. Just as research methods evolve to meet a particular field's need, methods of assessment develop in response to a discipline's or a profession's need. For occupational therapy evaluation, ipsative-referenced nonstandardized assessments are becoming more recognized and useful as individualized assessment instruments. In fact, Donnelly and Carswell (2002) reviewed the literature to report on individualized outcome measures that are client centered and concomitantly ipsative referenced.

WHY USE NONSTANDARDIZED TESTING?

Nonstandardized testing results in the collection of individuated information that can be traced to a single entity. Individuated evidence (e.g., fingerprints; DNA; a well-written, detailed performance observation) provides strong internal validity: The information collected is indicative of a person's uniqueness. Such ipsative information is considered an intrapersonal or "within-the-person" comparison.

If interpersonal (i.e., between-persons) comparisons are the goal, then occupational therapists need to use standardized assessments that have strong external validity. A standardized assessment allows comparison of a person's ability, behavior, performance, and so on with a standard (i.e., criterion) or a group (i.e., norm). The resulting information from many standardized assessments, however, is

TABLE 8.1.   Comparison of Nonstandardized and Standardized Assessment Characteristics

CHARACTERISTIC	NONSTANDARDIZED ASSESSMENT	STANDARDIZED ASSESSMENT
Focus	Ipsative referenced Individual, system Individualized, self	Norm referenced Criterion referenced
Personal	Intrapersonal	Interpersonal
Setting	Naturalistic	Laboratory controlled, prescribed
Type of evidence and examples	Individuated • DNA • Fingerprints • Performance observation • Ethnographic observation	Class • Blood type • Percentile rank • Standard score • Derived score
Data generated	Qualitative and quantitative	Primarily quantitative
Procedures	Less formal	Formal
Structure	Less structured	More structured
Clinical reasoning	Requires strong clinical reasoning for assessment and interpretation	Less dependent on clinical reasoning for administration and interpretation
Validity	Strong internal validity	Strong external validity

considered to be *class evidence:* classification within a category (e.g., blood type, perceptual–motor percentile). Class evidence does not offer the corresponding intrapersonal, within-the-person uniqueness provided by individuated evidence or ipsative reference.

Nonstandardized Testing in Occupational Therapy

In the history of occupational therapy, perspectives on assessments, evaluation, and intervention have evolved across different periods in the profession. For many years, the profession has tried to move away from traditional medical models of practice to focus on understanding the individualized, unique perspectives of occupation (i.e., an ipsative reference point); the dynamic systems of the person engaging and participating in occupations; and the environments in which the person performs the occupations. However, many aspects of occupational therapy service provision, particularly assessments, still focus on static protocols. Hinojosa (2007) pointed out that "occupational therapy practice has become less individualized and more routine, and that therapy becomes all about protocols, techniques and procedures" (p. 634). To be faithful to the principles and philosophy of occupational therapy, the profession emphasizes theory-driven and occupation-based practice, which may include more ipsative-referenced assessments. Coster (2008), in her Slagle Lecture focused on measurement challenges in practice, stated, "Instruments provide a way to extract pattern from the performance of an individual for some purpose" (p. 748).

Occupational therapists have used various assessments in everyday practice to justify reimbursement practices rather than looking at clients' individual and specific needs.

Using specific examples of cognitive assessments, Gillen (2013) in his Slagle Lecture asserted that many occupational therapy assessments are "originally and primarily adopted from other disciplines, not occupation based, contrived, novel, and two dimensional in a three-dimensional world" (p. 647). He further added that occupational therapy assessments must theoretically resemble everyday demands and not be dominated by artificially controlled, unnatural testing environments (Gillen, 2013). Similarly, Law et al. (2005) contended that in assessment, occupational therapists should focus on occupational performance (i.e., function) and analyze tasks, activities, and occupation. Moreover, they argued that best practice in assessment is centrally focused on occupational performance in everyday life. The focus on this area may not lend itself well to standardized assessments.

Many different paradigms in occupational therapy practice support the use of both standardized and nonstandardized assessments. Models and theories predict what occurs within the person and in the person's performance of occupations. Moreover, most describe how the environment influences occupational performance. Each of these models or theories then lends itself to the use of nonstandardized forms of assessment (see Table 8.2).

The *International Classification of Functioning, Disability and Health* (*ICF;* World Health Organization [WHO], 2001) has been the primary force for changing the focus of assessments from impairment to function. Norm-referenced, standardized assessments are intended to identify deficits or impairment. Nonstandardized assessments, such as skilled observation and semistructured interviews, aim to gather and interpret clients' occupational therapy performance.

The emphasis on performance (i.e., function) in the *ICF* calls for a *top-down assessment* approach in which

TABLE 8.2.   Examples of Occupational Therapy Conceptual Models and Perspectives on Nonstandardized Assessments

CONCEPTUAL MODEL	PERSPECTIVES ON ASSESSMENTS
Model of Human Occupation (Kielhofner, 2008)	"Nonstandardized assessments take advantage of natural circumstances that arise for learning about a client. They can be adapted to unfolding situations in therapy, and the occupational therapist gains conceptual answers to questions unanswered during the course of intervention" (Kielhofner, 2008, p. 157).
Ecological models: ■ Person–Environment–Occupation Model (Law et al., 1996) ■ Person–Environment–Occupation–Performance Model (Christiansen et al., 2015) ■ Ecology of Human Performance Model (Dunn, 2017)	The "evaluation process determines what features of the person, environment, and occupation support or interfere [with] occupational performance. [The] person is not viewed in isolation but is considered in terms of [the] environment where occupational performance takes place. Practice should not be confined to protocols but requires a thoughtful, reasoned and collaborative process of evaluation and intervention" (Brown, 2014, p. 499).
Occupational adaptation (Schultz, 2014)	Practice should be theory driven and include assessments that not only measure static outcomes but also assess the impact of intervention on the client's engagement in personally meaningful life roles. Occupational adaptation–based interventions target the client's increased adaptiveness, regardless of condition, as a primary outcome. Assessment and intervention are process oriented with an emphasis on the dynamic exchange that occurs between the therapist and the client (Schultz, 2014).

occupational performance and the environment and context of the performance are analyzed. ***Bottom-up assessment,*** however, focuses on clients' factors, skills, and capability. Nonstandardized assessments often use a top-down approach with a focus on occupational performance in areas such as ADLs, education, and work. Kielhofner (2008), using the Model of Human Occupation (MOHO), used different terminology to describe assessments that support his conceptual model; instead of the conventional terms *standardized* and *nonstandardized,* he used the terms *structured* and *unstructured.* ***Structured assessments*** have fixed procedures, specified guidelines for use, standardized administration procedures, and evidence of reliability and validity. ***Unstructured assessments*** use natural circumstances that arise to learn about a client.

Kielhofner (2008) recommended routinely using unstructured assessments in practice. To ensure dependability of unstructured forms of assessment, Kielhofner emphasized the importance of evaluating the contexts of occupational performance, triangulating or comparing the data gathered with other sources, and performing validity checks through proper and reasoned interpretation of data. Most MOHO assessments have protocols for administration as well as research on validity and reliability and thus could be categorized as structured assessments. However, MOHO assessments are ipsative referenced and thus are categorized as nonstandardized. To improve validity, occupational therapists may use the following actions before, during, and after assessment.

Before the assessment, ask

- Am I biasing this assessment in any way?

During the assessment, monitor the client's autonomic nervous system functioning.

- Is the person unduly stressed (sweating, repetitive behavior, self-stimulating, fast breathing, blanching)?
- Are the person's responses consistent? Does the message from the person's body language match the message from verbal statements?
- Are there signs of fatigue, frustration, or anger?

After the assessment, ask

- Was this a novel experience for the person?
- Did an event occur that could change the findings of the nonstandardized assessment?
- Were the responses average and typical of how the person usually functions?
- How can the outcomes of this assessment be corroborated?

Evidence-Based, Occupation-Based, Client-Centered Practice and Nonstandardized Testing

Evidence is at the center of evidence-based practice, a movement driving many health care disciplines. Tomlin and Borgetto (2011) developed a model of evidence-based practice for use in occupational therapy called the ***Research Pyramid,*** which puts descriptive research at its base and experimental, outcome, and qualitative research as its three sides. The added emphasis on the value of descriptive and qualitative studies in producing evidence addresses an essential component of occupational therapy practice:

clients' day-to-day experience (Tomlin & Borgetto, 2011). Cook (2001) highlighted the methods of inquiry in practice needed to capture the complex, multidimensional, and moving picture of clients during their daily engagement in occupations. Nonstandardized assessments can provide a dynamic picture of clients as they perform and engage in occupations in clinical and natural settings.

In a study on the use of standardized assessments by occupational therapists in the United States, pediatric therapists reported that standardized assessments were valued more highly in their practice setting than in adult practice settings (Piernik-Yoder & Beck, 2012). The study reported that occupational therapists practicing in adult settings tend to use nonstandardized assessments more than standardized assessments. One reason for this may be that the use of standardized assessments is required in schools. Occupational therapists in both adult and pediatric settings cite various reasons why they find standardized tests challenging to use. These reasons include the fast pace of the setting, high caseloads, amount of time available for assessments, and finding tests that accurately ascertain and portray clients' abilities and levels.

Occupation is the cornerstone of the occupational therapy profession. Scholars, educators, and practitioners have found, however, that occupational therapy practice has moved away from occupation-based practice (Che Daud et al., 2016; Reynolds et al., 2019). ***Occupation-based therapy*** means therapeutic interventions that use meaningful occupations designed specifically to meet a client's needs. To facilitate and maximize *occupation-based therapy,* an occupation-based assessment is essential in the occupational therapy process. Assessment is the first contact that occupational therapists have with people who receive service, and a top-down, occupational performance–focused, and individualized assessment is necessary to ensure occupation-based assessment. One excellent example of such assessment is the occupational profile. The American Occupational Therapy Association's (AOTA; 2017) Occupational Profile Template is available in Appendix A. The ***occupational profile*** is "a summary of a client's occupational history and experiences, patterns of daily living, interests, values, and needs" (AOTA, 2014, p. S13). Using the occupational profile, therapists can gather information from the client's perspective through a formal interview and casual conversation and develop individualized, client-centered, and occupation-based intervention.

Client-centered practice requires that occupational therapists understand each person's specific needs (Phipps & Foley, 2019). Consequently, assessments need to focus not only on measurable components that relate to occupational performance but also on subjective experience and observable qualities of people's participation in occupations (Law & Baum, 2005), which would thereby likely require at least one assessment that is ipsative referenced.

Controlling Bias and Nonstandardized Testing

The goal of any type of testing—standardized or nonstandardized—is to understand one or more aspects of the person being evaluated. To achieve this goal, evaluators are obligated to control for as much testing variance or bias as possible. The acronym *PIE* can help occupational therapists remember the three aspects of **testing bias**:

1. *Person*-related bias,
2. *Item* bias, and
3. *Environment* bias.

Case Example 8.1 illustrates controlling for PIE in a testing situation. In addition to the three aspects of bias, a certain unnaturalness occurs during the observation event itself, which can lead to testing variance and possible error.

Person-related bias

Person-related bias is the degree to which the assessment favors or is against the person. There are two types of person-related testing bias: (1) evaluator or rater bias and (2) test-taker bias. To determine actual occupational performance, evaluators must control for their expectations and rating tendencies that could result in error: severity or leniency, central tendency, and halo effect. **Severity or leniency** refers to how hard or easy a rater is when scoring the client. **Central tendency** refers to the tendency of a rater to score most items in the middle of the rating scale. **Halo effect** is the tendency of a rater to allow item rating to be influenced by other experiences or opinions that are not directly related to the test items (e.g., influence of age of the client when rating children lower in ability than adults on the same test, rating a client better than their actual performance because you believe they are trying their best).

For evaluators to gather critical information, the person being assessed must demonstrate genuineness in any performance and be a good historian (a person who provides the truth about a situation) when responding to questions. Remember that a good historian must have an adequate level of cognitive functioning.

Item bias

Item bias involves the degree to which the specific element being tested fits the actual occupation the test taker performs in real life. For example, a test of self-care may have an item related to combing hair and is biased against individuals who are bald. The relevance of the item to the occupation of the test taker is important within the context of testing. On occasion, tests of capacity may involve items that test if an individual has the capacity for certain tasks that an individual may never do in real life and the context for this type of testing should be clearly described to the client. For example, when using a test with nine holes and pegs that are commonly used for testing clients for dexterity, the person may never do this type of a task in real life and needs to be explained the rationale for the testing.

Environment bias

Environment bias concerns the degree to which the testing context matches the appropriate natural environment. For example, the clinic and home environment are very different for the performance of tasks and when a therapist is trying to assess the ability of an individual to perform a task in their own natural environment, setting up the clinic space as closely simulated to the person's home environment, including location of objects, distance, distractions, and available tools, may help reduce the bias due to the environmental context.

The outcomes (e.g., behaviors) of nonstandardized assessments must be double checked to make certain the findings are usual, typical, average, and representative (Brentnall & Bundy, 2009). Checking can be done by reviewing the data generated from the test with what is expected for the person's age and condition. Making nonstandardized testing as systematic as possible and controlling for bias can result in objective information that has great relevance to the client receiving occupational therapy services.

Organizing Structures and Nonstandardized Testing

Various naming systems (i.e., taxonomies) and theoretical approaches provide an organizing structure for evaluation, including the use of nonstandardized testing. AOTA (2014) provides a system that names the various aspects of the occupational therapy profession's domain of concern in the *Occupational Therapy Practice Framework: Domain and Process* (OTPF). Occupational therapists can use nonstandardized testing to assess the aspects of the OTPF that include areas of occupation, client factors, performance skills, performance patterns, and contexts and environment.

Related to the *OTPF*, the AOTA Occupational Profile Template is a means to organize supports and barriers to occupational engagement and is meant to be used in

---

CASE EXAMPLE 8.1. MR. O'NEIL: CONTROLLING TESTING BIAS

Mr. O'Neill is an 83-year-old widower who usually brushes his teeth alone in the bathroom of his home. Janet, an occupational therapist testing Mr. O'Neill's occupational performance of this task in a hospital setting, needed to control for all three aspects of PIE testing bias. To reduce testing error, both types of person bias would need extra attention: Janet would need to control for her expectations and rating tendencies and determine Mr. O'Neill's genuineness and historian abilities in his response to her questions about toothpaste container (manual squeeze or pump) and toothbrush (manual, battery operated, or electric). Janet's presence while observing Mr. O'Neill may result in him performing this seemingly mundane task differently than usual. By changing context—by observing Mr. O'Neill in his home—she could eliminate environment bias and most of the bias related to item and to person, especially to the person being tested. The variance corresponding to observer presence, however, would remain.

occupational therapy practice and education (AOTA, 2017). Currently, both the assessments that look at occupational engagement and the complete occupational profile are nonstandardized.

Nonstandardized assessments can be used on a global scale by using WHO's (2001) *ICF*. Globally, the *ICF* is used as a framework for disability, functioning, and health of individuals; its components can be assessed separately for individuals with any condition to allow consistency among the areas assessed within nonstandardized testing. Areas of the *ICF* that cover nonstandardized testing include assessment of a person's participation or involvement in a life situation, activity limitations or challenges a person may have in executing activities, participation restrictions or challenges a person may experience when engaged in life situations, and external and internal influences related to a person's functioning.

Occupational therapists can also use nonstandardized testing with theoretical approaches that have an organizing structure. For example, the Canadian Model of Occupational Performance and Engagement (CMOP–E; Canadian Association of Occupational Therapists [CAOT], 1997, 2002; Polatajko et al., 2007) provides a structure to allow assessment of person, environment, and occupation. Figure 8.1 compares three aspects of the CMOP–E (CAOT, 1997; Polatajko et al., 2007), *OTPF* (AOTA, 2014), and *ICF* (WHO, 2001): (1) life areas (occupation), (2) foundational components (body level), and (3) contextual factors. The content related to the essential components for assessing clients that are explained within the literature put forth by CAOT (1997, 2002), AOTA (2014), and WHO (2001) portray the value and importance of theory in the development and implementation of appropriate assessments.

Components of Nonstandardized Testing

When thinking about using a nonstandardized assessment, occupational therapists should consider three important components of such assessments: (1) elements, (2) operations, and (3) outcomes.

Elements of nonstandardized assessments

Elements of nonstandardized assessments refers to an assessment's characteristics, including its client centeredness, equipment and supplies, training, invasiveness, responsivity, needs, and cost. Nonstandardized assessments should incorporate consideration of and clinical reasoning about the following concerns:

- *Client-centered approach:* The client is a person or persons, group or population for whom the occupational therapy practitioner is providing services (Accreditation Council for Occupational Therapy Education®, 2018; AOTA, 2014).
- *Equipment:* The items needed are often highly portable and usually do not involve the purchase of additional supplies and equipment. Some standardized assessments require that buyers purchase additional equipment (e.g., a tricycle) not included in test kits.
- *Training:* Extensive training or certification for use is typically not required. For some standardized assessments,

costs are incurred not only to purchase the instrument but also for training in the use of the instrument.

- *Invasiveness:* Nonstandardized assessments are typically noninvasive and involve little risk.
- *Responsivity:* In cases in which the results of a standardized assessment might indicate that a client has reached a plateau, a nonstandardized assessment may be responsive enough to ascertain small outcome changes in the client's performance. In many cases, standardized instruments do not have enough sensitivity to detect small changes observed by occupational therapists.
- *Fulfills unmet need:* Nonstandardized assessments expand on the information obtained from standardized assessments and may be specific to a particular occupational performance aspect for which a standardized assessment does not exist.
- *Cost:* Many standardized assessment instruments are costly—after buying the initial assessment, individual test or scoring forms must often be purchased on an ongoing basis. The cost of nonstandardized assessments is typically much lower.

Operations of nonstandardized assessments

Operations of nonstandardized assessments refers to the manner of administering the assessment, including ease of administration, time, environment, ease of analysis, and reasoning.

- *Ease of administration:* The procedural steps in administering nonstandardized tests are usually straightforward compared with the complex procedures of some standardized tests.
- *Time:* Nonstandardized assessments take less time to administer than many standardized assessment instruments, although more time may be needed to document because of the need to select unique language to describe testing and test results.
- *Environment:* Nonstandardized assessments are typically conducted in the client's natural environment to help control for the environmental aspect of PIE testing bias. For example, observing a child in the classroom provides assessment information about a student in an environment that is natural to the child.
- *Ease of analysis:* Nonstandardized assessments do not have the complex scoring procedures typical of standardized assessments. Depending on the circumstances, topics, or data obtained, the analysis may take considerable time and may be multidimensional.
- *Reasoning:* Interpreting nonstandardized assessments may require considerable clinical expertise and analytic reasoning to provide an understanding of multiple data points.

Outcomes of nonstandardized assessments

Outcomes of nonstandardized assessments refers to the manner of administering assessments, including validity of findings for the client, control of PIE bias, validity of findings related to the natural environment, and the link between the outcomes of the nonstandardized assessment and theory. The specifics of these outcomes are as follows:

FIGURE 8.1. Comparison of the CMOP–E, *OTPF,* and *ICF.*

Model	Definition	Life Areas (Occupations)	Foundational (Body-Level) Components	Contextual Factors
ICF — Activities and Participation (Daily Life Area Domains)	Activity is the execution of a task or action by a person; participation is involvement in life situations.	Community, social, and civic life; Major life areas; Interpersonal interactions and relationships; Domestic life; Self-care; Mobility; Communication; General tasks and demands; Learning and applying	**Body Functions and Structures:** Skin and related structures; Neuromusculoskeletal and movement related; Genitourinary and reproductive; Digestive, metabolic, and endocrine; Cardiovascular, hematological, immunological, and respiratory; Voice and speech; Sensory; Mental	**Contextual Factors** — Personal factors; **Environmental Factors:** Services, systems, and policies; Attitudes; Support and relationships; Natural environment and human-made changes to the environment; Products and technology
OTPF — Occupation	Occupations are central to a client's identity and sense of competence and have particular meaning and value to the client.	Social participation; Leisure; Play; Work; Education; Rest and sleep; IADLs; ADLs	Performance patterns—groups and populations; Performance patterns—person; Performance skills; Client factors	**Context and Environment:** Virtual; Temporal; Social; Physical; Personal; Cultural
CMOP-E — Occupational Performance and Engagement	Occupations are composed of activities, which are made up of actions composed of voluntary movements.	Leisure; Productivity; Self-care	**Person:** Spirituality; Affective; Cognitive; Physical	**Environment:** Social; Cultural; Institutional; Physical

Note. ADLs = activities of daily living; AOTA = American Occupational Therapy Association; CMOP–E = Canadian Model of Occupational Performance and Engagement; IADLs = instrumental activities of daily living; *ICF* = *International Classification of Functioning, Disability and Health; OTPF* = *Occupational Therapy Practice Framework. Source.* Created by A. Luebben for "Nonstandardized Assessments" by C. B. Royeen, L. C. Grajo, and A. J. Luebben. In J. Hinojosa and P. Kramer (Eds.), *Evaluation in Occupational Therapy: Obtaining and Interpreting Data,* 4th Edition, p. 127. Bethesda, MD: AOTA Press. Copyright © 2014 by the American Occupational Therapy Association. Used with permission.

- *Validity of findings for the client:* Nonstandardized assessments capture the person's uniqueness, offering assessment results with strong internal validity for individual clients.
- *Control of PIE bias:* Nonstandardized testing offers opportunities to control for the person aspect of PIE testing bias, particularly evaluator or rater variance, by establishing rater reliability. A single occupational therapist can start with intrarater reliability by making sure to perform nonstandardized assessment methods the same way each time. Interrater reliability can be established across all therapists within a practice setting for commonly used nonstandardized testing methods. In fact, formalizing a system to ensure and document inter-rater reliability among therapists in a practice setting could serve to fulfill some requirements mandated by national agencies that accredit hospitals and clinics.
- *Validity of findings related to the natural environment:* Instead of testing performance on the basis of sterile conditions or contexts (sometimes associated with standardized assessment instruments), assessing behaviors that occur naturally in context can help control for the item aspect of PIE testing bias.
- *Link between outcomes of the nonstandardized assessment and theory:* The nonstandardized assessment should be administered and interpreted consistent with the conceptual framework, model, or frame of reference on which it is based so the therapist can decide whether the theoretical approach is a fit for the particular client.

WHEN TO USE NONSTANDARDIZED ASSESSMENT

Nonstandardized assessment is used throughout the occupational therapy process, both at the information-gathering stages of screening and evaluation and during intervention planning, intervention, and reevaluation. During the screening and evaluation process, therapists can use nonstandardized assessments to collect information for both parts of the *OTPF* evaluation process: the occupational profile and the analysis of occupational performance (AOTA, 2014). Even merely observing clients in their natural setting is considered nonstandardized assessment.

Using nonstandardized assessments is particularly common during screening, a time when occupational therapists collect information related to a potential client to determine the need for further evaluation and the possibility of intervention. Not intended as a comprehensive evaluation, *screening* provides preliminary information to determine whether further occupational therapy services are needed. Screening often involves observation and interview, two categories of a nonstandardized assessment. Nonstandardized screening in a school setting may consist of observing a student on the playground or interviewing the teacher to gather information related to the basis for occupational therapy referral and the background of the child. In an adult day care setting, an occupational therapist might perform a screening during a group craft activity to identify participants who are interested and have the functional capacity to participate in a gardening group.

During evaluation, the other initial information-gathering stage, occupational therapists use nonstandardized testing alone or in an integrated approach by using nonstandardized assessment methods to supplement standardized assessments. Although the recommendations and examples of nonstandardized assessments provided later in this chapter can be used for either screening or evaluation, the level of detail of certain assessments is more relevant to evaluation.

Occupational therapists can also use nonstandardized testing after the initial information-gathering stages: during intervention planning, intervention, and reevaluation. Occupational therapists interpret nonstandardized testing results to plan intervention and use nonstandardized methods (primarily observation, interview, and performance testing) to monitor progress during intervention. In reevaluation, occupational therapists compare the client's current performance with the initial results to gauge improvement. Nonstandardized testing can play a meaningful role in the area of reevaluation to determine the effectiveness of occupational therapy.

AOTA OCCUPATIONAL PROFILE TEMPLATE AS A GUIDE TO CHOOSING ADDITIONAL ASSESSMENTS

The purpose of the AOTA Occupational Profile Template is to understand the client's identified priorities and desired outcomes for therapy (AOTA, 2017). Information gathered from the occupational profile can assist therapists in deciding the most appropriate standardized and nonstandardized tests to use during assessment. The *OTPF* lists eight questions that a therapist can ask to efficiently develop a client's occupational profile (Exhibit 8.1). Remember that this approach is not norm-referenced in any way but uses an ipsative reference to identify the unique configuration of priorities for given clients and their family.

A few nonstandardized assessments can be used to provide a detailed occupational profile of a client. For pediatric clients, the Short Child Occupational Profile (SCOPE;

EXHIBIT 8.1.	Eight Important Areas to Cover When Using the AOTA Occupational Profile Template

1. Reasons for seeking services and concerns about performance of occupations and daily life tasks
2. Areas of perceived success and areas in which improvement is desired
3. The influence of environment or context in supporting or inhibiting performance
4. Occupational history
5. Values and interests
6. Daily life roles
7. Patterns of occupational engagement and perceived changes over time
8. Priorities and desired targeted outcomes, relative to occupational performance, participation, roles, and quality of life

Source. From "Occupational Therapy Practice Framework: Domain and Process (3rd ed.)," by American Occupational Therapy Association, 2014, *American Journal of Occupational Therapy, 68*(Suppl.), p. S13. Copyright © 2014 by the American Occupational Therapy Association. Adapted with permission.

Bowyer et al., 2008) can be used. For clients older than age 12 years, the Occupational Performance History Interview–II (OPHI–II; Kielhofner et al., 2004) can be used. (The SCOPE and OPHI–II are discussed in greater detail later in this chapter.)

USING NONSTANDARDIZED ASSESSMENTS

The appropriate and effective use of nonstandardized assessments requires occupational therapists to have a solid theoretical knowledge base and sound clinical reasoning, two of the three evidence-based practice approaches. Using nonstandardized assessment instruments appropriately and effectively depends on selecting and using assessments from four major categories: (1) observation, (2) interview, (3) questionnaire, and (4) occupational performance assessment. Table 8.3 provides questions and directions for effective use of nonstandardized assessments.

Recently, Maritz et al. (2018) analyzed occupational therapy models linking assessment and the *ICF*, an integration introduced in the first edition of this book and chapter. The more occupational therapy can link assessment and the *OTPF* to the *ICF*, the better therapists will be able to communicate clients' needs and goals.

Table 8.3 assists in ensuring that occupational therapists recognize the importance of using a theory, an evidence-based practice approach, an organizing taxonomy, triangulation of data, monitoring of the test taker issues of diversity, and establishing rapport.

The most common forms of nonstandardized assessment are observation and interview. The two remaining categories (occupational performance assessments and questionnaires) have less coverage in this chapter because observation is often used as a method of collecting occupational performance assessment information and interviews often include a questionnaire component.

Observation

Observation, which comes from the Latin *observo* (i.e., to watch, pay attention to, and take careful note of), has come to signify a systematic examination of some type of phenomenon. In occupational therapy, observation is probably the most powerful and common procedure for collecting knowledge for evaluation purposes. In fact, occupational therapists at all competence levels—novice to expert—include observation as an integral part of their assessment information-gathering repertoire. Thus, being able to observe and note critical pieces of information are important parts of an occupational therapist's toolkit for relevant assessment.

The following are examples of ways to observe phenomena (e.g., behaviors, activities, functions, participation, environments).

- Look at the posture, symmetry, and fluidity of motion while someone engages in mobility activities.
- Look at the posture, symmetry, and fluidity of motion while someone engages in any other type of activity.
- Examine a classroom for flow patterns, noise levels, and visual demands.
- Watch a person with a disability getting dressed in the morning at home or another appropriate site.
- Diagram the manner in which a person with a disability moves from one end of the occupational therapy clinic to the other while navigating around tables, people, and chairs.
- Observe a person interacting with others.

Although the process of observation involves visually sampling phenomena, other senses (e.g., hearing, smelling, touching) often provide additional information. For example, using vision alone to sample an environment such as a kitchen might involve a description of the physical layout, level of lighting, and efficiency of workstations. Additional sensory information about a kitchen—a lingering natural gas smell, sticky counters that hinder horizontal movement of pots to the stove, or a floor that is gritty with sand—may raise safety issues. For the purposes of this chapter, observation is synonymous with visual sampling and includes obtaining information through all senses. *Visual sampling* is a very powerful method of nonstandardized assessment.

Because of the nature of observation, occupational therapists must control for all three aspects of PIE assessment bias. Both types of the person aspect of PIE assessment bias must be controlled, particularly bias related to the evaluator. To control for the item aspect of PIE assessment bias, an occupational therapist must ensure that the specific element corresponds to the actual real-life occupation of the client being evaluated. Assessment of occupational performance conducted in a natural environment (e.g., the client's home, church, public library, social club) has built-in controls for the environmental aspect of PIE assessment bias.

Although not optimal, assessment of occupational performance also occurs in simulated contexts (e.g., clinic) when natural environments are not readily available. The validity of occupational performance assessment and its generalization to the natural environment are based on the match or fit of the simulated context to the natural environment. Test validity improves when a simulated context closely resembles the natural environment, increasing the probability that the client will be able to generalize skills practiced in the clinic to a natural setting such as home. In addition, therapists must account for the unnaturalness of the observation itself, which may lead to some testing variance and potential error in information gathering. Chapter 7, "Contextual Evaluation to Support Participation," describes the importance of context in evaluation in greater depth.

Occupational therapists use varying degrees of formality and structure to systematize the procedure of collecting evaluation information through observation. Information collected through observation can include nonnumerical descriptions of characteristics that are qualitative, measurable information resulting in numerical data that are quantitative, or a combination of qualitative and quantitative aspects. The systematic, procedural component of observation affects the degree of formality, level of structure, and balance of the qualitative and quantitative information.

Observations related to standardized assessments are frequently formal and structured because occupational therapists must follow specific protocols that were refined during instrument development. Results obtained through

TABLE 8.3.   Effective Use of Nonstandardized Assessments

QUESTION	DIRECTIONS
What theory is the assessment based on?	Base all information gathering on theory. Because theory and practice must be linked consistently, theory needs to provide the foundation for evaluation and intervention. Theoretical knowledge is 1 of 3 approaches to providing evidence-based practice.
How does the nonstandardized assessment relate to evidence-based practice?	Use an ipsative, client-centered approach to underpin nonstandardized information gathering. According to Ilott (2004), "The perspective of the patient, and their caregiver, is a critical component of experiential evidence, especially their views about what constitutes desirable or successful outcomes" (p. 348). Experimental evidence (the product of occupational therapy clinical reasoning) is 1 of the 3 approaches to providing evidence-based practice.
What organizing structure (i.e., taxonomy) is being used, and how is the nonstandardized assessment relevant?	Select the nonstandardized assessment method on the basis of its relevance to what is being measured and the organizing structure being used. For example, an occupational therapist using the *ICF* (WHO, 2001) would choose a method to assess either the 2 components of functioning and disability (activities and participation, body functions and structure) or the 2 components of contextual factors (environmental and personal factors). Another example is a therapist who uses the *OTPF* (AOTA, 2014) to assess areas of occupation, client factors, performance skills, performance patterns, context and environment, and activity demands.
How will the client be monitored during nonstandardized assessment?	Occupational therapists should be sensitive to client cues and be careful not to stress, fatigue, or invade the personal and cultural space of a client. Therapists can reschedule the session, take a break, or switch to a different information-gathering approach if client cues indicate a need for change.
What are the sources of nonstandardized assessments, and how are assessment data triangulated?	Use multiple assessments in evaluating a client. Although a therapist-designed checklist can offer some information about a person, documenting observations adds to the richness of the data collection. Using more than 1 assessment allows occupational therapists to triangulate the data collection process, fulfilling the goal of the nonstandardized assessment: determining the client's actual occupational performance.
How does nonstandardized assessment accommodate diversity and inclusion?	Respect the diverse nature of humans, who vary in gender, class, and cultural background. Sensitivity to diversity can be addressed by selecting nonstandardized assessments that allow for variation in client response. Nonstandardized assessments provide individuated evidence, not class evidence. When working with persons of diverse backgrounds, therefore, nonstandardized assessments may be the preferred method of evaluation to accommodate cultural differences and offer cultural sensitivity.
Are the findings valid?	Establish rapport with the client. An occupational therapist who is highly skilled in the interpersonal aspect of clinical areas is optimal. Regardless of the level of rapport established, the documentation of nonstandardized assessments must include information about the status of rapport to help readers interpret adequacy and accuracy of evaluation information.

Note. AOTA = American Occupational Therapy Association; *ICF* = *International Classification of Functioning, Disability and Health;* *OTPF* = *Occupational Therapy Practice Framework;* WHO = World Health Organization.

standardized assessments often start as qualitative information but are transformed into quantitative information: Observations are usually classified or ranked into categories, then assigned numerical values. The numerical values, based on observation of performance levels, factor into the scoring of the standardized assessment. For example, an occupational therapist watches Mark, an 8-year-old boy in second grade, string eight blocks within a 15-second time period. His performance is assigned a raw score of 8 (blocks), which correlates with a point score of 7 on the Manual Dexterity subtest of the Bruininks–Oseretsky Test of Motor Proficiency (Bruininks & Bruininks, 2005).

Without a routine systematic procedure, an observation is likely to be classified as informal and unstructured. For instance, an occupational therapist used an informal, unstructured approach to observation when he entered the home of Eunice, an 83-year-old widow who lived alone before hospitalization. The therapist watched her move from the foyer through the rooms and took notes for a home accessibility visit before her discharge. His observations probably included both qualitative and quantitative information (e.g., Eunice's motor and praxis skill performance as she reached for drinking glasses on a top shelf, the size and number of throw rugs on the

CASE EXAMPLE 8.2. MARK: OBSERVATION

Mark, a right-handed 8-year-old boy, used his left thumb and finger pads to hold a string (1 inch from the end) vertically 6 inches in front of his chest. With his right hand, he picked up three blocks at once, placing one block at a time on the tip of the string while retaining the other blocks fisted in his middle, ring, and little fingers. As Mark dropped one block on the string, he grasped the string tip (above the block) with his right thumb and index finger pads, allowing gravity to move the block vertically down the string. He then transferred the string back to his left thumb and finger pads to begin sliding another block onto the string.

The procedures developed during the standardization of the Manual Dexterity subtest of the Bruininks–Oseretsky Test of Motor Proficiency (Bruininks & Bruininks, 2005) resulted in observations about Mark that were formal, structured, and quantitative: Mark's raw score of 8 (blocks) equated to a point score of 7 for that subtest item. The supplemental nonstandardized assessment information, however, provided valuable unstructured and informal information that was qualitative in nature. On the basis of additional observations, the occupational therapist improved the richness of information related to Mark's ability to organize a task, sequence steps, and use strategies (in this case, a gravity-assist method).

---

floor, the time she required to move from the couch to the bathroom).

As procedures become more systematic and routine, observations become semiformal and semistructured. An occupational therapist who systematically works sequentially through a self-designed checklist as a guide to collecting observations is using a semiformal, semistructured approach. Although such assessment appears less official because there are no written guidelines, the expert therapist who has an established routine or habitual way of assessing persons demonstrating similar occupational patterns is also using a semiformal, semistructured approach.

Observations that are semiformal or informal and semistructured or unstructured are not necessarily inferior to formal, structured observation. Formal, structured observation (which is part of standardized assessments) is frequently a sterile procedure with resulting outcomes that can be different from what happens under customary conditions in a natural environment. In other words, standardized conditions in a prescribed setting may yield reliable information, but such information may not be truly valid for the person: Only the occupational therapist's clinical judgment can confirm the validity of assessment findings.

For example, a person may be able to transfer in a simulated clinic bathroom but may have difficulty transferring in the home bathtub if the shower nozzle is on the opposite side from that of the clinic shower. The clinic evaluation would provide documentation that the patient was successful in tub transferring.

Observation (i.e., visual sampling) that is less systematized often results in increased richness of information. Interestingly, formal, structured observation that is part of the information-gathering process for a standardized instrument is frequently augmented with less formal and structured observation. In Case Example 8.2, the occupational therapist makes additional observations about Mark.

Collection methods

To collect observation information, particularly in quantitative format, occupational therapists use four common methods: (1) event recording, (2) duration recording, (3) rate recording, and (4) time sampling. In occupational therapy, the most common methods of collecting information are event recording and duration recording.

Event recording. **Event recording** is the simplest of the four methods and provides a count of each occurrence of a specific type of phenomenon within a time frame or an evaluation period. In event recording, occupational therapists keep a tally of occurrences, resulting in an understanding of the frequency of a phenomenon. In Eunice's home accessibility evaluation, for example, an occupational therapist assisting in the decision of whether Eunice can return home to live alone could keep a tally of unsafe acts, a form of event recording, by counting the number of times Eunice slipped on a throw rug, used the towel bars in the kitchen and bathroom for stability in transitions, or steadied herself with both hands on the counter in preparation for reaching for a glass.

Duration recording. When occupational therapists use timing devices such as stopwatches or kitchen timers, they are performing **duration recording.** For a particular phenomenon (e.g., behavior, activity engagement), duration recording determines the length of time of an occurrence, the amount of time needed for completion, the length of time spent, or latency (the length of time a phenomenon is not observed). Using duration recording in Eunice's case, the occupational therapist could measure how much time she required to move from the driveway into the house, how long she spent moving from her foyer to the kitchen, and the length of time she needed to complete the task of getting a glass of tap water. The occupational therapist could also use latency duration recording by measuring the time interval between unsafe acts.

To use duration recording, the therapist must determine which "end" of the time scale is considered optimal by determining whether the focus is speed (a shorter time) or endurance (a longer time). For example, if the focus is speed, then the optimal end of the time scale is a low number of time units. In terms of speed, a person who assembled a five-piece work task in 10 seconds is three times faster than someone who took 30 seconds to assemble the same five-piece work task. If the focus of duration recording is endurance, then the optimal end of the time scale is a high number of time units.

For instance, when working on increasing attention to task (a type of endurance), a student who attended to task for 12 minutes without becoming distracted performed three times better than another student who was able to pay attention without distractions for only 4 minutes.

Rate recording. **Rate recording,** a combination of event and duration recording, is calculated by dividing frequency (event recording) by length of time (duration recording). Eunice's occupational therapist, who is primarily interested in determining whether she can return to living alone in her home, used event recording to keep a simple tally of the number of times she performed unsafe acts. A tally of one unsafe act provides little meaning unless the duration of the home accessibility evaluation is known. In the case of an evaluation lasting 15 minutes, the rate recording is calculated by dividing the event recording of unsafe acts (one act) by the duration recording of the evaluation (15 minutes).

In this instance, Eunice performed one unsafe act every 15 minutes. Extrapolating that information to a 24-hour day, allowing for 8 hours of sleep, Eunice had the potential for 64 unsafe acts per day and 448 unsafe acts per week. On this basis, the occupational therapist may recommend that it is not safe for Eunice to return home to live alone. One unsafe act during a 4-hour evaluation (1 per 240 minutes), however, results in an extrapolation of 4 possible unsafe acts per day and 28 potential unsafe acts per week.

Although 4 unsafe acts per day is better than 64, Eunice's occupational therapist would still need to determine whether it is safe for her to return to living home alone. In this case, the quantitative information generated by rate recording may not be enough to make a final recommendation. If her occupational therapist supplemented the rate recording with qualitative information that indicates all four unsafe acts during the visit occurred when Eunice tripped on a throw rug, a simple recommendation to remove the throw rugs would eliminate all 64 potentially unsafe acts per day predicted in the shorter evaluation as well as the four possible daily unsafe acts observed during the longer evaluation.

Time sampling. According to Ottenbacher (1986), **time sampling** (also called *scan sampling, instantaneous time sampling, discontinuous probe time sampling,* and *interval sampling*) "involves recording the state of a behavior at specific moments or intervals in time" (p. 71). This most sophisticated method of collecting observation data requires signaling specified intervals by a timer, recorded cues, or other means. The observation times are interspersed with intervals of no observation, which are usually used to record the results of preceding observation intervals. Time sampling can be used in combination with event recording, duration recording, or rate recording.

To apply time sampling to Eunice's case, her occupational therapist could use an audio recording indicating 5-minute observation times followed by 10-minute intervals of no observation to record the frequency (event recording) of unsafe acts within that observation interval. If the one unsafe act seen in the rate recording example earlier did not occur during the observation interval, then the occupational therapist would record observing no unsafe acts. As this example shows, time sampling (although a potent research strategy) can be time consuming and burdensome, and it has the potential to produce inaccurate information in practice settings.

A variation on the time sampling method is the combination of event occurrence and interval recording. In the preceding example, each minute during the 5-minute observation period can be divided into four intervals of 15 seconds each. Each 15-second interval is also divided into a 10-second observation period followed by a 5-second rest period. The observer is signaled by a timer at the beginning of each 10-second observation period to observe whether an operationally defined behavior occurs or not. The observer marks "yes" if the behavior occurs and "no" if the behavior does not occur. The duration of the behavior or the occurrence of the behavior at any other point during the 10-second observation interval is irrelevant in this case.

An example of an occupation-based observational assessment is the Short Child Occupational Profile (SCOPE (Bowyer et al., 2008). The SCOPE, based on the MOHO (Kielhofner, 2008), can be used to observe individual children or groups of children and provide a broad overview of their occupational participation. The SCOPE identifies a child's strengths and weaknesses and factors based on MOHO concepts that facilitate or restrict occupational participation and engagement.

Although not formally classified as an assessment, the Dynamic Performance Analysis (DPA; Polatajko et al., 2000) is an observation-based framework developed for the Cognitive Orientation to daily Occupational Performance (CO–OP) treatment approach (Polatajko & Mandich, 2004; Dawson et al., 2017). The DPA and CO–OP were developed on the basis of the CMOP–E. During client observations, occupational therapists use the DPA to analyze performer and performance requisites and identify sources of performance breakdown during participation and engagement in occupations.

Two other observational assessments, the Test of Playfulness (TOP) and the Test of Environmental Supportiveness (TOES; Skard & Bundy, 2008), are currently used in pediatric occupational therapy practice. Both the TOP and the TOES are considered ecological assessments; they are used to observe children ranging in age from 6 to 18 years during free play and identify person-related and environmental influences on children's playfulness.

Observation format

We have developed the following format to provide fundamental steps of observation-based nonstandardized assessment.

- *Step 1:* Describe the setting. Note whether the assessment is occurring indoors or outdoors; note whether the environment appears cluttered or uncluttered; note the number of people, animals, and objects in the setting; note the lighting, temperature, sounds or noise, and smells.
- *Step 2:* Assess the emotional and social tone of the setting and provide a label that connotes the feeling evoked. For example, is the setting safe? Peaceful? Chaotic?

- *Step 3:* Conduct an activity analysis by making note of activities and actions.
- *Step 4:* Reflect on how the community would view the ongoing activities (i.e., is the behavior acceptable in that community?)
- *Step 5:* Make note of how long the observation occurred and at what time of day.
- *Step 6:* Summarize findings.
- *Step 7:* Make an interpretation, including recommended actions, if necessary.

In rehabilitation departments, health care facilities, and clinics, skilled observation is often conducted by therapists by means of a homegrown observation checklist. In fact, the research literature has suggested that the chief reasons why occupational therapists choose specific assessments are their familiarity and availability at their worksites (Alotaibi et al., 2009; Grice, 2015). Although homegrown observation tools such as checklists can be valuable and practical in occupational therapy practice, ensuring acceptable reliability, that is, interobserver or interrater agreement, is key.

Interview

Interview refers to the process of inquiry during which one person asks another one or more questions. Virtually all occupational therapists use interviewing—and more often than not, nonstandardized interview methods—to collect information about almost every client from the very first moment of meeting. Interviews often begin with prompts (e.g., "Describe how you are doing," "Tell me how it has been going") that lead to follow-up probes or additional questions (e.g., "Tell more about that," "And what did you do then?"). Using prompts, probes, and questions such as these reveals a great deal to occupational therapists about clients' activities and participation in life and their challenges while engaging in life situations, including areas of occupation, client factors, performance skills, performance patterns, and contexts and environment (AOTA, 2014). The examples are open-ended questions, which are designed to elicit information and allow people being interviewed to express their own ideas and concerns without direction from the interviewer.

An alternative to open-ended questions is closed-ended questions, which have forced-choice options. An example of a forced-choice response format is selection of one item from an exclusive number of possible responses. Closed-ended questions are often found when specific information is required, such as asking people their age, or on questionnaires, a nonstandardized assessment category that is discussed later in this chapter.

Like observations, nonstandardized interviews vary in degrees of formality (formal, semiformal, or informal), structure (structured, semistructured, or unstructured), and information type (qualitative vs. quantitative). Generally, as a format becomes increasingly systematic, the interview assessment is correspondingly considered more formal and structured. Some interview assessments are not done in a systematic manner and are therefore considered semiformal and semistructured, offering an integrated approach to the collection of qualitative and quantitative information. *Structured interviews* can fall into the category of standardized testing if they have formal and structured procedures for the interview and scoring process. *Semistructured interviews* are usually aided with a list of interview questions. The list of questions ensures the interviewer covers all the topics, dimensions, and elements that are deemed to be important. The order of the listed questions can be altered or changed during the interview process. In addition, interviewers can ask probing questions and follow-up questions to gather in-depth information and clarify important topics and concepts during semistructured interviews. Semistructured interviews are more like conversations.

Unstructured interviews, however, are more like story telling. In unstructured interviews, interviewers do not have a list of interview questions. Rather, they have a roadmap and a basic understanding of the phenomena or concept that they intend to explore and examine. Unstructured interviews often start with open-ended questions such as:

- Please tell me. . . .
- What does . . . like?
- How do you . . . ?

Interviews factor heavily into occupational therapists' clinical reasoning process. For most occupational therapists, interviewing provides the foundation for three forms of clinical reasoning: narrative reasoning, interactive reasoning, and conditional processing. Occupational therapists use *interactive reasoning* (i.e., client-centered interchange) to piece together the fragments of a client's life story and the client's unique perspective (i.e., narrative reasoning) into a holistic pattern that guides interpretation and intervention planning. Therapists' conditional reasoning integrates their understanding of the client's perspective and the client's understanding of their actual abilities to allow for selection of the instruments and questions needed for the interview (Schell, 2014). Obtaining useful information during the data collection stage of an interview is contingent on controlling for item and person aspects of PIE assessment bias. Because interviews involve the interaction of two people, the evaluator and the person being assessed, both types of person-related assessment bias require close attention.

Interview guidelines

We view the following steps as those fundamental to interview-based nonstandardized assessments.

- *Step 1:* Tell me about yourself. Who are you?
- *Step 2:* What is the issue or problem?
- *Step 3:* Why is it an issue or problem?
- *Step 4:* When is it an issue or problem?
- *Step 5:* What areas do you see as your strengths?
- *Step 6:* How have you addressed the issue or problem in the past? How can I, as an occupational therapist, assist you with the problem?
- *Step 7:* Do you see a way that we can use your strengths in this process?

The series of questions provided in these steps may easily be adapted to switch the emphasis of the interview from a problem-based nonstandardized assessment to a different focus as needed.

Individualized interview assessments

Occupational therapy has several individualized interview assessments, including the OPHI–II (Kielhofner et al., 2004) and the COPM (Law et al., 1998, 2019). Both interview assessments are occupation centered, and each is based on a different conceptual model.

The OPHI–II (Kielhofner et al., 2004) is an ipsative-referenced assessment based on the MOHO (Kielhofner, 2008). It is an individualized, client-centered, semistructured interview that systematizes the collection of occupational history information that can be used in developing a person's occupational profile. Using the structure of the occupation-based OPHI–II to obtain client narratives, therapists help clients "integrate their past, present, and future into a coherent whole" (Kielhofner et al., 2004, p. 9). The OPHI–II, which is designed to allow flexibility while exploring a client's occupational life history, includes three scales: Occupational Identity, Occupational Competence, and Occupational Settings (Environment). Version 2.1 of the OPHI–II includes scale key forms (Kramer et al., 2008), designed using Rasch measurement, that convert Likert responses into interval measures. The OPHI–II manual (Kielhofner et al., 2004) has other reproducible forms, including the OPHI–II Clinical Summary Report Form and Life History Narrative Form.

The COPM (Law et al., 1998, 2019) is an ipsative-referenced assessment based on the CMOP–E. The COPM was designed to examine interactions among the person, environment, and occupation. A client-centered, occupation-based interview assessment, the COPM identifies problem areas in occupational performance, provides a rating of clients' priorities in occupational performance, evaluates performance and satisfaction relative to those problem areas, and measures changes in clients' perception of their occupational performance over the course of occupational therapy intervention (Law et al., 1998, 2019).

The COPM allows flexibility in interviewing clients. According to the COPM manual, "It is essential that therapists use their skills in interviewing, probing for full responses, validating assumptions and motivating respondents to obtain the most thorough and comprehensive assessment" (Law et al., 1998, p. 34). The test form provides additional directions:

> To identify occupational performance problems, concerns, and issues, interview the client, asking about daily activities in self-care, productivity, and leisure. Ask clients to identify daily activities which they want to do, need to do or [are] expected to do by encouraging them to think about a typical day. Then ask the client to identify which of these activities are difficult for them to do now to their satisfaction. (Law et al., 1998, p. 2)

Deceptively simple in appearance, the COPM is a powerful, time-saving assessment that gathers salient client-centered information. Exhibit 8.2 provides a SOAP note (**s**ubjective, **o**bjective, **a**ssessment, and **p**lan) for Sandy, a typical college student considered a member of the well population. Sandy is a right-handed, 21-year-old woman, a junior at a Midwestern university, and she lives in a campus apartment with three roommates. A business major, Sandy became engaged to an engineer in Alaska on Valentine's Day and plans to be married the week after graduation. The SOAP note for Sandy shows application of the COPM

and uses the COPM's Person–Environment–Occupation language.

Royeen et al. (2017) suggested a list of critical questions about what is meaningful to clients that should be included in client interviews. These questions were designed to get at the heart of *eudemonia,* an ancient Greek term that captures what makes life worth living for a client. Ten relevant questions that drive this aspect of eudemonic care can be administered to clients during nonstandardized occupational therapy assessment:

1. Participation in what occupations brings you happiness?
2. Participation in what occupations brings you joy?
3. Participation in what occupations gives you meaning?
4. Participation in what occupations gives you pleasure?
5. Participation in what occupations gives you satisfaction?
6. What are you not doing that you used to do that brought you pleasure?
7. What do you find fun?
8. What occupations in which you engage contribute to irritability, aggressiveness, apathy, and/or sexual dysfunction?
9. Is there sadness during your participation in occupations?
10. What could improve your quality of life?

Again, these questions are only recommended and should be selectively woven in at appropriate times during the overall assessment process. This requires skill, tact, timing, and sensitivity on the part of the occupational therapist.

Questionnaires

Questionnaires are used to collect information during the evaluation process, and they include self-report measures that a client or caregiver completes with paper and pencil or instruments administered via electronic devices such as computers. Because this type of assessment can be completed with or without an occupational therapist present, selection of completion method may help control for person-related PIE assessment bias that involves the evaluator. Questionnaires have the potential to control for person-related assessment bias, depending on whether the client or caregiver is a good historian, can read and comprehend the information requested, has the requisite motor skills (using a writing instrument or a computer), and makes appropriate decisions among choices. Medical histories that people complete in a medical setting are an example of questionnaires that document a person's past.

Questionnaires are usually indirect measures of behavior, that is, they reflect the client's perception, rather than direct measures. Indirect measures inherit certain characteristics and weakness such as the unknown linkage between perception and behavior and social desirability in responding to questions.

In occupational therapy, the Occupational Self Assessment (OSA; Baron et al., 2006), which is based on the MOHO (Kielhofner, 2008), is one example of an ipsative-referenced questionnaire. The OSA was "developed to assess the MOHO concepts of occupational competence and value for occupation through self report" (Kramer et al., 2008, p. 173). This individualized, client-centered questionnaire consists of two primary self-assessment forms: (1) OSA Myself and (2) OSA My Environment. The OSA

EXHIBIT 8.2. Occupational Therapy Initial Evaluation: The SOAP Note for Sandy

S: Sandy indicated that she was relieved to be working on her occupational performance (OP), saying her "life is such a mess." She said that she can't seem to get anything done, is failing her business law course, and forgets simple things.

O: On the Canadian Occupational Performance Measure (COPM), a client-centered, interview-based assessment instrument that detects self-perceived change in OP over time, Sandy identified 9 OP problems. Of these, 2 (22%) were in self-care (taking too long in morning routine and forgetting to brush teeth); 5 (56%) were in productivity (decreased time management skills because of high levels of electronic social networking, misplacing homework, getting unorganized easily, running out of gas, and falling asleep in business law class); and 2 (22%) were in leisure (paying high communication bills and having no fun at all). Using the importance scale (COPM–I), Sandy prioritized her 5 most critical OP problems and then rated her performance (COPM–P) and satisfaction (COPM–S) for each. The table below lists Sandy's COPM scores, which indicate overall decreased performance and satisfaction levels associated with 2 underlying person components related to cognition: (1) time management and (2) organizational skill difficulties.

OP PROBLEM	COPM–I SCORE	COPM–P SCORE	COPM–S SCORE
Time management	10	2	1
Homework	10	3	2
Brushing teeth	9	4	3
Organizational skills	9	3	3
Paying bills	8	2	2
COPM Total Score (average)	**9.2**	**2.8**	**2.2**

Note. COPM–I = Client's perceived importance; COPM–P = Client's perceived performance score; COPM–S = Client's satisfaction with performance score. COPM–I, COPM–P, and COPM–S scales consist of a 1–10 rating, with 10 indicating the optimal level of each.

A: Rapport was established, and testing indicated that Sandy is a good historian, so the results of this evaluation reflect a reliable and valid estimate of Sandy's OP at the current time. Use of the COPM showed functional deficits in Sandy's OP related to self-care, productivity, and leisure performance and satisfaction, secondary to inadequate time management and organizational skills. Sandy's problem list consists of the 5 OP problems listed in the previous table. Sandy, who has excellent potential for improvement, would benefit from skilled occupational therapy to improve her OP through compensatory strategies.

P: Sandy is to be seen for 45-minute sessions semiweekly for 2 weeks for skilled occupational therapy instruction in compensatory time management and organizational strategies. By discharge, Sandy will exhibit independent use of these strategies, demonstrating improved self-care, productivity, and leisure performance and satisfaction as evidenced by improvements in COPM–P and COPM–S reevaluation scores compared with initial COPM–P and COPM–S scores. The table below lists Sandy's long- and short-term goals.

OP PROBLEM	SHORT-TERM GOAL (1 WEEK)	LONG-TERM GOAL (BY DISCHARGE)
Time management	Decrease electronic social networking to a scheduled 5 times per day.	Decrease electronic social networking to a scheduled 3 times per day.
Homework	Place finished homework for 1 course in an expandable folder.	Place finished homework for all courses into color-coordinated expandable folders.
Brushing teeth	Brush teeth 1 time per day.	Brush teeth 2 times per day.
Organizational skills	Organize work related to school.	Organize work related to school and personal life.
Paying bills	Decrease monthly communication bill by $20.	Decrease monthly communication bill by $50.

helps clients establish priorities for change, which translate into intervention goals. Included with the assessment are reproducible forms for planning and implementing goals and showing progress and outcomes.

Occupational Performance Assessments

Standardized and nonstandardized assessments can be subdivided into performance-based and non–performance-based assessments. Performance-based assessments are direct measures, and non–performance-based assessments

are indirect measures. Occupational performance assessments are different from questionnaires. With respect to performance assessments, occupational therapists use their activity analysis skills as a means of collecting information about how a client carries out a task in context rather than relying on self-report. From a nonstandardized perspective, observation is a primary assessment in the collection of data related to occupational performance. Therefore, occupational therapists who use this method of collecting information must control for the three aspects of PIE assessment bias. In addition, the occupational therapist must take into account the unnaturalness of the observation itself, which can lead to testing variance.

Examples of nonstandardized occupational performance assessment include activities such as cooking lunch in a kitchen, buttering a piece of toast while seated at a dining table, changing the sheets on a bed, or creating a pinch pot out of clay. Occupational performance assessment can be based on the client's real-time performance of predetermined criteria such as making a sandwich, operating a stove efficiently and safely, moving within a room or from one room to another, or preparing a space for completion of a specified craft project. In this situation, the client demonstrates an aspect of occupational performance that is rated qualitatively and quantitatively by the occupational therapist.

SUMMARY AND FUTURE DIRECTIONS

Both nonstandardized and standardized assessments are important in occupational therapy. Standardized assessments must be used in restricted and prescribed conditions, which often impose sterile or artificial conditions on the client. Moreover, standardized assessment instruments sometimes provide little usable information related to the occupational therapy domain of concern. Nonstandardized assessments, however, produce ipsative-referenced results that may offer stronger internal validity and more sensitivity than information obtained through standardized instruments.

In the era of evidence-based, client-centered, and occupation-based occupational therapy practice, occupational therapists should consider nonstandardized assessment as a sound method to gather rich information about clients, and they are challenged to improve the reliability and validity of nonstandardized assessments. Any assessment—standardized or nonstandardized—should be used in a systematic way to provide consistency and to control for all three aspects of PIE assessment bias. Making the nonstandardized assessment process as systematic as possible should provide equally valid results every time the assessment is used, regardless of the person conducting the evaluation. Nonstandardized assessments can be used alone to effectively gather information during evaluation. For various reasons, a nonstandardized assessment may be the only way an occupational therapist can perform a particular evaluation.

An optimal method of data collection uses nonstandardized and standardized assessments in an integrated approach. Integration of nonstandardized assessment offers ipsative-referenced information about individual clients to supplement information from standardized assessments that compare clients' performance with criterion-referenced standards or with norm-referenced peer groups.

To use nonstandardized assessments appropriately and effectively, occupational therapists must have a solid theoretical knowledge base and sound clinical reasoning, two of the three evidence-based practice approaches. Therapists who want to implement evidence-based practice should consider Ilott's (2004) reminder that all sources of evidence (empirical research, experiential evidence, and theoretical knowledge) are equally valid.

Finally, there is a view in current practice that use of standardized assessments strengthens occupational therapists' role in evidence-based practice, yet the use of standardized assessments is believed to be as low as 26% (Romli et al., 2019). In addition, the use of occupation-based instruments is relatively scant in contrast to the use of assessments that focus on the impairment level of function (Romli et al., 2019). Thus, the field of occupational therapy is challenged to develop more and better occupation-based assessments, both standardized and nonstandardized, that focus on occupational engagement and participation.

QUESTIONS

1. What is the role of theory in nonstandardized assessment?
2. What is the role of clinical reasoning in nonstandardized assessment?
3. What are three actions the occupational therapist can take during nonstandardized assessment that incorporate PIE to ensure the evaluation's validity?
4. What are three clinical situations in which nonstandardized assessment would be appropriate? Why?
5. When does a standardized assessment become nonstandardized?
6. What are the benefits and drawbacks of evaluating clients in their natural environment (e.g., home, work, school)?
7. What are the benefits and drawbacks of evaluating clients in a specialized intervention environment (e.g., hospital clinic, outpatient rehabilitation center)?

REFERENCES

Accreditation Council for Occupational Therapy Education (2018). 2018 Accreditation Council for Occupational Therapy Education (ACOTE®) standards and interpretative guide. *American Journal of Occupational Therapy, 72*(Suppl. 2), 7912410005. https://doi.org/10.5014/ajot.2018.72S217

American Occupational Therapy Association. (2014). Occupational therapy practice framework: Domain and process (3rd ed.). *American Journal of Occupational Therapy, 68*(Suppl.), S1–S48. https://doi.org/10.5014/ajot.2014.682006

American Occupational Therapy Association. (2017). AOTA occupational profile template. *American Journal of Occupational Therapy, 71*, 7112420030. https://doi.org/10.5014/ajot.2017.716S12

Alotaibi, N. M., Reed, K., & Nadar, M. S. (2009). Assessments used in occupational therapy practice: An exploratory study. *Occupational Therapy in Health Care, 32*, 302–318. https://doi.org/10.3109/07380570903222583

Anastasi, A., & Urbina, S. (1997). *Psychological testing* (7th ed.). Upper Saddle River, NJ: Prentice Hall.

Baron, K., Kielhofner, G., Iyenger, A., Goldhammer, V., & Wolenski, V. (2006). *A user's manual for the Occupational Self Assessment (OSA; Version 2.2).* Chicago: Model of Human Occupation Clearinghouse.

Bowyer, P., Kramer, J., Ploszaj, A., Ross, M., Schwartz, O., Kielhofner, G., & Kramer, K. (2008). *A user's manual for the Short Child Occupational Profile (SCOPE).* Chicago: Model of Human Occupation Clearinghouse.

Brentnall, J., & Bundy, A. C. (2009). The concept of reliability in the context of observational assessments. *OTJR: Occupation, Participation and Health, 29,* 63–71. https://doi.org/10.3928/15394492-20090301-01

Brown, C. (2014). Ecological models in occupational therapy. In B. A. B. Schell, G. Gillen, & M. E. Scaffa (Eds.), *Willard and Spackman's occupational therapy* (12th ed., pp. 494–504). Philadelphia: Lippincott Williams & Wilkins.

Bruininks, R. H., & Bruininks, B. D. (2005). *BOT-2: Bruininks–Oseretsky test of motor proficiency (second edition) examiner's manual.* Circle Pines, MN: American Guidance Service.

Canadian Association of Occupational Therapists. (2002). *Enabling occupation: An occupational therapy perspective.* Ottawa: CAOT Publications.

Canadian Association of Occupational Therapists. (1997). *Enabling occupation: An occupational therapy perspective.* Ottawa: CAOT Publications.

Che Daud, A., Judd, J., Yau, M., & Barnett, F. (2016). Barriers of occupation-based intervention. *Asia Journal of Quality of Life, 1*(4), 1–10. https://doi.org/10.21834/ajqol.v1i4.12

Christiansen, C. H., Baum, C. M., & Bass, J. (2015). *Occupational therapy: Performance, participation, and well-being* (4th ed.). Thorofare, NJ: Slack.

Cook, J. (2001). Qualitative research in occupational therapy. In J. V. Cook (Ed.), *Qualitative research in occupational therapy: Strategies and experiences* (pp. 3–9). Albany, NY: Delmar.

Coster, W. J. (2008). Eleanor Clarke Slagle Lecture—Embracing ambiguity: Facing the challenge of measurement. *American Journal of Occupational Therapy, 62,* 743–752. https://doi.org/10.5014/ajot.62.6.743

Dawson, D. R., McEwen, S. E., & Polatajko, H. J. (Eds.). (2017). *Cognitive Orientation to daily Occupational Performance in occupational therapy: Using the CO–OP Approach™ to enable participation across the lifespan.* Bethesda, MD: AOTA Press.

Donnelly, C., & Carswell, A. (2002). Individualized outcome measures: A review of the literature. *Canadian Journal of Occupational Therapy, 69,* 84–94. https://doi.org/10.1177/000841740206900204

Dunn, W. (2017). Ecological Model of Occupation. In J. Hinojosa, P. Kramer, & C. B. Royeen (Eds.), *Perspectives on human occupation: Theories underlying practice* (pp. 207–236). Philadelphia: Lippincott Williams & Wilkins.

Gillen, G. (2013). Eleanor Clarke Slagle Lecture—A fork in the road: An occupational hazard. *American Journal of Occupational Therapy, 67,* 641–652. https://doi.org/10.5014/ajot.2013.676002

Grice, K. O. (2015). The use of occupation-based assessments and intervention in the hand therapy setting—A survey. *Journal of Hand Therapy, 28,* 300–308. https://doi.org/10.1016/j.jht.2015.01.005

Hinojosa, J. (2007). Becoming innovators in an era of hyperchange. *American Journal of Occupational Therapy, 61,* 629–637. https://doi.org/10.5014/ajot.61.6.629

Ilott, I. (2004). Challenges and strategic solutions for a research emergent profession. *American Journal of Occupational Therapy, 58,* 347–352. https://doi.org/10.5014/ajot.58.3.347

Kielhofner, G. (2008). *A Model of Human Occupation: Theory and application* (4th ed.). Baltimore: Lippincott Williams & Wilkins.

Kielhofner, G., Mallinson, T., Crawford, C., Nowak, M., Rigby, M., Henry, A., & Walens, D. (2004). *A user's manual for the Occupational Performance History Interview* (OPHI–II; version 2.1). Chicago: Model of Human Occupation Clearinghouse.

Kramer, J., Kielhofner, G., & Forsyth, K. (2008). Assessments used with the Model of Human Occupation. In B. J. Hemphill-Pearson (Ed.), *Assessments in occupational therapy mental health: An integrative approach* (2nd ed., pp. 159–184). Thorofare, NJ: Slack.

Law, M., Baptiste, S., Carswell, A., McColl, M. A., Polatajko, H., & Pollack, N. (1998). *Canadian Occupational Performance Measure* (3rd ed.). Ottawa: CAOT Publications.

Law, M., Baptiste, S., Carswell, A., McColl, M., Polatajko, H., & Pollock, N. (2019). *Canadian Occupational Performance Measure* (5th ed., rev.). Altona, MB: COPM, Inc.

Law, M., & Baum, C. (2005). Measurement in occupational therapy. In M. Law, C. Baum, & W. Dunn (Eds.), *Measuring occupational performance: Supporting best practice in occupational therapy* (2nd ed., pp. 3–20). Thorofare, NJ: Slack.

Law, M., Baum, C. M., & Dunn, W. (2005). Occupational performance assessment. In C. H. Christiansen & C. M. Baum (Eds.), *Occupational therapy performance: Participation and well being* (3rd ed., pp. 3–17). Thorofare, NJ: Slack.

Law, M., Cooper, B. A., Strong, S., Stewart, D., Rigby, P., & Letts, L. (1996). The Person–Environment–Occupation Model: A transactive approach to occupational performance. *Canadian Journal of Occupational Therapy, 63,* 9–22. https://doi.org/10.1177/000841749606300103

Maritz, R., Baptiste, S., Darzins, S. W., Magasi, S., Weleschuk, C., & Prodinger, B. (2018). Linking occupational therapy models and assessments to the ICF to enable standardizing documentation of functioning. *Canadian Journal of Occupational Therapy, 85,* 330–341. https://doi.org/10.1177/0008417418797146

Ottenbacher, K. J. (1986). *Evaluating clinical change: Strategies for occupational and physical therapists.* Baltimore: Williams & Wilkins.

Phipps, S., & Foley, K. (2019). Understanding client-centered practice. In K. Jacobs & G. McCormack (Eds.), *The occupational therapy manager* (6th ed., pp. 243–250). Bethesda, MD: AOTA Press.

Piernik-Yoder, B., & Beck, A. (2012). The use of standardized assessments in occupational therapy in the United States. *Occupational Therapy in Health Care, 26,* 97–108. https://doi.org/10.3109/07380577.2012.695103

Polatajko, H. J., & Mandich, A. (2004). *Enabling occupation in children: The Cognitive Orientation to daily Occupational Performance (CO–OP) approach.* Ottawa: CAOT Publications.

Polatajko, H. J., Mandich, A., & Martini, R. (2000). Dynamic performance analysis: A framework for understanding occupational performance. *American Journal of Occupational Therapy, 54,* 65–72. https://doi.org/10.5014/ajot.54.1.65

Polatajko, H., Townsend, E., & Craik, J. (2007). Canadian Model of Occupational Performance and Engagement (CMOP-E). In E. A. Townsend & H. J. Polatajko (Eds.), *Enabling occupation II: Advancing an occupational therapy vision of health, well-*

being, and justice through occupation (pp. 22–36). Ottawa: CAOT Publications.

Reynolds, M., Volkmer, K., Jewell, V., & Russell, M. (2019, June). Creative solutions to implementing occupation-centered practice in skilled nursing facilities. *OT Practice,* pp. CE1–CE9.

Romli, M. H., Yunus, F. W., & Mackenzie, L. (2019). Overview of reviews of standardized occupation-based instruments for use in occupational therapy practice. *Australian Journal of Occupational Therapy, 66,* 428–445. https://doi.org/10.1111/1440-1630.12572

Royeen, C. B., Stein, F., Murtha, A., & Stambaugh, J. (2017). Eudemonic care: A future path for occupational therapy? *Open Journal of Occupational Therapy, 5*(2). https://doi.org/10.15453/2168-6408.1301

Schell, B. A. B. (2014). Professional reasoning in practice. In B. A. B. Schell, G. Gillen, & M. E. Scaffa (Eds.), *Willard and Spackman's occupational therapy* (12th ed., pp. 384–397). Philadelphia: Lippincott Williams & Wilkins.

Schultz, S. (2014). Theory of occupational adaptation. In B. A. B. Schell, G. Gillen, & M. E. Scaffa (Eds.), *Willard and Spackman's occupational therapy* (12th ed., pp. 527–540). Philadelphia: Lippincott Williams & Wilkins.

Skard, G., & Bundy, A. (2008). Test of playfulness. In L. D. Parham & L. S. Fazio (Eds.), *Play in occupational therapy for children* (2nd ed., pp. 71–93). St. Louis: Mosby Elsevier.

Tomlin, G., & Borgetto, B. (2011). Research Pyramid: A new evidence-based practice model for occupational therapy. *American Journal of Occupational Therapy, 65,* 189–196. https://doi.org/10.5014/ajot.2011.000828

Wilkinson, G. W., Sager, A., Selig, S., Antonelli, R., Morton, S., Hirsch, G., & Lee, C.R. (2017). No equity, no triple aim: Strategic proposals to advance health equity in a volatile policy environment. *American Journal of Public Health, 107*(S3), S223–S228. https://doi.org/10.2105/AJPH.2017.304000

World Health Organization. (2001). *International Classification of Functioning, Disability and Health.* Geneva: Author.

Psychometric Properties Related to Standardized Assessments: Understanding the Evidence for Reliability, Validity, and Responsiveness

Namrata Grampurohit, PhD, OTR/L, and MJ Mulcahey, PhD, OTR/L, CLCP, FASIA

9

CHAPTER HIGHLIGHTS

- New terminology
- Defining the construct
- Levels of measurement
- Standardization of assessments
- Psychometric studies
- Understanding correlations and the correlation coefficient
- Psychometric properties: validity and responsiveness
- Finding literature on psychometric properties
- Validity as a unitary concept
- Theoretical foundations of psychometric analyses: Classical Test and Item Response Theories

KEY TERMS AND CONCEPTS

- Ceiling effect
- Classical Test Theory
- Coefficient α
- Computer adaptive test
- Concurrent validity
- Construct
- Construct-irrelevant variance
- Construct-related evidence
- Content validity
- Convergent validity
- Correlation
- Correlation coefficient
- Criterion-related evidence
- Cronbach's α
- Divergent validity
- Errors
- Face validity
- Factor analysis
- Factors
- Floor effect
- Internal consistency

- Interrater reliability
- Interval level
- Intraclass correlation
- Intrarater reliability
- Item characteristic curve
- Item Response Theory
- Known-groups validity
- Latent traits
- Level of measurement
- Minimal clinically important difference
- Minimal detectable change
- Nominal level
- Ordinal level
- Parallel forms
- Pearson product–moment correlation coefficient
- Predictive validity
- Psychometric properties
- Psychometric studies
- Psychometrics

- Rasch model
- Rater severity
- Ratio level
- Recalibration
- Reliability
- Reliability coefficient
- Responsiveness
- Score band of uncertainty
- Sensitivity
- Spearman's rank correlation coefficient
- Specificity
- Standard error of measurement
- Standardized assessments
- Test blueprint
- Test–retest reliability
- Theories of measurement
- Unidimensionality
- Unified view of validity
- Validity

INTRODUCTION

Clinical reasoning and decision making in occupational therapy are based on information or data gathered during an evaluation. This information must be appropriate for the decision to be made, and occupational therapists must know how to use it and what inferences can reasonably be drawn from it. Information gathered systematically using standardized assessments facilitates decision making because the properties that support their appropriate usage are rigorously examined through research methods.

Occupational therapy assessments allow the measurement of complex phenomena such as people's traits, abilities, knowledge, and skills, as well as the environments in which they live. These phenomena are not easily observed and are thus referred to as *latent traits*. Objective measurement of

https://doi.org/10.7139/2020.978-1-56900-596-5.009

constructs is done using a tool, instrument, or questionnaire that generates numerical data. The numerical data generated by a standardized tool can be used for comparisons, prediction, or screening only if the tool's properties have been systematically tested for accuracy and validity. The science of construction and validation of standardized behavioral instruments is known as *psychometrics.*

NEW TERMINOLOGY

The properties of the interpretation and use of scores are examined in the process of validation and are referred to as *psychometric properties* or *measurement properties.* The understanding of psychometric properties has advanced in recent years and is now recognized as a characteristic of score interpretation. Current literature on validity theory has clarified that tests themselves are not valid or invalid; only score inferences and interpretations are valid or invalid (Kane, 2013). For example, it is most appropriate to refer to an intraclass correlation coefficient (ICC) of .92 as the evidence for the test–retest reliability of scores on the Performance scale of the Canadian Occupational Performance Measure (COPM; Law et al., 2019) for adults with ankylosing spondylitis (Kjeken et al., 2005), and it would be inaccurate to refer to it as the test–retest reliability of the COPM. In other words, it is incorrect to refer to a test or measure as being valid or reliable. However, it is correct to state that the scores of a test are reliable and that they are a valid indicator of the construct the test measures. This chapter uses this updated terminology.

The terms *tests, instruments, tools, scales, measures,* and *assessments* are used interchangeably in the literature in the context of assessment tools used to measure a behavior, ability, or trait. The term *outcome measure* is used in reference to a measure that is used to track outcomes. This chapter specifically and this book more broadly also uses these terms interchangeably to refer to various types of assessment scales. The terms used to describe the psychometric properties of the two measurement theoretical systems—Classical Test Theory (CTT) and Item Response Theory (IRT)—are distinct. The traditional understanding of psychometric properties in the occupational therapy literature is based on the older CTT system. The newer terminology related to IRT methods requires readers to familiarize themselves with new concepts.

This chapter provides a broad overview of psychometric properties, described using classical methods, and it includes a brief description of concepts and terms used in IRT. The three types of psychometric properties—reliability, validity, and responsiveness—are discussed in detail.

WHAT IS THE CONSTRUCT?

The *construct* is the ability assessed by the test. Most standardized tests explicitly state the construct being measured in the test manual or in publications about the test. An understanding of the operational definition of the construct is essential for any examiner using an assessment. For example, the construct being assessed with the Executive Function Performance Test (EFPT; Baum et al., 2008) is higher-level cognitive function in everyday life. An examiner would not be able to use the EFPT as a test of memory. Although memory retention and recall are needed for the tasks, the test is not designed to allow interpretation solely for memory. Other tests, such as the Wechsler Memory Scale–Revised (Wechsler, 1987), may be closely aligned with the construct of memory and be better suited to assess that construct. If therapists do not find standardized assessments that match the constructs they need to measure, they can use systematic observation with a nonstandardized structured assessment and include a detailed record of administration and interpretation in their documentation. (See Chapter 8, "Nonstandardized Assessments.")

LEVELS OF MEASUREMENT

Measurements are not the same as the constructs they measure. For example, a score on a cognitive test is not the same thing as cognition. Hence, if therapists want to draw conclusions based on their measurements, they must understand the relationship between the construct and the measurement. The way in which numbers are assigned to measure a behavior or trait is called the *scale of measurement* or *level of measurement.*

There are four levels of measurement (Figure 9.1):
1. ***Nominal level.*** The nominal level of measurement consists of names or labels used to identify categories, for example, yes-or-no responses to questions or right or left handedness. The categories are mutually exclusive and can be counted for frequency or proportion types of mathematical operation.
2. ***Ordinal level.*** Ordinal-level measurement consists of rank-ordered categories based on a defined characteristic and with a greater than–less than relationship. Many rehabilitation measures belong to this category, for example, Likert-type scales that use such anchors as *strongly disagree, disagree, agree,* and *strongly agree.* Another example is the scale used in manual muscle testing: 5, 4, 3, 2, 1, and 0. The interval between the numbers assigned to the scale are ordered from greater to lesser strength. However, the difference between 3 and 2 is not always

FIGURE 9.1. Levels of measurement.

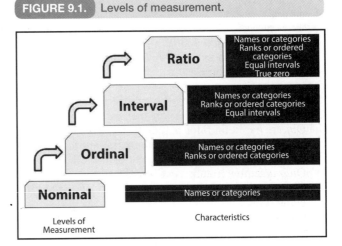

Source. N. Grampurohit. Used with permission.

the same for each person and it is not the same as the distance between 5 and 4. Moreover, one person with a strength of 5 may not necessarily be the same as another person with a strength of 5. Frequencies or proportions are the preferred type of mathematical operations used with ordinal-level measurement.

3. *Interval level.* The hallmark of interval-level measurement is that the distance between the units is equal. A body temperature scale is an example of interval-level measurement in which the unit used is degrees Celsius or degrees Fahrenheit and the distance between 100° and 101° Fahrenheit is the same as that between 98° and 99° Fahrenheit. Moreover, beyond frequencies, mathematical operations such as multiplication can be performed. For example, a mathematical formula can be applied to convert body temperature in Fahrenheit to body temperature in Celsius. Another example of an interval-level scale is a grip dynamometer reading, which can be converted from pounds to kilograms and vice versa.

4. *Ratio level.* The ratio level of measurement includes a true or absolute zero point that represents the absence of the characteristic being measured. Common examples are height, weight, or range of motion. All mathematical and statistical calculations can be performed with ratio-level measurement, which is highly desirable.

It is also important to note the hierarchy of the levels. The most superior among them is ratio-level measurement, which builds on and includes all three preceding levels of measurement: category names, ordered categories, and equal intervals, with the addition of a true zero.

Occupational therapists may choose to measure the same construct at different levels. For example, manual muscle strength can be graded at a nominal level as present or absent, at an ordinal level as 0–5 manual muscle strength grading, at an interval level as dynamometer reading in kilograms or pounds, and at a ratio level as counts of the number of fibers in the muscle. When comparing CTT and IRT, the levels of measurement are superior in IRT-based measures; IRT-based measures use an interval-level scale, which allows for statistical analysis of the data they provide.

ASSESSMENT STANDARDIZATION

Standardized assessments have published guidelines that outline the standard procedures for their administration and scoring. The scores generated through standard administration can support the reasons why an occupational therapist chooses to use the assessment for a client because the assessment properties for that particular use may have been studied and demonstrated. A standardized assessment provides:

- *Objectivity:* Definitions of the setup, test items, and scoring of responses can reduce the examiner's bias and personal influence.
- *Quantification:* Total scores and subscale scores generate numerical data that can quantify the skill or behavior being tested.
- *Communication:* Interprofessional communication among team members and documentation for payers are enhanced with the use of standardized tests.
- *Data analysis:* Standardized tests make available for analysis person-level or group-level data that can be used in program evaluation, outcome studies, and secondary data analysis.

A standardized assessment is an instrument that has undergone rigorous psychometric analysis to examine its intended purpose and use. Results of psychometric studies are made available to examiners, and a review of an assessment's psychometric properties tells them how accurate the test scores are with repeated administrations (i.e., evidence of test–retest reliability) and between different therapists treating the patient (i.e., evidence of interrater reliability) and whether the test measures what it was intended to measure (i.e., evidence of validity). Administration and scoring guidelines for standardized assessments are included in their manuals and in other publications, along with normative data, if applicable. Suggested interpretations, use, and limitations are also provided.

PSYCHOMETRIC STUDIES

Research studies designed to examine an assessment's measurement properties are referred to as *psychometric studies* or *methodological studies.* The design of psychometric studies can vary, and their methodological quality can be evaluated using critical appraisal tools. Critical appraisal tools help test administrators to systematically evaluate a psychometric study for qualities that are hallmarks of rigorously conducted research. One example of a standard critical appraisal tool that can be used with psychometric studies is the Consensus-based Standards for the Selection of Health Measurement Instruments (COSMIN; Mokkink et al., 2010).

A high-quality psychometric study has the following characteristics, based on the COSMIN criteria:

- An adequate sample size for the study supported by sample size calculations
- A description of missing data for items and how missing data were handled in the analyses
- Subscale analysis presented separately if a scale has more than two domains or dimensions, each with its own subscale score
- No design flaws—for example, a lack of reporting on the stability of the function being measured between two administrations (test and retest) when examining test–retest reliability
- Appropriate reporting by the authors of statistical information relevant to the measurement property such as reporting measures of variance and confidence intervals
- Hypotheses formulated before data collection—for example, in an examination of convergent validity, the magnitude and direction of correlation between two measures is hypothesized before data collection and the results then confirm or refute the hypothesis
- Consideration of language and cultural adaptations.

UNDERSTANDING CORRELATIONS AND THE CORRELATION COEFFICIENT

Correlation is frequently used in reliability and validity statistics. *Correlation* is the degree of association of two random variables. A brief introduction is provided here to enable the reader to understand the remainder of this chapter. Readers are referred to textbooks on research methodology for an extensive explanation of this topic (Howell, 2014; Portney & Watkins, 2009).

Correlation indicates only the relationship between measures, not causality. A variable external to the two variables may be the cause of the relationship. For example, the self-reported negative impact of stroke as measured by the Stroke Impact Scale and self-reported hand function impairment as measured by the *ABILHAND* have a moderate positive correlation (Wang et al., 2011). This correlation does not mean that reduced stroke impact causes reduced hand function, nor does it mean that reduced hand function causes reduced stroke impact. Moreover, depression can affect both variables as an external factor (Penta et al., 2001), as well as the outcome.

The *correlation coefficient,* or *r,* is a test statistic that indicates the degree of relationship between two measures. Correlation coefficients can range from −1.00 to 1.00. A correlation of 0, the midpoint of the continuum between the two extremes, indicates no relationship between the two variables. As one moves toward the ends of the continuum, the magnitude or strength of correlation increases. In other words, the relationship between the two variables becomes stronger as the correlation coefficient approaches either −1.00 or 1.00. A positive correlation is an association between two variables going in the same direction. As one increases, the other also increases. Positive correlations are coefficients ranging from greater than 0 to 1.00. A negative correlation is an inverse association between two variables. As one variable increases, the other decreases. Negative correlations are coefficients ranging from less than 0 to −1.00.

Positive and negative represent only the direction of the relationship; they have nothing to do with the strength of the relationship. For example, in Figure 9.2A, the positive correlation indicates only the direction of the relationship between pain scores and anxiety scores. Higher pain scores are correlated with higher anxiety scores and vice versa. To understand the relationship, it is also important to know what higher scores mean for the given measure. In this example, higher scores on the anxiety scale indicate more anxiety. In Figure 9.2B, the negative correlation indicates an inverse relationship between pain scores and quality-of-life scores.

The numerical value of the correlation coefficient indicates the strength of the relationship. The higher the value, the greater the strength of the relationship. For example, when interpreting the strength of the relationship in Figure 9.2B, the absolute value .90 is considered without the negative sign. In a good-quality psychometric study, the correlational hypotheses are set before the start of the study, or a priori, to allow meaningful interpretation. When r is squared, r^2 explains to what extent the variance of one variable explains the variance of the second variable. For example, in Figure 9.2B, r^2 is .81, meaning that anxiety explains 81% of the variance in pain. The remaining 19% variance in pain remains unexplained.

p Values and the Correlation Coefficient

The probability level, or *p,* measures the significance of a relationship. The significance of a relationship should not be confused with the strength of the relationship (discussed in the previous section). Significance testing tells one how likely or unlikely for measures to be correlated, given the null hypothesis that there is no relationship in the population. The smaller the obtained *p* value, the more significant the relationship (in contrast to the strength of the relationship, in which a larger correlation coefficient indicates a stronger relationship). Typically, the *p* value is set before the study, or a priori, for the purpose of hypothesis testing.

It is important to note that the strength of a relationship can be strong and but not significant (Taylor, 1990). Conversely, a relationship can be weak but significant. For small samples, it is easier to produce a strong correlation coefficient by chance; hence, one needs to pay attention to the *p* value to appropriately interpret the correlation. However, for large samples, it is easier to produce statistical significance, and one needs to pay attention to the strength of the correlation coefficient to appropriately interpret it. A strong and significant relationship is desirable, as is the case with the two examples shown in Figure 9.2 ($p < .001$).

Interpreting correlation coefficients varies with the type of correlational statistic and the context of measurement. It is not an all-or-none condition. For example, diagnostic or decision-making assessments may require a higher strength of correlation with the findings, and a descriptive assessment may consider a lower strength of correlation to be acceptable for its measurement purposes.

There are many types of correlation coefficients, each with its own mathematical formula (Mukaka, 2012). Only the three types of correlation coefficient most commonly reported in psychometric studies are described here.

1. *Pearson product–moment correlation coefficient.* This is a common parametric correlation statistic, reported as *r.* Its use is appropriate when both variables are normally distributed. The accepted standard for interpretation (Crist, 2014) is as follows:
   - .90–.99: high and preferred but not frequently observed
   - .80–.89: satisfactory or adequate
   - .70–.79: weak or minimally acceptable
   - Less than .70: caution—inadequate or unacceptable.
2. *Spearman's rank correlation coefficient.* This nonparametric statistic is reported as ρ. Its use is appropriate when one or both variables are skewed or ordinal and robust when extreme values are present. Interpretation is the same as for Pearson's *r.*
3. *Intraclass correlation.* This type of correlation is frequently used and is preferred for test–retest, interrater, or intrarater reliability because it reflects both correlation and agreement. It is described as ICC(2,1). The numbers in parentheses represent the type of statistical model used. In ICC(2,1), Model 2 is used, where the raters are representative of other similar raters. ICC(3,1) is recommended for intrarater reliability when no generalization is intended. Note that ICCs give a slightly lower numerical value than Pearson's *r* or Spearman's ρ. The accepted standard for interpretation (Andresen, 2000) is as follows:
   - .75 or higher: strong and preferred
   - .40 to less than .75: moderate or adequate
   - Less than .40: weak or inadequate or unacceptable.

FIGURE 9.2. Examples of Pearson product–moment correlations: (A) Pearson's $r = 0.91$ and (B) Pearson's $r = -.90$. The positive correlation in A indicates that as pain increases, anxiety increases. The strength of this relationship is .91, indicating strong correlation between pain and anxiety. The negative correlation in B indicates that as pain increases, quality of life decreases. The strength of this relationship is .90, indicating strong correlation between pain and quality of life.

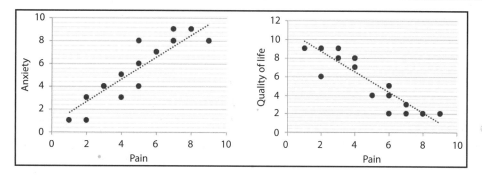

Source. N. Grampurohit. Used with permission.

TABLE 9.1. Basic Statistical Terms Used in Measurement

TERM	DESCRIPTION
Correlation	Degree of relationship between two sets of scores; implies association but not causality
Correlation coefficient	Statistical indicator that quantifies the degree of relationship
Psychometrics	Science of measuring; test statistics provide evidence of the measurement quality
Reliability	Degree of precision of a score
Test score	Score obtained on an instrument
Test statistic	Reported statistical numerical value from an analysis that represents results
Validity	Degree to which an instrument measures the construct it is designed to measure
Responsiveness	Ability of the scores on an instrument to detect change as a result of an intervention

The statistical terms used in measurement are described in Table 9.1.

PSYCHOMETRIC PROPERTIES

Understanding psychometric properties is essential for appropriate selection and use of standardized assessments. The conceptualization of measurement properties has evolved over the decades. The traditional view of properties as separate entities such as construct validity, concurrent validity, or content validity has changed to a unified view of validity (Messick, 1989). The *unified view of validity* integrates content, criteria, and consequences under the umbrella of construct validity and considers reliability, validity, and responsiveness under the umbrella of construct validity evidence. We have divided our discussion of psychometric properties into (1) reliability, (2) validity, and (3) responsiveness, the three most important properties that occupational therapists must understand. Although this classification is used for ease of understanding, readers must consider reliability and responsiveness not as distinct from validity but as integrated into the unified view

of validity. The unified view of validity considers reliability and responsiveness as aspects within the umbrella of validity according to the most current understanding of psychometric properties. The first prerequisite for an assessment is reliability or error-free measurement. Without reliability, one cannot have confidence in the scores and therefore cannot draw conclusions that are based on the scores. The second prerequisite is validity or appropriateness, meaningfulness, and usefulness of conclusions based on the scores. The third prerequisite, which applies to assessments that are used as outcome measures, is responsiveness, or the ability to detect change.

Measurement Reliability

Reliability is the precision or accuracy of the measurement procedures. There are two main ways to express reliability: (1) standard error of measurement and (2) reliability coefficients. The *standard error of measurement* indicates the variability in measurement. The *reliability coefficient* indicates the consistency and reproducibility of the scores. Both ways of expressing reliability are mathematically related;

an increase in the reliability coefficient corresponds to a decrease in the standard error of measurement. Evidence of reliability is a necessary precondition for examination of validity. As noted earlier, reliability and validity in the traditional literature are now viewed as contributors to the unified concept of construct validity. To support the claims about clients' abilities that occupational therapists make on the basis of the client's performance on assessment tools, therapists are encouraged to detail the reliability of a measure in their documentation.

Standard error of measurement

Standard error of measurement (*SEM*) is a measure of score instability. Statistically, it is the standard deviation of the distribution of errors in measurement (Thorndike & Thorndike-Christ, 2010). On repeated assessment of the same person under the same conditions, any variations in score are considered *errors.* When calculating *SEM,* the distribution of errors around the true score is examined for its standard deviation. The value of *SEM* is in the units of the assessment; it answers the question, "How closely does the assessment score approximate the true score of a test taker?" (Kubiszyn & Borich, 2013).

The *SEM* derived through a psychometric study should be available in the published literature or test manual. Occupational therapists can use the *SEM* to determine the accuracy of an individual score. The *SEM* enables therapists to have confidence a client's score as a measure of the client's real performance or ability rather than random error.

For example, the *SEM* for the Mini-Mental State Examination (MMSE; Folstein et al., 2020) is 2.4 points for older adults age 65 years without dementia (Jacqmin-Gadda et al., 1997). Occupational therapists using the MMSE would take the *SEM* of 2.4 into account when interpreting the score obtained by a person without dementia. For a 65-year-old person, an MMSE score of 23 out of 30 would fall in the range of mild cognitive impairment, but the therapist would exercise caution and consider the test taker's true score to fall in the range of 20.6 to 25.4 (total score of 23 ± *SEM* of 2.4). This range is referred to as the *score band of uncertainty.* Therapists' interpretation of MMSE scores would also depend on how these scores are used. For example, if the scores were used for high-stakes decision making such as employment or discharge from the hospital, therapists would prefer to have a high level of confidence in them.

Test–retest reliability

Test–retest reliability is a measure of the stability of scores on an assessment. It is calculated by having the same examiner administer the assessment to the same person under the same conditions on two occasions. If the scores on a test are stable or highly reliable, readministration of the test under the same conditions should yield the same or similar scores. The time between repeated measurements is an important consideration when retesting; it should not be so short that test takers remember their responses or are fatigued by repeated testing or so long that other factors such as time of day, natural recovery, development, or effect of medicines influence test scores.

Occupational therapists often note test–retest reliability when using tests to measure outcomes of their intervention because they want to be certain that the test scores are stable enough to pick up the effect of the intervention and are not easily influenced by external factors. In a test with stable scores, reliability coefficients across repeated administrations will be high. ICC is the commonly reported coefficient for test–retest reliability.

Parallel forms or equivalence

In situations when memory and practice on a test can influence a client's performance, such as on tests of cognition, parallel forms of a test are designed for repeated measurement. With *parallel forms,* item wording, presentation, or order is changed across the two forms of the test, but item difficulty is maintained. When using tests with parallel forms, equivalence between the two forms is important to examine. Occupational therapists should look at the reliability of the scores on parallel forms to ascertain whether it is adequate, particularly if the test is to be used as an outcome measure to determine intervention effectiveness.

For example, the Montreal Cognitive Assessment (MoCA; Nasreddine et al., 2005) uses parallel forms of the test for screening for cognition. When using the MoCA as an outcome measure (Costa et al., 2014), therapists need to know that the evidence for parallel forms validity is strong, as indicated by the reliability coefficient of .83 between the original MoCA and Alternate Version 2 and of .92 between the original MoCA and Alternate Version 3 (Costa et al., 2012) for mild cognitive impairment.

Intrarater reliability

The stability of scores on a test for the same rater across repeated measurements is referred to as *intrarater reliability.* All the criteria related to test–retest reliability apply in this case; in addition, the same rater is involved in test administration. It is greatly influenced by training, competency in using the assessments, use of standardized procedures, and clarity in scoring.

Occupational therapists need to recalibrate for frequently and infrequently used assessments because their skills vary over time. *Recalibration* includes, but is not limited to, studying standard procedures of administration and scoring, review and feedback on the fidelity of administration, and statistical recalibration of computer-generated scores for rater severity. *Rater severity* is the variability in administration and scoring that can make a rater score a client too easily or too harshly. Newer measurement methods use statistical techniques to account for rater severity in the calculation of the final score.

Interrater reliability

The stability of scores across different raters is referred to as *interrater reliability.* Training and adherence to published standards for a standardized assessment should produce similar scores across different raters. However, this is not always the case. Any type of performance, ability, or behavior testing involves variation in rater styles. Thus, therapists need information on the interrater reliability of tests. This information is particularly relevant in settings in which different practitioners are seeing the same client, such as the acute care setting or clinical settings in which occupational therapists complete the initial assessment but occupational therapy assistants complete follow-up assessments. In these instances, an assessment with greater interrater reliability would be preferred.

Internal consistency

Internal consistency is a type of reliability that provides information about a measure's internal structure. It is the degree of agreement between items in a measure that measure a single or unidimensional construct. In determining internal consistency, the person is tested only once, as opposed to twice or more, as with test–retest or interrater reliability, which are the preferred reliability measures. The statistical procedures used to derive internal consistency include the split-half reliability method and the interitem reliability method.

The split-half reliability method involves splitting the test into halves, each of which consists of equivalent items. The correlation between the two equivalent halves is computed as the split-half reliability coefficient. However, this method has been critiqued because of the arbitrary nature of splitting items and variability of the coefficients on the basis of the type of split.

The interitem reliability method involves computing the correlation between items on a test that measure the same construct. The Kuder–Richardson formula is used to compute item-to-total-score correlations for tests when the responses are dichotomous (e.g., yes–no); the correlations are reported as Kuder–Richardson Formula 20 (*KR20*) or Kuder–Richardson Formula 21 (*KR21*). *KR20* ranges from 0 to 1 and is interpreted similarly to coefficient α. **Coefficient α** is a statistic commonly used when response scales are polytomous (e.g., Likert-type scales such as *strongly agree, agree, disagree,* and *strongly disagree*). It is interpreted as follows:

- *.80 or higher:* strong and preferred
- *Less than .80 and greater than .70:* moderate and acceptable
- *Less than .70:* weak.

Coefficient alpha is highly sensitive to the number of items and sample size. The more items a test has, the greater the value of coefficient α. A very high value of coefficient α, such as .98 or .99, can suggest that test items are too closely related and indicates redundancy among them. Redundancy is not a desired quality in a test; each part of the test must measure a different aspect of the same construct or ability.

Caution about coefficient α. The use of coefficient α as the only psychometric property supporting the use of a test is strongly discouraged. Therapists must use caution and consider other indicators of reliability (e.g., test–retest or interrater reliability) to support the claims made in their documentation regarding a test's reliability. Readers are referred to Sijtsma's (2009) critique of coefficient α for a detailed explanation of its lack of usefulness in psychometrics. We discourage its overemphasis, and our sole purpose for including it in this chapter is to enable therapists

to understand articles and summaries in which this property is reported and to exercise caution in its interpretation.

Unidimensionality. Internal consistency assumes that only one construct is being measured. However, measures used in occupational therapy frequently measure more than one construct or are multidimensional. These constructs are referred to as *dimensions* within a measure. A measure is said to be unidimensional when all the items on a test measure a single construct; **unidimensionality** is also a property of a test's internal structure. Unidimensionality is commonly derived by factor analysis using CTT methodology, which is described later in this chapter. Information about unidimensionality can be very helpful to therapists in explaining the phenomenon being assessed. For example, with factor analysis, two dimensions can be observed for an upper extremity (UE) test—gross and fine movement functions. This will come as no surprise to clinicians who work with people with UE impairment. However, the evidence from the literature that this test captures these two dimensions can be helpful in documenting the client's performance.

Measurement Validity

Validity of test scores provides support that the assessment measures the construct of ability, behavior, or trait that it claims to measure. Valid test scores add credibility to assessment-based decisions.

Reliability is a necessary property but not sufficient as evidence of a measure's usefulness. To be useful, a test's scores need to be accurate, as measured by reliability indicators, and aligned with underlying theory and evidence as measured by validity indicators. Validity indicators can be in the form of a relationship to other similar constructs (convergent evidence), no relationship to dissimilar constructs (divergent evidence), adequate item content to cover the entire construct (content-related evidence), ability to differentiate between different levels of the trait (known-groups discrimination), being able to predict another trait (prediction-related evidence), and other variables or traits not influencing the test. Occupational therapists commonly use certain categories of validity evidence, outlined in Table 9.2.

Face- and content-related evidence of validity

The acceptability of a test to occupational therapists and clients may depend on what the test "looks like," also known as **face validity**. The appearance of reasonable test items, wording, and concepts can be important to the engagement of clients and therapists in the assessment process. Face validity cannot be empirically tested; however, qualitative information about the measure gained from stakeholders in the test development phase should be reported in the literature.

Content validity is the extent to which test items represent the construct being tested. It goes beyond face validity to examine the degree to which the underlying theory or mechanism explains and the test items truly assess the breadth of the construct. Content validity appears simple to establish, but it requires extensive thought regarding

TABLE 9.2.   Types of Validity, Reliability, and Responsiveness Evidence

TYPE	DESCRIPTION
Reliability	
Standard error of measurement	Amount of inconsistency or unreliability in the scores obtained on an instrument
Test–retest reliability	Measure of a test score's stability when using the same version of an instrument over 2 testing occasions under the same conditions
Parallel forms, or equivalence	Stability between scores obtained on two versions of the same instrument
Intrarater reliability	Stability of scores on an instrument when using the same rater across repeated measurements
Interrater reliability	Stability of scores on an instrument when using different raters
Internal consistency	Degree of agreement between items in a measure that measure a single or unidimensional construct
Validity	
Face- and content-related evidence	*Face-related evidence:* the appearance of test items in relationship to the purpose of the test *Content-related evidence:* the extent to which the test items represent the construct being measured
Criterion-related evidence of validity	Relationship of the scores on an instrument to an external criterion
Concurrent validity	Correlation of the scores on a measure with those on an existing measure, typically the gold standard used to measure the construct
Predictive validity	Ability of scores on the measure to predict future abilities or outcomes
Construct-related evidence of validity	Relationship between the underlying theory of the construct and the scores on an instrument
Convergent validity	Correlation of scores on an instrument with certain other measures that may be similar to the construct or closely associated with the construct
Divergent validity	Scores on the instrument diverge from those of other measures with a different construct and demonstrate a low correlation
Known-groups validity	Ability of a measure to differentiate between distinct groups of people such as those with and without the condition or with high and low levels of the trait
Factors	Different aspects of a construct that are distinct enough to be identified through factor analysis methods; a single measure may have many
Responsiveness	
Minimal detectable change	Change in scores beyond the measurement error of the instrument
Minimal clinically important difference	Change in scores that results in substantial gains in the person that are meaningful
Floor and ceiling effects	*Floor effect:* when the scores on a measure are not able to detect a change at the lower level of ability *Ceiling effect:* observed when the scores are not able to detect a change in the higher ability level
Sensitivity and specificity	*Sensitivity:* ability of test scores to correctly detect a condition or impairment with high accuracy *Specificity:* ability of the test scores to correctly reject those people who do not have the condition or impairment

the definition of the construct and the theoretical basis for design of the test items.

For example, the Nine-Hole Peg Test (Oxford Grice et al., 2003) is commonly used and recommended as part of the NIH Toolbox® in testing the UE function of clients with stroke. Although occupational therapists are quite familiar with this test because of its quick administration, its face and content validity have not been systematically reported in the literature. The test's origin as a work-related assessment used to determine war veterans' job-related skills further demonstrates its lack of face and content validity for people with neurological conditions. Although therapists' familiarity with the test causes them to overlook evidence for face and content validity, clients who are not familiar

with the test can question the reasonableness of its use to determine UE functional level.

Considering what therapists know about neurological conditions and their underlying anatomy and physiology, the construct of the Nine Hole Peg Test does not align with the concepts of motor control, spasticity, coordination or midline orientation that form the basis of assessing most neurological conditions. Therapists will note that the construct of the Nine-Hole Peg Test is purely related to dexterity, including speed in handling pegs. The lack of alignment of the Nine Hole Peg Test with neurological impairments is further clarified by examining the scoring of the Nine-Hole Peg test: Using a stopwatch, therapists calculate the time taken to place small pegs. Performance of this task is only one small aspect of UE function within the larger construct that can include reaching for objects, manipulating large and small objects, turning, or unimanual versus bimanual tasks. Therapists need to carefully consider a measure's face and content validity before making assessment-based decisions for clients.

To analyze content validity, test developers frequently use a test blueprint. A *test blueprint* is a table of specifications for the test that lays out the content to be covered in testing the construct; items covering that content are intentionally developed with a team of stakeholders. The blueprint provides a detailed breakdown of the percentage of items from each subcategory that should be included in the final draft of the assessment. Theory, evidence, experience, or the desired goal of the test supports the distribution of items.

For example, the National Board for Certification in Occupational Therapy (NBCOT®) examination is derived from a test blueprint that allocates the number of items to be included on the exam. The blueprint lays out the percentage of time stakeholders reported spending in activities such as evaluation and intervention in a national study of entry-level practice. Therefore, the assessment's content validity is established by confirming whether it reflects current practice. NBCOT continues to investigate practice trends and update the test blueprint with the current standards. Content validity is reported using quantitative methods such as the content validity ratio and content validity index. The higher the statistic and the closer it is to 1, the better the content validity. However, a qualitative study of content validity with agreement among stakeholders that the items are essential and represent the construct can provide sufficient content-related evidence.

Criterion-related evidence of validity

The correlation of scores on a measure with those on a well-established external measure is referred to as *criterion-related evidence.* There are two types of criterion-related evidence, concurrent and predictive, that are determined by when in the study design the measurement of the external criterion occurs.

Concurrent validity. **Concurrent validity** refers to congruency, or the correlation of scores on the measure with those on an existing measure, typically known as the gold standard. However, determining the gold standard in occupational therapy has been challenging because the profession is relatively new and literature establishing standardization of measures is limited. The concurrent validity of scores on a measure is determined to be adequate when the correlation between the measure and another standard or legacy measure used in practice is high.

- *Greater than .6:* excellent
- *.31–.59:* adequate
- *Less than .30:* poor or inadequate.

Predictive validity. **Predictive validity** refers to the ability of scores on a measure to predict future abilities or outcomes. Occupational therapists are frequently interested in tests that help with decision making to predict some future outcome. The correlation between the scores on a measure

at one point in time and scores on another criterion variable in the future indicate predictive validity. Predictive validity correlation coefficients are interpreted similarly to concurrent validity criteria. Statistical tests such as regression are also used to establish predictive validity. When receiver operating curve analysis is used to find the area under the curve (AUC) to establish predictive validity, the statistic is interpreted as follows:

- *AUC .9 or greater:* excellent
- *AUC .7–.89:* adequate
- *AUC less than .7:* poor.

Construct-related evidence of validity

Construct-related evidence refers to how well a measure conforms to the construct. The relationship between the underlying theory of the construct and scores on the measure establishes evidence. For example, a handwriting test has items that assess quality and speed of handwriting and is based on the theory that speed and quality of writing can change after occupational therapy intervention. The construct-related evidence for this theory can then include an examination of the pre–post change in test scores after occupational therapy intervention. However, if the theory states that handwriting development is related to a child's grasp and the test measures grasp patterns, then construct-related evidence could include an examination of change in grasp patterns by age and the test's ability to distinguish children of different ages on the basis of grasp pattern.

Construct-irrelevant variance is the variability in scores brought about by factors that are not related to the construct but that can directly influence the construct during measurement. For example, when using a patient-report outcome measure, the client's cognition, literacy, and cultural background can introduce construct-irrelevant variance.

The unified theory of validity considers that all psychometric properties inform construct validity and should be considered as all encompassing. Readers are encouraged to take a broad approach to viewing construct validity in the light of current literature. In this chapter, for the purpose of understanding the concepts, we present convergent, divergent, and known-groups validity as types of construct validity, reflecting the traditional way of conceptualizing construct validity.

Convergent validity. **Convergent validity** occurs when the construct represented by the score on a measure correlates highly with scores on certain other measures that may be based on a similar construct or one closely associated with it. Unlike concurrent validity, comparisons are not made with a gold-standard measure. The interpretation of the validity coefficient for convergent validity is similar to that for predictive validity. A very high correlation between two similar tests of a construct can mean that administration of both tests is not needed because they measure the same thing.

Divergent validity. Alternatively, **divergent validity** occurs when scores on a measure show low correlation with other measures of dissimilar constructs. For example, the scores on a measure of shoulder function will show low correlation with those on a measure of walking, an unrelated construct.

Known-groups validity. **Known-groups validity** reflects a measure's ability to differentiate between distinct groups. Known-groups validity is also referred to as *discriminant validity*. A test that can discriminate among known groups can be thought of as measuring the construct in a valid manner. For example, a test of balance should be able to differentiate between people with and without balance deficits. The known-groups hypotheses are set up before data collection for the measurement study, and statistical tests of significance are applied during analysis.

Factor analysis. **Factors** are the different constructs measured by a single measure. For complex behaviors, a test may consist of items measuring different aspects of the construct that are distinct enough to be identified by factor analysis. **Factor analysis** is a statistical procedure used to determine the extent to which shared variance exists between items. Items with shared variance load together as one factor and each factor loads separately on a test. For example, the Geriatric Depression Scale (Yesavage et al., 1983) has a five-factor structure: Anxiety, Dysphoric Mood, Cognition, Hopelessness, and Withdrawal–Apathy–Vigor (Adams et al., 2004). Factor analysis can be done to explore the number of underlying factors or to confirm the predicted factors.

Measurement Responsiveness

Responsiveness is the ability of the scores on a measure to indicate change as a result of an intervention. Responsiveness is a critical characteristic of an outcome measure. Occupational therapists are primarily interested in selecting outcome measures that are sensitive to change. They are also interested in quantifying the magnitude of change to document progress for the client, organization, or payers. Thus, measures need to not only detect change but also indicate the amount of change produced by an intervention. Therapists need to carefully select assessments to be used as outcome measures.

Minimal detectable change

Minimal detectable change is the change in scores beyond measurement error that a test can detect. For example, for the Stroke Impact Scale's (Duncan et al., 1999) ADL/IADL subscale, the standard error of measurement is 6.3 (Lin et al., 2010); thus, a change score of 6.3 or less from admission to discharge for a client with stroke would not qualify as a change because it is within the bounds of the test's measurement error. Lin et al. (2010) determined minimal detectable change for the Stroke Impact Scale by calculating the real change for individual patients with 95% confidence. A minimal detectable change score of 17.3 or greater from admission to discharge would qualify as change because the minimal detectable change for this instrument is estimated to be 17.3 (Lin et al., 2010).

Minimal clinically important difference

Minimal clinically important difference (MCID) is the change in scores beyond measurement error, and typically beyond minimal detectable change, that results in substantial gains by the person that are meaningful to the person or family. For example, the MCID for the Stroke Impact Scale's Hand Function subscale is 17.8 points for people with chronic stroke (Lin et al., 2010). A score of 17.8 or greater is considered a clinically meaningful change for the client and would be a desirable outcome after occupational therapy intervention.

Floor and ceiling effects

Floor and ceiling effects refer to the lack of detection of change at the lower and upper ranges of the construct, respectively. A **floor effect** is observed when the scores on a measure are not able to detect between changes at the lower level of the ability or trait being tested. This effect may be due to a lack of items representing the lower ability level. Conversely, a **ceiling effect** is observed when the scores are not able to differentiate between changes at the higher ability level.

In the interpretation of floor and ceiling effects, a conservative estimate of 15% and a liberal estimate of 20% are considered acceptable (Andresen, 2000). For example, for the Stroke Impact Scale's Hand Function subscale, Duncan et al. (1999) reported floor effects in 40% of those with moderate stroke and in 2% of those with mild stroke. The same study reported the reverse trend: ceiling effects in 15% of those with mild stroke and 5% of those with moderate stroke. Thus, one can interpret the floor effects for moderate stroke as unacceptable for this scale, and the scale should be used with caution for those with moderate stroke.

Sensitivity and specificity

Sensitivity is the ability of the test scores to correctly identify people with a condition or impairment with high accuracy. **Specificity,** however, is the ability of the test scores to correctly identify those people who do not have the condition or impairment. Sensitivity and specificity criteria apply to tests that screen for or detect conditions or impairments. For example, the MMSE is used to detect cognitive impairment; for community-dwelling individuals, its sensitivity is reported to be 85% and its specificity is reported to be 86% (Mitchell, 2009). Readers are referred to a detailed discussion of sensitivity and specificity by Classen and Velozo (2018).

FINDING LITERATURE ON PSYCHOMETRIC PROPERTIES

Although the original research literature is the best source of evidence for therapists, more efficient sources of information are available. These sources include systematic reviews on outcome measures, databases such as the Rehabilitation Measures Database (https://www.sralab.org/rehabilitation-measures), recommendations by national organizations such as the American Occupational Therapy Association, and the National Institutes of Health Common Data Elements Repository. Chapter 3, "Assessment Identification and Selection," provides a list of such databases and recommendations to aid therapists in the selection of measures. Other types of psychometric properties not discussed in this chapter can be found in other sources such as Classen and Velozo (2018).

VALIDITY AS A UNITARY CONCEPT

All validity is construct validity, a "unitary" concept, according to modern validity theory (Messick, 1994). Instead of viewing content, criterion, and construct as distinct types of validity, they are considered to be sources of evidence that inform the unitary construct validity (Figure 9.3). Five sources or types of construct validity evidence are recommended for reporting in occupational therapy (Brown, 2010):

1. *Test items cover adequate content to measure the construct being examined.* This type of validity aligns with content validity in the older system.
2. *Responses of test takers fit the construct to be examined.* The type of validity aligns with construct validity in the older system.
3. *Internal structure reflects relationships between test items that match the construct being examined.* This type of validity aligns with construct validity in the older system.
4. *Relationships to other variables or tests are as the examiner expects.* This type of validity aligns with concurrent and predictive validity in the older system.
5. *Consequences of testing occur as expected, and unanticipated outcomes are reported.* The previous conceptualizations of validity lacked this new area of focus.

THEORETICAL FOUNDATIONS OF PSYCHOMETRIC ANALYSES

Psychometric analyses are based on theories that dictate their conceptual foundations, assumptions, and principles. These theories are referred to as *theories of measurement*.

Occupational therapists reading the published literature on psychometrics need to understand the different ways in which articles report psychometric properties. Knowledge of the theories of measurement helps therapists understand the different reporting styles and improves understanding of the psychometric properties.

The origins of psychometric theories come from educational measurement, later applied to psychological measurement and only recently applied to measures in occupational therapy. The test statistic is an indicator that describes the measurement property (e.g., ***Cronbach's α*** is a test statistic for the measurement property of internal consistency reliability). Theoretical assumptions form the basis of the equations used to derive a test statistic. Two main theories are used in psychometrics (Figure 9.4). The oldest of the two is the CTT, which has been used for more than 90 years.

Classical Test Theory

CTT is also called the *true score model* (Kline, 2005). It assumes that each person has an innate true score on any given test and that the true score and random error together make up the observed score for a person on the test. CTT is represented as $X = T + E$, where X is the observed score, T is the true score, and E is the random error.

For example, assume that a client with stroke scores 50 out of a total Fugl–Meyer Assessment UE motor score of 60 (Fugl-Meyer et al., 1975). The score of 50 is the observed score for this client. According to the assumptions of the CTT, this observed score is composed of the client's true score and random error. If the client's true score was lower than what was observed, then the observed score can be represented as 50 (observed score) = 49 (true score) + 1 (error). The less random error a measure has, the more the observed score reflects the true score. The true score is a

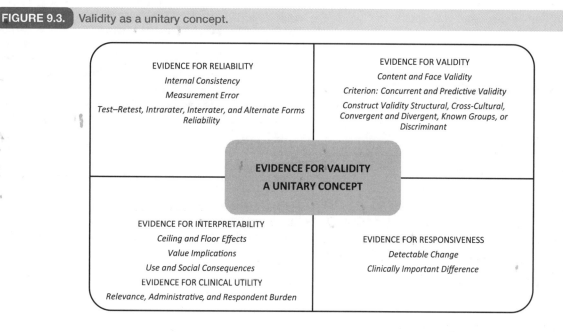

FIGURE 9.3. Validity as a unitary concept.

EVIDENCE FOR RELIABILITY
Internal Consistency
Measurement Error
Test–Retest, Intrarater, Interrater, and Alternate Forms Reliability

EVIDENCE FOR VALIDITY
Content and Face Validity
Criterion: Concurrent and Predictive Validity
Construct Validity Structural, Cross-Cultural, Convergent and Divergent, Known Groups, or Discriminant

EVIDENCE FOR VALIDITY
A UNITARY CONCEPT

EVIDENCE FOR INTERPRETABILITY
Ceiling and Floor Effects
Value Implications
Use and Social Consequences
EVIDENCE FOR CLINICAL UTILITY
Relevance, Administrative, and Respondent Burden

EVIDENCE FOR RESPONSIVENESS
Detectable Change
Clinically Important Difference

FIGURE 9.4.   Theoretical basis of psychometric analyses.

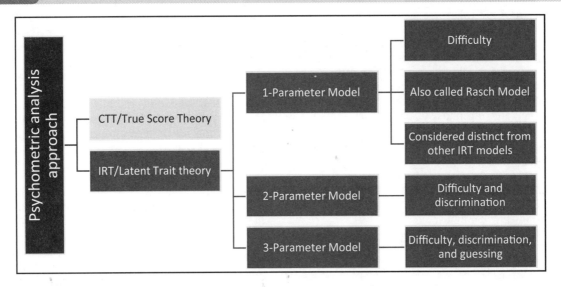

Note. CTT = Classical Test Theory; IRT= Item Response Theory.

hypothetical score that can never be calculated. The *SEM* is the standard deviation of the distribution of random errors around the true score.

Another assumption of CTT is that true scores are measured at an interval level and are normally distributed. Interval-level measures have scores with equal intervals. Many rehabilitation measures use Likert-type scales (e.g., the Numeric Pain Scale is an 11-point scale that ranges from 0 to 10); only a few instrumented measures use an interval-level unit of measurement (e.g., the Jamar dynamometer, which measures in pounds or kilograms). Test developers convert scores or combine scales to meet these assumptions. Thus, following the guidelines set forth in the test manual for standard administration and conversion of scores reduces random error and is essential for appropriate use of the test scores.

Item Response Theory

IRT is also called *latent trait theory* and is newer than CTT. The conceptual foundations of this theory lie in the relationship between a person's performance on individual items and the person's performance on the overall measure. IRT analyses are at an item level, as opposed to CTT, where the analyses are at the level of the total score or subscale scores. The response to each item provides information about the person's ability.

The ability of a person is represented by theta (θ). The person's ability is the probability of endorsing or responding positively to that dichotomous item. The higher the person's ability, the higher their probability of responding positively to the item. For example, for fatigue–ability, θ is the probability of responding positively to the item "Did you have problems with extreme tiredness or fatigue in the past week? Please say yes or no," based on the person's fatigue level. For example, the higher the person's fatigue,

the higher the person's probability of responding "yes" to this item is—a higher θ. The probability that a person not experiencing fatigue would respond "yes" to this item is very low, so the person's θ would be very low.

Statistical models are used in IRT to determine the ability of the person. Theta is expressed in units called logits. *Logits* are a logarithmic transformation of the ratio of the probability of endorsing or responding positively to an item and of not endorsing or responding positively to the item. Logits are typically converted to a user-oriented scale such as a *T* score for ease of understanding.

The statistical models used in IRT can be dichotomous (e.g., yes–no response), polytomous (e.g., multiple response options), or specialized. The dichotomous models are classified as one-parameter (1PM), two-parameter (2PM), and three-parameter (3PM) models. The 1PM model is commonly used and is also referred to as the ***Rasch model.*** The Rasch model is distinct from the other IRT models and is also referred to as *Rasch analysis* or *Rasch Measurement Theory.* The parameter of interest in the Rasch model is item difficulty. The 2PM model includes an additional discrimination parameter and requires a large sample size. The 3PM model consists of an additional guessing parameter and is commonly used in educational tests in which examinees can guess the answers; it is rarely applied in health-related outcomes because it is difficult to assume that guessing is involved.

Figure 9.5 shows what is referred to as an ***item characteristic curve*** and shows the three parameters of a single dichotomous item. When a 1PM model is used, the other two parameters are assumed to be constant. The parameter of difficulty is represented on the *x*-axis, the parameter of discrimination is represented by the slope, and the parameter of guessing is represented by the lower asymptote toward the tail of the *S*-shaped curve.

The terminology used to describe measurement properties in IRT can be different from that used in CTT. For

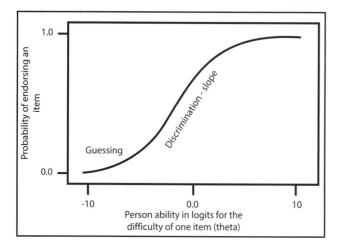

FIGURE 9.5. Item characteristic curve showing the three parameters of difficulty, discrimination, and guessing.

Source. N. Grampurohit. Used with permission.

Note. Probability of endorsing an item refers to the probability of responding positively to an item.

example, internal consistency using the test statistic Cronbach's α is reported in the traditional CTT approach; however, psychometric studies using the Rasch (1PM) model report person separation reliability, which is interpreted similarly to Cronbach's α, for which .80 or above is acceptable. Cronbach's α is also reported in psychometric studies when using an IRT approach.

A computer adaptive test (CAT) uses the IRT model. In a CAT, each item acts as its own mini-test. The CATs focus on *SEM* to assess the reliability of measurement. When a person answers the first item, the *SEM* is calculated and provides an estimate of that person's true score. Each subsequent item improves the estimate and reduces the *SEM* to increase precision. The test is complete after the desired precision is achieved, and only a few items may be needed to get to the best estimate with a low *SEM*. Although the most commonly encountered CATs are found in education (e.g., the Graduate Record Examination or Standardized Achievement Test), they are also used in health care to obtain patient-reported outcomes. The most notable ones are the Patient-Reported Outcomes Measurement Information System (PROMIS®) instruments (https://www.healthmeasures.net/explore-measurement-systems/promis) and, in occupational therapy, the Pediatric Evaluation of Disability Inventory Computer Adaptive Test (Coster et al., 2016).

SUMMARY

Occupational therapists need to have foundational knowledge of psychometric properties and their interpretation. Therapists should consider the most current evidence and best practices in assessment and measurement when selecting, using, and interpreting measures with a careful review of their psychometric properties.

QUESTIONS

1. How might you define *construct* within the context of assessment scales? For example, what is the construct being assessed by the Canadian Occupational Performance Measure (Law et al., 2019)?
2. What are the four levels of measurement? Define each level of measurement and provide an example from an assessment.
3. What is a psychometric study? What are the hallmarks of a good quality psychometric study?
4. Explain to your colleague or peer, the different types of correlation coefficients reported in psychometric studies. What is the difference between the strength of a correlation and the statistical significance of correlation?
5. What is the difference between reliability and validity? Can an assessment be reliable but not valid? Can an assessment be valid but not reliable? What is the clinical relevance of using a reliable assessment? What is the clinical relevance of using a valid assessment?
6. How does the traditional psychometric approach of classical test theory differ from the modern approach of item response theory?

REFERENCES

Adams, K. B., Matto, H. C., & Sanders, S. (2004). Confirmatory factor analysis of the Geriatric Depression Scale. *Gerontologist, 44,* 818–826. https://doi.org/10.1093/geront/44.6.818

Andresen, E. M. (2000). Criteria for assessing the tools of disability outcomes research. *Archives of Physical Medicine and Rehabilitation, 81*(12, Suppl. 2), S15–S20. https://doi.org/10.1053/apmr.2000.20619

Baum, C. M., Connor, L. T., Morrison, T., Hahn, M., Dromerick, A. W., & Edwards, D. F. (2008). Reliability, validity, and clinical utility of the Executive Function Performance Test: A measure of executive function in a sample of people with stroke. *American Journal of Occupational Therapy, 62,* 446–455. https://doi.org/10.5014/ajot.62.4.446

Brown, T. (2010). Construct validity: A unitary concept for occupational therapy assessment and measurement. *Hong Kong Journal of Occupational Therapy, 20,* 30–42. https://doi.org/10.1016/S1569-18611070056-5

Classen, S., & Velozo, C. A. (2018). Critiquing assessments. In B. A. B. Schell & G. Gillen (Eds.), *Willard and Spackman's occupational therapy* (13th ed., pp. 391–405). Baltimore: Wolters Kluwer.

Costa, A. S., Fimm, B., Friesen, P., Soundjock, H., Rottschy, C., Gross, T., . . . Reetz, K. (2012). Alternate-form reliability of the Montreal Cognitive Assessment screening test in a clinical setting. *Dementia and Geriatric Cognitive Disorders, 33,* 379–384. https://doi.org/10.1159/000340006

Costa, A. S., Reich, A., Fimm, B., Ketteler, S. T., Schulz, J. B., & Reetz, K. (2014). Evidence of the sensitivity of the MoCA alternate forms in monitoring cognitive change in early Alzheimer's disease. *Dementia and Geriatric Cognitive Disorders, 33,* 95–103. https://doi.org/10.1159/000351864

Coster, W. J., Kramer, J. M., Tian, F., Dooley, M., Liljenquist, K., Kao, Y. C., & Ni, P. (2016) Evaluating the appropriateness of a new computer-administered measure of adaptive function for children and youth with autism spectrum disorders. *Autism, 20*(1), 14–25. https://doi.org/10.1177/1362361314564473

Crist, P. (2014). Reliability and validity: The psychometrics of standardized assessments. In J. Hinojosa & P. Kramer (Eds.), *Evaluation in occupational therapy: Obtaining and interpreting data* (4th ed., pp. 143–160). Bethesda, MD: AOTA Press.

Duncan, P. W., Wallace, D., Lai, S. M., Johnson, D., Embretson, S., & Laster, L. J. (1999). The Stroke Impact Scale Version 2.0. Evaluation of reliability, validity, and sensitivity to change. *Stroke, 30,* 2131–2140. https://doi.org/10.1161/01.STR.30.10.2131

Folstein, M. F., Folstein, S. E., & McHugh, P. R. (2020). *Mini-Mental State Examination.* Lutz, FL: PAR, Inc. Available at https://www.parinc.com/Products/Pkey/237

Fugl-Meyer, A. R., Jaasko, L., Leyman, I., Olsson, S., & Steglind, S. (1975). The post-stroke hemiplegic patient: A method for evaluation of physical performance. *Scandinavian Journal of Rehabilitation Medicine, 7,* 13–31.

Howell, D. C. (2014). *Fundamental statistics for the behavioral sciences* (8th ed.). Belmont, CA: Wadsworth/Cengage Learning.

Jacqmin-Gadda, H., Fabrigoule, C., Commenges, D., & Dartigues, J. F. O. (1997). A 5-year longitudinal study of the Mini-Mental State Examination in normal aging. *American Journal of Epidemiology, 145,* 498–506. https://doi.org/10.1093/oxfordjournals.aje.a009137

Kane, M. (2013). Validating the interpretations and uses of test scores. *Journal of Educational Measurement, 50,* 1–73. https://doi.org/10.1111/jedm.12000

Kjeken, I., Dagfinrud, H., Uhlig, T., Mowinckel, P., Kvien, T. K., & Finset, A. (2005). Reliability of the Canadian Occupational Performance Measure in patients with ankylosing spondylitis. *Journal of Rheumatology, 32,* 1503–1509. Retrieved from http://www.jrheum.org/content/32/8/1503

Kline, T. (2005). Classical Test Theory: Assumptions, equations, limitations, and item analyses. In T. Kline (Ed.), *Psychological testing: A practical approach to design and evaluation* (pp. 91–105). Thousand Oaks, CA: Sage.

Kubiszyn, T., & Borich, G. D. (2013). *Educational testing and measurement: Classroom application and practice* (10th ed.). New York: Wiley.

Law, M., Baptiste, S., Carswell, A., McColl, M., Polatajko, H., & Pollock, N. (2019). *Canadian Occupational Performance Measure* (5th ed., rev.). Altona, MB: COPM, Inc.

Lin, K. C., Fu, T., Wu, C. Y., Wang, Y. H., Liu, J. S., Hsieh, C. J., & Lin, S. F. (2010). Minimal detectable change and clinically important difference of the Stroke Impact Scale in stroke patients. *Neurorehabilitation and Neural Repair, 24,* 486–492. https://doi.org/10.1177/1545968309356295

Messick, S. (1989). Meaning and values in test validation: The science and ethics of assessment. *Educational Researcher, 18*(2), 5–11. https://doi.org/10.2307/1175249

Messick, S. (1994). The interplay of evidence and consequences in the validation of performance assessments. *Educational Researcher, 23,* 13–23. https://doi.org/10.3102/0013189X023002013

Mitchell, A. J. (2009). A meta-analysis of the accuracy of the mini-mental state examination in the detection of dementia and mild cognitive impairment. *Journal of Psychiatric Research, 43,* 411–431. https://doi.org/10.1016/j.jpsychires.2008.04.014

Mokkink, L., Terwee, C., Knol, D., Stratford, P., Alonso Caballero, J., Patrick, D., . . . De Vet, H. (2010). The COSMIN checklist for evaluating the methodological quality of studies on measurement properties: A clarification of its content. *BMC Medical Research Methodology, 10,* 22. https://doi.org/10.1186/1471-2288-10-22

Mukaka, M. M. (2012). A guide to appropriate use of correlation coefficient in medical research. *Malawi Medical Journal, 24,* 69–71.

Nasreddine, Z. S., Phillips, N. A., Bédirian, V., Charbonneau, S., Whitehead, V., Collin, I., . . . Chertkow, H. (2005). The Montreal Cognitive Assessment, MoCA: A brief screening tool for mild cognitive impairment. *Journal of the American Geriatrics Society, 53,* 695–699. https://doi.org/10.1111/j.1532-5415.2005.53221.x

Oxford Grice, K., Vogel, K. A., Le, V., Mitchell, A., Muniz, S., Vollmer, M. A. (2003). Adult norms for a commercially available Nine Hole Peg Test for finger dexterity. *American Journal of Occupational Therapy, 57*(5), 570–573. https://doi.org/10.5014/ajot.57.5.570

Penta, M., Tesio, L., Arnould, C., Zancan, A., & Thonnard, J. L. (2001). The ABILHAND questionnaire as a measure of manual ability in chronic stroke patients: Rasch-based validation and relationship to upper limb impairment. *Stroke, 32,* 1627–1634. https://doi.org/10.1161/01.str.32.7.1627

Portney, L. G., & Watkins, M. P. (2009). *Foundations of clinical research: Applications to practice* (3rd ed.). Upper Saddle River, NJ: Pearson/Prentice Hall.

Sijtsma, K. (2009). On the use, the misuse, and the very limited usefulness of Cronbach's alpha. *Psychometrika, 74,* 107–120. https://doi.org/10.1007/s11336-008-9101-0

Taylor, R. (1990). Interpretation for the correlation coefficient: A basic review. *Journal of Diagnostic Medical Sonography, 6*(1), 35–39. https://doi.org/10.1177/875647939000600106

Thorndike, R. M., & Thorndike-Christ, T. (2010). *Measurement and evaluation in psychology and education* (8th ed.). Boston: Pearson Education.

Wang, T., Lin, K., Wu, C., Chung, C., Pei, Y., & Teng, Y. (2011). Validity, responsiveness, and clinically important difference of the ABILHAND questionnaire in patients with stroke. *Archives of Physical Medicine and Rehabilitation, 92,* 1086–1091. https://doi.org/10.1016/j.apmr.2011.01.020

Wechsler, D. (1987). *Wechsler Memory Scale–Revised.* San Antonio: Psychological Corporation.

Yesavage, J. A., Brink, T. L., Rose, T. L., Lum, O., Huang, V., Adey, M. B., & Leirer, V. O. (1983). Development and validation of a geriatric depression screening scale: A preliminary report. *Journal of Psychiatric Research, 17,* 37–49. https://doi.org/10.1016/0022-3956(82)90033-4

Scoring and Interpreting Results

10

Namrata Grampurohit, PhD, OTR/L, and MJ Mulcahey, PhD, OTR/L, CLCP, FASIA

CHAPTER HIGHLIGHTS

- Scoring
- Survey scores versus standardized assessment tool scores
- Essential statistical concepts for scoring and interpretation
- Rating scales
- Hand scoring versus computerized scoring
- Norm-referenced versus criterion-referenced test scores
- Converted scores
- Total versus subscale scores
- Screening tools and cutoff scores
- Sharing scores with clients and families

KEY TERMS AND CONCEPTS

- Age equivalents
- Bimodal distribution
- Central tendency
- Checklist
- Computer adaptive tests
- Computer-based scoring
- Converted scores
- Criterion-referenced tests
- Cutoff scores
- Developmental age
- Grade equivalents
- Graphic, pictorial, or visual analog scale
- Hand scoring
- Interpretation
- Interquartile range
- Interval level of measurement
- Likert scale
- Local norm groups
- Logit
- Mean
- Median
- Mode
- Multiple norm groups
- National norm groups
- Nominal level of measurement
- Normal curve
- Normal distribution
- Normative group
- Norm-referenced tests
- Norms
- Obtained scores
- Ordinal level of measurement
- Percentile
- Percentile rank
- Psychometric properties
- Quartiles
- Q-sort
- Range
- Rating scales
- Ratio level of measurement
- Raw scores
- Response scales
- Scale of measurement
- Screening tool
- Semantic differential scale
- Special norm groups
- Standard deviation
- Standard score
- Standardized assessment tool
- Stanine
- Survey
- *T* score
- Variability
- Variance
- *z* score

INTRODUCTION

Occupational therapists use scores generated by assessment instruments to measure constructs, traits, behaviors, or phenomena. The end goal of using a measurement tool is to generate scores that can be used to report information, compare data across conditions and people, and determine individual-level change and effect or group-level aggregate information. Scores can be useful, but they also can be misused if they are not calculated accurately or are not interpreted in ethical and appropriate ways.

When an occupational therapist gets a score of 80 out of 100 for a client with shoulder pain after a fall, the therapist needs to answer multiple questions to interpret this score—that is, to ascertain what *80* means. Was this score obtained using a standardized measure of shoulder function? Does the client have poor function or good function? Does a higher score mean better shoulder function or more shoulder impairment? Can this score be used to compare the client to other clients with shoulder problems to determine (or make a claim) that this client has more shoulder impairment than another person with a shoulder problem or than a healthy person? Scores themselves do not tell therapists anything unless they know how the scores behave. Scores need to be interpreted to give them meaning and context.

At the foundation of this understanding are the psychometric properties described in Chapter 9, "Psychometric Properties Related to Standardized Assessments." *Psychometric properties* provide evidence for the different ways scores can be used for a certain population or condition or behavior. For example, if a client's scores on a test are to be used to monitor outcomes over time, the psychometric properties of interest would be test–retest reliability to determine the consistency of scores measured repeatedly, construct validity to determine whether the scores truly measure the targeted outcome, and responsiveness to quantify the degree of change in scores needed to claim a change in the behavior or trait. The application of knowledge required to give meaning to assessment scores is called *interpretation*. Occupational therapists' confidence in the accuracy of scores and their ethical use are important components of an evaluation that will help in developing an intervention or discharge plan for clients.

This chapter describes the process of and concepts in scoring and interpreting the results of assessment instruments. It outlines the differences between scores generated by surveys and standardized assessment tools, the essential statistical concepts required for scoring and interpretation, types of rating scales and scoring methods, the difference between norm-referenced and criterion-referenced test scores, use of converted scores and total versus subscale scores, and use of screening tools and cutoff scores. Finally, guidance is provided for sharing scores with clients and families.

SCORING

The goal of *scoring* is to transform observed or self-reported performance on a test into an accurate, meaningful, and defensible interpretation that can contribute to clinical reasoning and provide objective assessment data for problem solving, intervention and discharge planning, and communication with team members and payers. Figure 10.1 illustrates the stepwise progression of the scoring process.

FIGURE 10.1.   Scoring process.

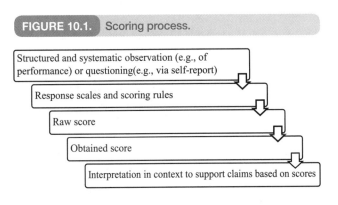

The first step an occupational therapist takes toward accurate scoring is a systematic and structured process of observing behaviors or asking questions. The therapist then scores the behavior or response using scoring rules and *response scales,* which are a set of options provided to the therapist to rate the behavior—for example, scoring daily activity independence using the response scale 0 = *dependent*, 1 = *partially dependent*, and 2 = *independent*. *Raw scores,* which are the original unaltered scores obtained by simply adding the individual item-level scores often are then transformed into *obtained scores* (sometimes called *derived scores* or *converted scores*), which are scores converted or adjusted linearly or non-linearly. Obtained scores can be of several types, such as percentiles or standard scores. This transformation is done to take into account normative data—for example, for development in children or aging in older adults. Transformation tables are provided in the assessment manual or published articles. Standard scores can be compared across different assessments because their interpretation is mostly consistent.

Occupational therapists should choose assessments that report standard scores to conform to standardization, value, and appropriate use. Certainly, the ability to complete all these steps is dependent on the test development procedures and published protocols. Because these vary greatly for rehabilitation measures, therapists should select measures for which test development information is available, standard scores can be reported, and score interpretation is discussed within the manual or published literature.

SURVEY SCORES VERSUS STANDARDIZED ASSESSMENT TOOL SCORES

Surveys and assessment tools can both generate scores. It is important for occupational therapists to differentiate between scores from a *standardized assessment tool,* in which individual item scores have meaning, and scores from a nonstandardized *survey,* in which individual items or aggregate scores are used primarily for statistical analysis and are not meaningful by themselves. Surveys should be used as nonstandardized assessments and not as standardized measures, even if they provide a score. Exhibit 10.1 further delineates the differences between surveys and standardized assessment tools and scores.

A detailed instrument development methodology is used to develop standardized measures so that scores can be used for validated purposes such as screening, assessment of performance, or prediction of discharge. Instrument development and measurement research information can be found in other sources such as Velozo et al. (2012) and Furr and Bacharach (2014).

ESSENTIAL STATISTICAL CONCEPTS FOR SCORING AND INTERPRETATION

Understanding basic statistical concepts, particularly related to scoring and interpretation, is essential for occupational therapists to appropriately use tests and

EXHIBIT 10.1. Comparison of Standardized Measure Scores and Nonstandardized Survey Scores

STANDARDIZED MEASURE SCORES	NONSTANDARDIZED SURVEY SCORES
Scores can be used to make claims about a client that are supported by the relevant literature.	Scores cannot be used to make claims about a client.
Measure is unidimensional; total and subscale scores each reflect measurement of a single, unique construct.	Measure is multidimensional; it can include multiple questions and need not generate a total score. Item-level data can also be used.
Scores can be compared across other assessments and may be normed.	Scores cannot be compared across other assessments or clients and are not normed.
Psychometric data are available to support the measure's reliability, validity, and responsiveness.	No or limited psychometric data are available for the measure; face and content validity may be reported with an informal methodology.
Measure is developed intentionally by instrument developers.	Measure is developed by survey experts for a research or program evaluation study.
Scores can be used for individual- and group-level statistical analysis.	Scores can be used for individual- and group-level statistical analysis.
Scores can be used for describing a phenomenon, screening, assessing, comparing, and measuring outcomes.	Scores can be used to describe or understand a phenomenon.

measurements. Evidence-based practice also demands that therapists have a firm grasp of statistical concepts to understand psychometric articles and systematic reviews that contribute to the evidence. This chapter provides only a conceptual understanding of selected statistics relevant to the evaluation process. Readers are advised to consult more thorough textbooks for a deeper discussion of statistical concepts (e.g., Portney & Watkins, 2009).

Levels of Measurement

Numbers assigned to behaviors or traits are referred to as a *scale of measurement* or *level of measurement*. There are four levels of measurement: (1) nominal, (2) ordinal, (3) interval, and (4) ratio (see Table 10.1 for examples). The *nominal level of measurement* is the simplest and consists of names or labels used to identify categories (e.g., yes or no). The *ordinal level of measurement* involves rank-ordered categories (e.g., manual muscle grading of 5, 4, 3, 2, 1, and 0). The *interval level of measurement* involves units of measurement with

equal distances between them (e.g., body temperature measured in degrees Celsius or Fahrenheit). The *ratio level of measurement* involves interval scales with a true zero indicating absence of the characteristic (e.g., range of motion in degrees). All mathematical and statistical calculations can be performed with ratio-level measurement; therefore, it is highly desirable. See Chapter 9 for a detailed discussion and examples of levels of measurement.

Measures of Central Tendency

Central tendency is the typical value for a distribution or the center of a distribution and occasionally referred to as an average. Mean, median, and mode are the three indicators of central tendency. *Mean* ($\bar{x}$) is the average value calculated with the formula

$$\bar{x} = \frac{\sum x}{n},$$

TABLE 10.1. Levels of Measurement

LEVEL OF MEASUREMENT	ASSESSMENT EXAMPLE	SCALE
Nominal	Caregiver Strain Index (Robinson, 1983)	Yes–no response format for 13 questions related to stressful caregiver experiences.
Ordinal	Parkinson's Disease Activities of Daily Living Scale (Hobson et al., 2001)	5-point ordinal scale of 1 = *no difficulty*, 2 = *mild difficulty*, 3 = *moderate difficulty*, 4 = *high difficulty*, and 5 = *extreme difficulty* for one question: "Describe how your Parkinson's disease has affected your day-to-day activities in the last month."
Interval	Pinch dynamometer (Jansen et al., 2008)	Pinch strength in pounds. The score of 0 does not necessarily reflect a complete absence of strength in the hand muscles.
Ratio	Range of joint motion (Classen & Velozo, 2019)	Goniometer measurement of movement in degrees. The score of 0° reflects the complete absence of motion at the joint.

where Σx is the sum of all available scores and n is the total number of scores in the sample. The mean is usually preferred because each score contributes to the calculation, but it is greatly affected by extreme scores. Interval- and ratio-level data can be represented with the mean.

Median (x̃), the second most frequently encountered measure of central tendency, evenly divides the population in half, with 50% of values above and 50% below it. The median is favored over the mean when extreme scores are present and also for ordinal-level data. Calculating the median score involves the following steps:

1. Order the scores from low to high.
2. Select the middle score that divides the group equally.
3. If there are an even number of scores, then the median is the average of the two center-most scores.
4. If there are an odd number of scores, then the median is the middle score.

Mode is the most frequently occurring score. If two scores occur most frequently, it is a **bimodal distribution.** Mode is the least frequently encountered measure of central tendency and is used only when an important point is being made regarding interpretation of the results.

Normal Curve and Normal Distribution

A *normal curve* is a specific type of bell-shaped curve illustrating the *normal distribution,* in which most of the scores fall in the middle of the scale and progressively fewer fall at the extremes (Figure 10.2). The appeal of the normal curve is that its characteristics are constant and predictable for statistical purposes. As shown in Figure 10.2, the curve is smooth, symmetrical, and bell shaped. The mean, median, and mode all have the same value. In theory, the tails (i.e., extremes) of the curve can go on infinitely and approach, but never quite touch, the baseline. The standard shape of the curve allows determination of the proportions under the curve; 68.26% of the area of the normal distribution is bound by one standard deviation, 95.45% by two standard deviations, and 99.74% by three standard deviations.

Variability

Variability is the spread of scores around a measure of central tendency and provides information on how widely spread the scores are in the distribution. Variability is important because small variability indicates greater accuracy in scores. However, no variability is not desirable because it indicates a larger problem with testing; individuals usually vary in their ability, so no variability would indicate a poorly designed item that is very hard or very easy, resulting in all individuals answering it the same way. The four indicators of variability commonly used are (1) standard deviation, (2) variance, (3) range, and (4) interquartile range.

Standard deviation is the square root of the variance and accompanies the mean. It is a powerful statistic because it is influenced by all scores in the data. If ordinal-level data are collected for item-level scores, however, mean and standard deviation should not be used for reporting because the data are not sophisticated enough to warrant this mathematical application. The formula for calculating the standard deviation (*SD*) is

---

FIGURE 10.2.   Normal distribution and standard scores.

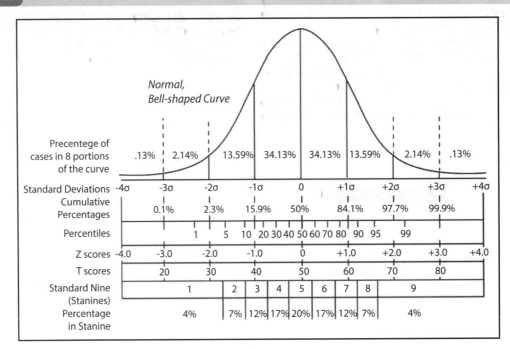

$$SD = \sqrt{\frac{\Sigma(x - \overline{x})^2}{n - 1}},$$

where x is the obtained score, $\Sigma(x - \overline{x})^2$ is the sum of squares of the difference between individual scores and the mean, and is the total number of scores.

Variance (s^2) is the squared standard deviation, shown by the formula

$$s^2 = \frac{\Sigma(x - \overline{x})^2}{n - 1},$$

where x is the obtained score, $\overline{x}$ is the mean, $\Sigma(x - \overline{x})^2$ is the sum of squares of the difference between individual scores and the mean, and is the total number of scores.

Range is the easiest measure of variability to calculate. Range is obtained by subtracting the lowest score (min) from the highest (max).

Interquartile range is the difference between the first and third quartiles and accompanies the median. *Quartiles* divide a distribution into four equal parts, or quarters, and three quartiles exist for any data set, Q1, Q2, and Q3. The quartiles correspond to percentiles at 25%, 50%, and 75%. The 50th percentile is the median value or midpoint of the distribution. Interquartile range (IQR) is shown by the formula

$$IQR = Q3 - Q1,$$

where *Q1* is the first quartile and *Q3* is the third quartile.

RATING SCALES

Rating scales are response scales that provide an ordinal level of measurement where the choices for response to an item are ordered categories that are increasing or decreasing in intensity/severity. The rating scale for test items can be completed by the occupational therapist (i.e., performance-based), the client (i.e., patient-reported or self-reported), the caregiver (i.e., proxy-reported), or a measuring instrument (i.e., instrument-based). The different types of rating scales used in measures are summarized in Table 10.2.

HAND SCORING VERSUS COMPUTERIZED SCORING

Test developers may offer more than one method for scoring, including hand scoring and computerized scoring.

TABLE 10.2. Types of Rating Scales

RATING SCALE	APPLICATION	EXAMPLE
Graphic, pictorial, or visual analog scale	Clients are asked to choose from among images that depict the trait being assessed.	Faces with expressions corresponding to pain levels in the Wong–Baker Faces Pain Rating Scale (https://wongbakerfaces.org) Five-star quality rating
Checklist	Clients are provided a list of characteristics and asked to mark a dichotomous response.	*Present* or *absent* *Yes* or *no*
Q-sort	Clients are asked to sort a series of objects, pictures, or words into categories.	Riverside Behavioral Q-set Version 3.11 has a set of 64 statements that can be sorted to describe the behavior that is being described by the respondent (Funder et al., 2000).
Semantic differential scale	Two opposing qualities or adjectives are provided, and clients are asked to rate where they fall on the continuum.	For a self-image scale, clients rate where they think they are on the following continuum: Ugly _ _ _ _ _ _ _ Beautiful 1 2 3 4 5 6 7
Likert scale	*Frequency:* Clients are asked how often they perform a task or behavior being assessed.	*Never, rarely, sometimes, always, often,* or *don't know*
	Agreement: Clients are asked to select the response that reflects their level of agreement.	*Strongly agree, agree, neutral, disagree,* or *strongly disagree*
	Forced choice: Clients are asked to choose among response options that do not include a neutral response, such as *don't know* or *not sure*	*Impossible, very difficult, somewhat difficult,* or *not at all difficult*
	Comparative scale: Clients are asked to select a response in comparison to other variables.	On the COPM, clients rate their level of performance and satisfaction with performance of specific occupations, and the two ratings are compared.
	Ranking scale	On the COPM, clients rank the priority of identified occupations in their lives.

Note. COPM = Canadian Occupational Performance Measure (Law et al., 2019).

Hand scoring is the most commonly encountered method; occupational therapists manually calculate the scores with simple mathematical operations such as adding, subtracting, multiplying, dividing, or using a chart to find corresponding values. The Jebsen Hand Function Test (Jebsen et al., 1969) is an example of a hand-scored assessment; therapists use a scoring form to record raw scores, and then compare them to normative scores to aid in interpretation (Sears & Chung, 2010). Occupational therapists using a hand-scored assessment should allow adequate time during test administration to convert raw scores to standard scores as described in the test manual or published literature; scoring should be part of therapists' orientation or training for the test.

In *computer-based scoring,* individual test item information is entered into the test website or downloaded test software and scored automatically. A computer-based test is any test for which data are entered on a computer and a score automatically generated using Excel or test software.

In recent years, computers are increasingly used for adaptive administration of tests. *Computer adaptive tests* have an algorithm built into the software that enables test items to be administered on the basis of a prior response. The software presents an item of medium difficulty and, depending on the client's response, next presents an item of higher or lower difficulty consistent with the client's knowledge or ability. Computer adaptive tests work like standardized educational assessments (e.g., Graduate Record Examination) and can be limited to 10–15 items that help achieve precise measurement. For example, for a mobility assessment, a client who responds that they cannot walk will not be presented any stairs-related items, and the next item presented will be of lower difficulty. This tailoring makes item administration highly relevant to individual clients and reduces the number of items to be administered. Examples of computer adaptive tests are the Patient-Reported Outcomes Measurement Information System (PROMIS®; Hong et al., 2016), the Neurological Quality of Life measurement system (Cella et al., 2011), the Spinal Cord Injury–Functional Index/Assistive Technology (Jette et al., 2015), and the Cerebral Palsy Profile of Health and Function (Grampurohit et al., 2019).

PROMIS, a widely used system of health measures, allows item responses to be recorded either on paper-based forms or using a computer app, tablet, or Research Electronic Data Capture (REDCAP) data collection software. Data are uploaded to the assessment center website, which automatically generates scoring information (https://www.healthmeasures.net/explore-measurement-systems/promis). PROMIS measures are also available as computer-adaptive tests. Like some other tools, PROMIS is available as an Epic module that a facility can make available to therapists; Epic is health information software used by health care organizations to manage clients' health records (Epic Systems Corp., Verona, WI). G-code severity modifiers, which are required for Medicare claims, are also available for PROMIS and other tools and may be helpful in score interpretation.

NORM-REFERENCED VERSUS CRITERION-REFERENCED TEST SCORES

Interpretation of *norm-referenced tests* involves comparing clients' scores to those of a well-defined group, referred to as the test's *normative group* or *sample*. *Norms* are a group of scores generated by large-scale test administration to healthy people or to population-specific groups for whom the test was developed or who are likely to use the test. Norms are published in the test manual or literature to allow therapists to compare the obtained scores to aid in interpretation of the scores. Normative data are assumed to approximate the normal distribution.

Normative groups can be of the following types:

- *Multiple norm groups* enable comparisons of a client's score to the scores of multiple different groups. For example, client scores on a vocational readiness inventory can be compared to norms of several different occupational groups.
- *Local norm groups* are sometimes used to establish norms that are more representative of a specific local, typical population. For example, if the demographics of a community are different from those of the normative sample for a test, local norms can be established to enable more useful comparisons. Establishing local norms is a complex process, but one that can be undertaken in collaboration with a psychometrician.
- *National norm groups* are representative of a country's population. Although national norms are desirable and meaningful, many test developers do not provide this information. In addition, national norms may not be appropriate for use with language and cultural adaptations of tests, which should use normative samples representative of the population of interest.
- *Special norm groups,* also referred to as *fixed reference groups,* are groups of people with a unique condition that influences performance. For example, the norm groups for the Developmental Test of Visual Perception include not only a sample of healthy people but also a special group of people who are hard of hearing (Hammill et al., 2014). Developmental and mental age norms are also developed using special norm groups.

To interpret clients' scores using norms, the clients' characteristics should be similar to those of the norm group to which they are being compared. Occupational therapists should describe in their report the type of normative group used in the comparison.

Interpretation of *criterion-referenced tests* involves comparing clients' scores to a predetermined set of performance criteria. Cut scores are often used for determining proficiency level or performance category and need to be applied for a valid interpretation of scores. The normal curve and distribution do not apply to criterion-referenced test interpretation.

In pediatric practice, for example, children's growth is compared to that of a normative sample of the same age group. However, for children with disabilities such as cerebral palsy, normative data do not provide useful comparisons because these children's developmental trajectory is altered (Griffiths et al., 2018). Likewise, to measure function in children with conditions such as spinal cord injury, developmental trajectory typically is not applicable. Thus, criterion-referenced tests are preferred in outcome measurement for children with developmental and physical disabilities because they eliminate the impact of scores emphasizing differences from a normative sample.

CONVERTED SCORES

Converted scores are a set of scores with the same mean and standard deviation that allow them to be compared across individuals and referred to as *standard scores, scaled scores, or obtained scores*. Raw scores are converted to standard scores to enable interpretation (U.S. Department of Labor, Employment and Training Administration, 1999). Table 10.3 provides an overview of the different types of converted scores. Conversion of scores is particularly important for assessments in which the individual item responses are on a nominal or ordinal scale. Simply stated, the standard score is a weighted score that takes into account normative data and errors. Stanines are standard scores first developed by the military for aptitude testing to identify candidates who were capable of serving successfully. Educational testing was the next to adopt standard scores.

A *percentile* is a cumulative percentage score used with norm-referenced tests. It represents the area under the normal curve as shown in Figure 10.1 and indicates the percentage of people who scored above and below the client. *Percentile rank* explains the relative standing of the client among members of the normative group. Percentile ranks are considered better than grade or age equivalents because they enable comparisons with children in the same grade or adults in the same age or reference group. The Peabody Developmental Motor Scales (Tavasoli et al., 2014) use percentiles for reporting gross motor, fine motor, and total motor composite scores.

Stanine scores are standard scores on a nine-point scale and are also referred to as *standard nines* because the normal distribution is divided into nine segments, with 5 as the mean and a standard deviation of 2. Stanines are always expressed as whole numbers, making their reporting easy to understand; this simplicity also means that detailed information about a client is lost because of the nine broad segmented levels that would otherwise be available through, for example, a 100-point scale. A stanine score of 9 is in the top 4% of scorers, and a score of 1 is in the bottom 4%. The Otis–Lennon School Ability Test is an example of a test that uses stanines, among other types of score reporting (Otis & Lennon, 2019).

Grade equivalents are established by testing normative samples of students at each grade level. Individual students' scores are compared to these norms to identify the grade level they are currently demonstrating. **Developmental age or age equivalents** are determined in a similar way; the student's score is compared to norms for specific ages and matched to the appropriate developmental age.

Grade and age equivalents have been controversial because they are not standard scores. Raw score comparisons are not a valid representation, particularly when

TABLE 10.3. Types of Converted Scores

SCORE	DEFINITION	EXAMPLE
Percentile	Scores indicate what percentage of the normative group scored above and below the client's score.	A client's score falls in the 80th percentile or third quartile, indicating that 80% of test takers scored below and 20% scored above the client.
Percentile rank	Scores indicate the client's standing in comparison with the normative group, usually of the same grade or age.	A client whose score is in the 80th percentile has a percentile rank of 80 among peers in the client's grade or age range.
Stanine	Scores are assigned on a scale from 0 to 9, where the mean is 5 and the SD is 2. Scores are always expressed as a whole number.	A client with a stanine score of 9 is in the top 4% of the normative group.
Grade equivalent	Scores indicate the grade level the student is currently exemplifying.	A student with a grade equivalent of 5.2 demonstrates proficiency at the fifth-grade level of performance.
Age equivalent	Scores indicate the developmental age the client is currently exemplifying.	A child with an age equivalent of 2 years demonstrates proficiency at the 2-year level of performance.
z score	Scores are related to the normal distribution, where the mean is 0 and the SD is 1. z scores can have negative values.	A client with a z score of 0.5 is within 1.0 SD for the test or 0.5 SD above the mean.
T score	Scores are related to the normal distribution, where the mean is 50 and the SD is 10.	A client with a T score of 30 is 2 SD below the mean for the test.
Logit	Scores are linear and express the odds of success of the client on any given item, where the average item difficulty is 0. Conversion of logits to a T score can improve the client's understanding of the score.	Items with higher scores are easier and those with lower (including negative) scores are harder for a client.

Note. SD = standard deviation.

children's grade and age equivalents are used. One issue is the quick progression in development in younger age groups, reflected in larger changes with larger raw scores, making grade and age equivalents a poor marker of clinical outcome. Another problem with grade equivalents in particular is the lack of translation across schools because of variations in curricula and expectations that result in differing demands and opportunities across schools.

The most commonly used standard scores are the z score and the T score. (Note that the T score in psychometrics is different from the t statistic obtain on the inferential t test.) They are easy to compute when the mean and standard deviation are available from the test manual or literature. Clients may find T scores easier to understand than z scores because T scores have only positive values.

The **z score** reflects the distance the score falls above or below the mean and is computed with the formula

$$z = \frac{x - \bar{x}}{SD},$$

where x is the obtained or raw score, $\bar{x}$ is the mean score for the test, and SD is the standard deviation. For example, a client age 60 scores 25 seconds with the right hand on the Nine Hole Peg Test (Mathiowetz, Weber, et al., 1985). The table of norms for this client's age group shows a mean of 17.86 and a standard deviation of 2.39 (Oxford et al., 2003). The score would be computed as follows:

$$z = \frac{25 - 17.86}{2.39} = \frac{7.14}{2.39} = 2.99.$$

The z score for this client is 2.99. Another way of saying this is, "The client's score is more than two standard deviations above the mean" or "The client's score is very extreme, greater than two standard deviations away from the mean." An important consideration for interpretation in this example is the fact that on the Nine Hole Peg Test, higher scores indicate worse dexterity (Mathiowetz, Weber et al., 1985). Therefore, the interpretation would be, "the client's scores on the Nine Hole Peg Test indicate extremely low dexterity, greater than two standard deviations away from the mean for that age."

Another advantage of the z score is the ability to compare performance on two different tests. For example, the same client is administered the Box and Blocks Test, another test of coordination, which measures the number of blocks the client places in the box in 1 minute; the lower the score, the worse the performance (Mathiowetz, Volland et al., 1985). The 60-year-old client scores 55 blocks on the test in 1 minute. The table of norms (Mathiowetz, Weber et al., 1985) indicates that the right hand normative mean for his age is 71.3 blocks with a standard deviation of 8.8 blocks. The z scores would be computed as follows:

$$z = \frac{55 - 71.3}{8.8} = \frac{-16.3}{8.8} = -1.85$$

The client's z score on the Box and Blocks test of -1.85 is consistent with results for the Nine Hole Peg Test (i.e., low performance). In addition, comparison of the two z scores indicates that the client has greater problems with manipulating smaller objects because the z score for the Nine Hole Peg Test (2.99) is more extreme (i.e., further from zero) than that for the Box and Blocks Test (–1.85). Standard scores enable comparisons across tests that would not otherwise be comparable using raw scores.

The **T score** is a standard score with as mean of 50 and a standard deviation of 10. The T score is easier to understand than the score because there are no negative values. The T score is computed with the formula

$$T = z\,(10) + 50,$$

where is the score, 10 is the standard deviation, and 50 is the mean. For the client in the example, using the formula yields a T score of 79.9 for the Nine Hole Peg Test and 31.0 for the Box and Blocks Test. These results match the scores, but because the understanding of scores parallels the understanding of percentages, clients with a literacy or cognitive level adequate to understand percentages can understand the occupational therapist's explanation of their test results.

Logit is defined as the standard score with a natural logarithm of the odds $\frac{p}{1-p}$ where p is the proportion of endorsing a response on an item. Logit is the linear unit that expresses the odds of endorsement (for multiple choices) or success (for yes or no) on any given item. The modern measurement method of item response theory provides scores in logits. The scale is centered around 0, which is the average item difficulty. Higher scores indicate easier items, and lower scores indicate harder items. Item-level analysis can be obtained in a score report, as can the person measure (i.e., the score a person obtains as opposed to an item measure, which is the difficulty level for an item). The person measure in logits can be interpreted as the standard total score. Because logit scores are harder to interpret, it is best practice for test developers to provide a T score conversion for easier application.

TOTAL VS. SUBSCALE SCORES

Occupational therapists are frequently presented with the dilemma of using subscale scores versus total scores. Subscale scores are the scores obtained for each subscale of the test and total score is the overall single score for the test (e.g., Montreal Cognitive Assessmnt [MOCA] (Nasreddine, et al., 2005) has seven subscales, each with its own score and it also provides an overall total score). The purpose of the test and the instructions in the manual should guide therapists in making this decision. If the available information is inadequate, a cautious approach would be to use subscale scores that are applicable to one specific dimension of interest and could be more meaningful to interpret than the total score. Therapists should conduct a thorough review of available tests to find one that presents little ambiguity related to scoring and score interpretation. The burden of test administration includes the scoring challenges a test presents, and therapists need to evaluate these challenges prior to test selection.

SCREENING TOOLS AND CUTOFF SCORES

A *screening tool* is a brief assessment used to identify at-risk individuals for further evaluation. *Cutoff scores* are specific score ranges that indicate the potential presence or absence of a disease, condition, or impairment. It. The psychometric properties to consider for screening tools are the validity in terms of sensitivity, specificity, and predictive value. Tests not developed specifically for screening would not have these properties established for valid use in screening. Screening tools can be norm referenced or criterion referenced, and cutoff scores can take the formats of percentiles, *T* scores, *z* scores, or logits. The use of standard scores is best practice when making high-stakes decisions on the basis of cutoff scores.

SHARING SCORES WITH CLIENTS AND FAMILIES

Although the score conversion process is intended to improve the communication of results to clients and families, in reality occupational therapists must address many barriers to make communication of results with clients and families a common practice. First, therapists must themselves develop comfort and self-efficacy in obtaining and interpreting test scores, which requires time and practice. Second, therapists must understand the needs of the client and determine whether the test provides meaningful information that needs to be shared. Third, therapists must understand the correct use of and value to be placed on the measure, requiring self-reflection on clinical practice. Inappropriate and unethical practices can result from using a measure for a purpose unintended by the test developers. For example, if a test is meant to be used for screening, its use for evaluating outcomes and clinical change is inappropriate. Therapists must engage clients in the testing process for best client-centered care in the following ways:

- Inform the client about the test to be administered and its purpose.
- Consider situational, environmental, and personal issues that may result in test bias.
- Administer the test in a standardized manner.
- Score the test, interpret the results, and document the results.
- Discuss the test administration process, scores, and your interpretation of results with clients and appropriate stakeholders, including families.
- Gather feedback regarding the test process and results from the client to inform future testing.

SUMMARY

Occupational therapists need to understand the process of scoring and interpretation. Essential statistical concepts can provide an understanding of the types of scores and the meaning that can be attributed to them. Therapists can assertively share assessment results with team members, payers, clients, and families if they have a thorough understanding of scores and their interpretation.

QUESTIONS

1. What are the advantages of standardized outcome measures over non-standardized surveys?
2. Why is it important to control for error in scoring tests? Give an example of how the errors in scoring might influence the scores you assigned to a client's performance or that might influence the client's response on a questionnaire.
3. Calculate the mean, median, and mode for the following set of test scores: 8, 1, 3, 14, 35, 5, 4, 8, 9, 10, 11, 2, 10, 9, 8, 7, and 6. Plot these scores on a graph and label the mean, median, and mode. Remove the score of 35 and redo the exercise. What happened to the measures of central tendency? What is the clinical relevance of this exercise?
4. What are cut-off scores? Do you use any screening tools in your setting that have cut-off scores? What is the interpretation associated with the cut-off score for that screening tool?
5. Why is it important to share scores with clients and families? Are there instances where this will not be feasible in your setting?

REFERENCES

Cella, D., Nowinski, C., Peterman, A., Victorson, D., Miller, D., Lai, J.-S., & Moy, C. (2011). The neurology quality-of-life measurement initiative. *Archives of Physical Medicine and Rehabilitation, 92*(10 Suppl.), S28–S36. https://doi.org/10.1016/j.apmr.2011.01.025

Classen, S., & Velozo, C. A. (2019). Critiquing assessments. In B. A. B. Schell & G. Gillen (Eds.), *Willard and Spackman's occupational therapy* (13th ed., pp. 390–412). Philadelphia: Wolters Kluwer.

Funder, D. C., Furr, M. R., & Colvin, R. C. (2000). The Riverside Behavioral Q-sort: A tool for the description of social behavior. *Journal of Personality, 68,* 451–489. https://doi.org/10.1111/1467-6494.00103

Furr, R. M., & Bacharach, V. R. (2014). *Psychometrics: An introduction* (2nd ed.). Thousand Oaks, CA: Sage.

Grampurohit, N., Slavin, M., Ni, P., Kozin, S., Jette, A., & Mulcahey, M. (2019). Sensitivity of the Cerebral Palsy Profile of Health and Function: Upper-extremity domain's sensitivity to change following musculoskeletal surgery. *Journal of Hand Surgery, 44,* 274–287. https://doi.org/10.1016/j.jhsa.2018.12.007

Griffiths, A., Toovey, R., Morgan, P. E., Spittle, A. J. (2018). Psychometric properties of gross motor assessment tools for children: A systematic review. *BMJ Open, 8*(10), e021734. https://doi.org/10.1136/bmjopen-2018-021734

Hammill, D. D., Pearson, N. A., & Voress, J. K. (2014). *Developmental Test of Visual Perception* (3rd ed.). Austin, TX: Pro-Ed.

Hinojosa, J., & Kramer, P. (2014). *Evaluation in occupational therapy: Obtaining and interpreting data* (4th ed.). Bethesda, MD: AOTA Press.

Hobson, J. P., Edwards, N. I., & Meara, R. J. (2001). The Parkinson's Disease Activities of Daily Living Scale: A new simple and brief subjective measure of disability in Parkinson's disease. *Clinical Rehabilitation, 15*, 241–246. https://doi.org/10.1191/026921501666767060

Hong, I., Velozo, C. A., Li, C.-Y., Romero, S., Gruber-Baldini, A. L., & Shulman, L. M. (2016). Assessment of the psychometrics of a PROMIS item bank: Self-efficacy for managing daily activities. *Quality of Life Research, 25*, 2221–2232. https://doi.org/10.1007/s11136-016-1270-1

Jansen, C., Niebuhr, B. R., Coussirat, D. J., Hawthorne, D., Moreno, L., & Phillip, M. (2008). Hand force of men and women over 65 years of age as measured by maximum pinch and grip force. *Journal of Aging and Physical Activity, 16*, 24–41. https://doi.org/10.1123/japa.16.1.24

Jebsen, R. H., Taylor, N., Trieschmann, R. B., Trotter, M. J., & Howard, L. A. (1969). An objective and standardized test of hand function. *Archives of Physical Medicine and Rehabilitation, 50*(6), 311–319.

Jette, A. M., Slavin, M. D., Ni, P., Kisala, P. A., Tulsky, D. S., Heinemann, A. W., . . . Williams, S. (2015). Development and initial evaluation of the SCI-FI/AT. *Journal of Spinal Cord Medicine, 38*, 409–418. https://doi.org/10.1179/2045772315Y.0000000003

Law, M., Baptiste, S., Carswell, A., McColl, M. A., Polatajko, H., & Pollock, N. (2019). *Canadian Occupational Performance Measure* (5th ed., rev.). Ottawa, ON: COPM, Inc.

Mathiowetz, V., Volland, G., Kashman, N., & Weber, K. (1985). Adult norms for the Box and Block Test of manual dexterity. *American Journal of Occupational Therapy, 39*, 386–391. https://doi.org/10.5014/ajot.39.6.386

Mathiowetz, V., Weber, K., Kashman, N., & Volland, G. (1985). Adult norms for the Nine Hole Peg Test of finger dexterity. *OTJR: Occupation, Participation and Health, 5*, 24–38. https://doi.org/10.1177/153944928500500102

Nasreddine, Z. S., Phillips, N. A., Bédirian, V., Charbonneau, S., Whitehead, V., Collin, I., . . . Chertkow, H. (2005). The Montreal Cognitive Assessment, MoCA: A brief screening tool for mild cognitive impairment. *Journal of the American Geriatrics Society, 53*, 695–699. https://doi.org/10.1111/j.1532-5415.2005.53221.x

Otis, A., & Lennon, R. (2019). *Otis–Lennon School Ability Test* (8th ed.). London, UK: Pearson Education.

Oxford, G. K., Vogel, K. A., Le, V., Mitchell, A., Muniz, S., & Vollmer, M. A. (2003). Adult norms for a commercially available Nine Hole Peg Test for finger dexterity. *American Journal of Occupational Therapy, 57*, 570–573. https://doi.org/10.5014/ajot.57.5.570

Portney, L. G., & Watkins, M. P. (2009). *Foundations of clinical research: Applications to practice* (3rd ed.). Upper Saddle River, NJ: Pearson/Prentice Hall.

Robinson, B. C. (1983). Validation of a Caregiver Strain Index. *Journal of Gerontology, 38*, 344–348. https://doi.org/10.1093/geronj/38.3.344

Sears, E. D., & Chung, K. C. (2010). Validity and responsiveness of the Jebsen–Taylor Hand Function Test. *Journal of Hand Surgery, 35*, 30–37. https://doi.org/10.1016/j.jhsa.2009.09.008

Tavasoli, A., Azimi, P., & Montazari, A. (2014). Reliability and validity of the Peabody Developmental Motor Scales–second edition for assessing motor development of low birth weight preterm infants. *Pediatric Neurology, 51*, 522–526. https://doi.org/10.1016/j.pediatrneurol.2014.06.010

U.S. Department of Labor, Employment and Training Administration. (1999). *Using, scoring, and interpreting assessment instruments.* Retrieved from https://hr-guide.com/data/G366.htm

Velozo, C. A., Seel, R. T., Magasi, S., Heinemann, A. W., & Romero, S. (2012). Improving measurement methods in rehabilitation: Core concepts and recommendations for scale development. *Archives of Physical Medicine and Rehabilitation, 93*(8 Suppl.), S154–S163. https://doi.org/10.1016/j.apmr.2012.06.001

Interpretation and Documentation of the Evaluation Process

Rondalyn V. Whitney, PhD, OTR/L, FAOTA, and Wendy E. Walsh, PhD, OTR/L

11

CHAPTER HIGHLIGHTS

- Interpretation
- Solving a patient mystery through review of documentation
- Applying a theoretical rationale
- Accounting for testing bias
- Synthesizing multiple data points
- Defending evaluation results
- Documentation
- Types of evaluation documentation
- Guidelines for documentation of occupational therapy

KEY TERMS AND CONCEPTS

- Accessibility
- Confidentiality
- Data, Assessment, and Plan (DAP) note
- Discharge documentation
- Discharge summary
- Discrepancy analysis
- Documentation
- Evaluation report
- Family Educational Rights and Privacy Act of 1974
- Formative evaluations
- *Guidelines for Documentation of Occupational Therapy*

- Health Insurance Portability and Accountability Act of 1996
- Initial documentation
- Interpretation
- Narrative documentation
- Patient Protection and Affordable Care Act of 2010
- PERFORM Templates
- Periodic reassessment
- Person–Item–Environment (PIE)
- Privacy
- Progress documentation
- Progress notes
- Reassessment process

- Reassessment report
- Reevaluation
- Relevant, Understandable, Measurable, Behavioral, Achievable (RUMBA) note
- Security
- Screenings
- Subjective, Objective, Assessment, and Plan (SOAP) note
- Summative evaluation
- Synthesis of multiple data points
- Template-based documentation
- Testing bias
- Theoretical rationale

INTRODUCTION

Interpretation, a critical element of the evaluation process, refers to the extraction of meaning from data collected through quantitative (i.e., standardized) and qualitative (i.e., nonstandardized) methods. Accurate interpretation of data is required for using inductive and deductive reasoning to inform service delivery decisions, a process fundamental to evidence-based intervention planning. The section on interpretation includes information on factors that contribute to the transition from evaluation to intervention planning, including applying a theoretical framework, accounting for testing bias, synthesizing multiple data points, and defending evaluation results.

Documentation tells a story, and like storytelling, the process of documentation involves discovery of new ideas and new connections between concepts, creates new perspectives, and ultimately empowers thought through the written word. Whereas scholarly writing tells the story of your research, professional documentation tells the story of a client's experiences with occupational therapy. In many ways, documentation follows a conventional narrative structure, including who the main character (the client) is, what problems the client needs to solve, what the narrator (the occupational therapist) observes (measures) about the client, and how the client's problems will be solved (i.e., intervention plan) or that you have made a difference worthy of reimbursement (i.e., a discharge summary).

The section on documentation discusses the purposes and types of evaluation documentation, style and settings, data gathering and storage formats, health information privacy and confidentiality, accessibility and security

https://doi.org/10.7139/2020.978-1-56900-596-5.011

concerns, and helpful recommendations for writing effective documentation.

INTERPRETATION

Interpreting evaluation results is a primary part of the occupational therapist's job. Although many standardized assessment instruments have computer applications that score a client's performance and are advertised as capable of interpreting scores, interpretation of scores within the client's contexts is the principal realm of occupational therapists. Interpreting evaluation information is an art that requires theoretical knowledge, clinical reasoning, reflection, and practice. The results of standardized assessments are useful in documenting the presence and degree of deficits clients experience. However, occupational therapists must correctly interpret the results to assess how functional deficits might interfere with the performance of everyday skills and occupations. When interpreting data, therapists include interpretation and recommendations. This is the section of the report where the examiner's comments, suggestions for interventions, and discussion of test validity are documented.

Solving a Mystery Through a Case Review

Consider the mystery story of **Logan,** a boy age 5 years who attended preschool. **Amy,** a pediatric occupational therapist, received an impassioned plea from Logan's parents for an evaluation for their son. The parents disclosed that another therapist had performed an evaluation 4 months previously and had concluded that Logan was not eligible for direct occupational therapy services and that, as a boy, "he just doesn't want to write."

Amy reviewed the documentation and noted that the previous therapist had administered the Peabody Developmental Motor Scales (PDMS–2; Folio & Fewell, 2000). Logan's Fine Motor Quotient, shown in Table 11.1, indicated average performance and was the basis for the direct service ineligibility decision. However, Logan's parents reported behaviors that indicated he was experiencing challenges in typical developmental tasks for children of his age. When asked to write letters, numbers, or his name during classroom instruction, and when required to open and close his lunchbox and containers at lunchtime, Logan had begun to display tantrums and to run out of the room, and recently he had bitten his teacher.

TABLE 11.1.   Logan's Fine Motor Subscale Scores on the Peabody Developmental Motor Scales

SUBSCALE	STANDARD SCORE	PERCENTILE	PERFORMANCE
Grasping	5	5	Very poor
Visual–Motor Integration	13	84	Superior
Fine Motor Quotient	94**	36**	Average

Note. ** indicates average performance.

The mystery of Logan's behavior and his ineligibility for services deepened when Amy looked at Logan's scores. Amy's detective work focused on Logan's PDMS–2 scores and revealed that the testing procedures had been adequate, but the mystery was why Logan scored as average when his Grasping subtest score showed limited ability to grasp objects (e.g., pencils, cups, crayons, close zippers). The original therapist had noted in the documentation that during testing, Logan refused to hold the marker ("it's slimy"), was unable to button or unbutton buttons in the time allowed ("they're itchy"), and refused to engage in a nonstandardized assessment of touching thumb to fingers (he did not watch the demonstration). The mystery seemed to lie in the interpretation of the PDMS–2 results.

Discrepancy analysis

Any significant discrepancy between findings on related subtests offers clues about the client's day-to-day functional capacity. In Logan's case, Amy noted a discrepancy in his scores on two PDMS–2 subtests that was useful in generating a hypothesis regarding his performance.

Logan's Grasping score was in the 5th percentile, yet his Visual–Motor Integration score was in the 84th percentile. As operationalized in the PDMS–2 scoring criteria, these two scores were combined to yield Logan's Fine Motor Quotient, which indicated "average" performance. In fact, Logan's ability to perceive visual information was well above that of most of his peers, but his ability to grasp and manipulate items was well below that of most of his peers. Children with a high Fine Motor Quotient are described in the test manual as "good with their hands," but this was clearly not the case for Logan. Amy deduced that the previous therapist had provided an incomplete interpretation of the PDMS–2 findings.

Occupational therapists should be suspicious when one section of a test (i.e., subtest score) is much higher than another, related subtest score, especially when such scores are averaged. When a wide difference is present, explanations such as testing error, distraction, or subject error (i.e., inattention, poor attitude, or lack of motivation) should be considered. Importantly, taking an average of two scores that vary widely is not to be understood as a meaningful "average." Fortunately, examiner manuals may provide guidance for how to address this type of discrepancy. The PDMS–2 manual recommends conducting a discrepancy analysis to identify whether, when, and to what degree a variance in scores is important and how this information should influence the therapist's interpretation and plan for intervention.

Discrepancy analysis is a step-by-step examination of a between-subtest and between-quotient variance that involves consultation of a table of significance. This information enables therapists to interpret whether differences between scores are meaningful and significant. Table 4.4 in the PDMS–2 manual provides data necessary to assess whether a difference between subtest scores is beyond that which would be accounted for by chance or other factors such as subject error or environmental factors. In Logan's case, the threshold (i.e., difference score) for a meaningful discrepancy is 2, meaning that if the scores on two subtests differ by 2 or more points, the composite of the two scores should be considered suspect.

Amy's interpretation of Logan's scores

Amy concluded that Logan did not require a reevaluation, but the previous evaluation report needed reinterpretation. Exhibit 11.1 shows what Amy wrote in her report.

Occupational therapists are detectives (figuratively) who search for clues, test hypotheses, interpret findings, draw conclusions, and disseminate discoveries. So "solving mysteries" is an appropriate metaphor for the practice of evaluation in occupational therapy. Therapists use data-driven assessment to solve the mystery of why a client is struggling to fully participate in the occupations of his or her role (in Logan's case, the role of student).

Logan's previous occupational therapist failed to follow the primary directive of evaluation: Tests don't diagnose; people do. Basing decisions solely on a test result is ill advised; test scores are only one type of observation necessary to inform a clinical hypothesis. It would also have been helpful if she had included his parents' or teachers' concerns about his performance when coming to her conclusions. Amy was suspicious of the fine motor composite score, whereas the original therapist was not. Amy followed the clinical reasoning that a child who was behaving as Logan was might have more of a story to tell than not liking to write. Her sleuthing took her back to the data gathering and manual to guide interpretation.

Logan's case illustrates occupational therapists' responsibility to form a hypothesis about the cause of a problem given the test results, rather than considering the test results alone to provide the hypothesis. Accurate assessment interpretation combines data about the child, the child's contextual factors, the testing environment, and the test outcomes.

Next steps for Logan

Although the previous occupational therapist had determined that Logan was ineligible for direct service intervention, Amy applied the theoretical foundation of developmental theory; accounted for testing bias (indicated by the wide gap between scores on the two subscales); considered the meaning of data when data points are contradictory; and reevaluated the standardized assessment results, guided by advanced clinical knowledge and intuition. Amy questioned the common use of norms based on age to determine developmental delay and eligibility for occupational therapy services. After analyzing Logan's two reports, Amy returned to the examiner's manual to seek guidance for unusual findings—in this case discrepancy in scores resulting in what seemed to be a result that failed to match her clinical intuition. She provided a new evaluation report justifying Logan's eligibility for direct services using a persuasive narrative to tell the story of a child who was overwhelmed by the difficulties he faced when asked to perform seemingly simple tasks, and she used a deductive approach to decision making about intervention planning. Ultimately, Amy solved a mystery for Logan's family and wrote a developmentally appropriate intervention plan that had the potential to close the gap between Logan's current performance and his potential.

Applying a Theoretical Rationale

Assessments are usually based on a theoretical perspective or rationale. In best practice, occupational therapists choose an assessment based on the theoretical rationale that they think will work best with a client. To consistently link theory and practice, evaluation and intervention planning must be grounded in theory; occupational therapists use theory to organize thinking and begin the clinical reasoning process.

Selecting an appropriate theoretical rationale to guide evaluation and treatment comes after careful consideration of the client. This includes a review of the referral and presenting problems, a discussion with significant others about the problem (parents and teachers in the case of a child, and

---

EXHIBIT 11.1.   Amy's Documentation of Logan's Reinterpreted Assessment Scores

Logan used his dominant (right) hand for all fine motor tasks on the Peabody Developmental Motor Scales (PDMS–2; Folio & Fewell, 2000). A composite score was derived for Logan's Grasping and Visual–Motor Integration subtest scores, indicating that Logan's fine motor skills were "average" for his age level (5 years). However, Logan's scores on the two subtests are highly discrepant, and the PDMS–2 manual provides guidance for conducting a discrepancy analysis to determine the significance of the difference in these subtest scores (Folio & Fewell, 2000, p. 34).

Logan's standard score of 5 on the Grasping subtest reflects "very poor" performance, whereas his standard score of 13 on the Visual–Motor Integration subtest reflects "superior" performance. When these two subtest scores are converted to the Fine Motor Quotient, the result is interpreted as "average" performance. This finding, however, masks the challenges Logan experiences with occupations related to task performance, and the discrepancy analysis determined this difference was significant. His superior skills in recognizing visual–spatial information (e.g., replicating shapes, connecting dots) are not supported by his below-average skills in using the small muscles of his hands to perform fine motor tasks such as drawing, cutting, and grasping. This gap between skills is a likely explanation for Logan's observed frustration, avoidance, and nonadaptive behavior.

A review of the examiner's notes indicates that the PDMS–2 tasks related to grasping should have been considered unscorable because of subject error, evident in clinical observations of Logan's avoidance and inattention behaviors that further support the significance of the discrepancy.

The clinical hypothesis is that Logan will benefit from developing greater tolerance of sensations and participating in activities to foster develop of the muscles in his hands. These activities will support Logan's development in the area of grasp, promote adaptive strategies for frustration tolerance, and increase his ability to use his gifts related to visual–motor integration in occupations related to school, home, and play. Intervention aimed to improve grasping patterns will allow Logan to take advantage of his strong visual–motor skills in school. Closing the gap early will support Logan's ability to participate in the general curriculum and prevent maladaptive behaviors (avoidance) currently exhibited. A short course of intervention (six sessions and a home program to improve functional hand use) is recommended, together with three consultation sessions with the teacher as Logan completes this academic year.

with an adult when they agree to the therapist talking with significant others), and an observation of the client when performing tasks. Administering an occupational profile may also be helpful in choosing a theoretical perspective through the identification of areas of importance to the client and specific supports and barriers to occupational performance. An appropriate *theoretical rationale* guides the complete evaluation and intervention, identifying methods for measuring treatment outcomes.

In the case of Logan, Amy determined a developmental approach was the most the most appropriate theoretical rationale based on observations and the previous assessment used (the PDMS–2), which uses developmental theory. Amy used clinical reasoning to assess Logan's problem and determined it to be a developmental delay. Using this theoretical perspective allowed Amy to identify the expected performance for Logan's age, his current performance, and interventions that might close the gap.

Accounting for Testing Bias

The goal of testing is to determine the actual performance of the person being evaluated, but testing bias can influence an evaluation and must be accounted for. *Testing bias* may be, in part, cultural bias such as when testing is applied to a specific group that has not been used in developing the normative data of the test. Testing bias can also occur when the person giving the test does not adhere to test specifications such as giving prompts, modifies items on the test, presents an item totally unfamiliar to the client, or gives the assessment in a distracting or inappropriate environment. Optimal conditions are not always possible, but occupational therapists should strive to control for as much testing bias as possible. When any change in the testing specifications or the environment is a barrier to accurate assessment of performance, therapists must include this in the evaluation report.

When thinking about bias, occupational therapists must consider the *person-item-environment (PIE)*; the acronym can be a helpful reminder of these three important considerations for bias (discussed in Chapter 8, "Nonstandardized Assessments"). Amy ruled out *person* for several reasons: Logan had been observed by people who were familiar to him; his previous therapist had selected the PDMS–2, a widely used assessment instrument that was age appropriate for Logan; and his family appeared to be accurate reporters and good historians. She ruled out *environment* because Logan was familiar with the facility where his evaluation was conducted. Amy's suspicions therefore centered on *item*, and she used the test manual to determine how to reinterpret the item data she had received. For more information on avoiding bias in testing and accommodating diversity in testing, see Chapter 13, "Addressing Diversity in Occupational Therapy Assessment."

Synthesizing Multiple Data Points

To interpret assessment findings, summarizing multiple data points is not enough. Occupational therapists must engage in *synthesis of multiple data points,* which refers to evaluating and putting data together in a meaningful way. This involves making certain that the qualitative

and quantitative information collected during evaluation provide a holistic and accurate picture of the client's occupational performance. Failure to do so can result in misinterpretation of the data. Occupational therapists are highly valued because of their ability to accurately synthesize the evaluation data to develop a targeted and effective intervention plan.

Logan's story demonstrates how easily interpretation of data points can go awry. The previous therapist had based the direct service ineligibility decision on the age equivalent for Logan's Fine Motor Quotient but not for the component subtest scores. Age equivalents present substantial potential for misinterpretation when used to determine service delivery and should be interpreted with caution. For example, assessing a child age 6 months using a developmental assessment makes perfect sense. However, if that child had been born at 24 weeks gestation, the chronological age would need to be adjusted, and this step should be included in the report.

Occupational therapists understand reporting normalized standard scores, but they may have difficulty interpreting just what they mean. Therapists also need to understand that raw scores alone cannot take the place of the professional reasoning that is required to look at all the data and not just the raw score. Logan's initial report appeared to describe detailed clinical observations of Logan but actually used the language of individual test items from the assessment instrument. The clinical observations that are seen need to be synthesized with an understanding of the individual test items so that a comprehensive picture of the child can be effectively presented in the report. Interpretive guides for individual test items are often found in test manuals and can be helpful.

Amy gave Logan's parents a document that included reconstructed raw scores, hand-calculated standard scores, interpretations of all derived scale scores, and a narrative report with important clinical observations of Logan. Amy told the family that the original reports included raw scores and enough data to reevaluate, which indicated good practice on the part of the previous therapist. Amy could determine that the raw scores and individual percentiles for performance better explained Logan's developmental function. Amy compared Logan's performance with children in his age group, synthesized what this information said about Logan's ability to perform school-based tasks, and issued a new eligibility determination. He was eligible for direct services because he had serious developmental delays that were evident in the previous evaluation document but previously unrecognized because Logan's previous therapist summarized but did not synthesize the test findings into an accurate interpretation.

Defending Evaluation Results

Even when occupational therapists have finalized and disseminated the evaluation report, the job is not done. The report, which lives forever in records, must be defensible. Logan's original report did not meet this criterion; Amy's sleuthing revealed that Logan had been denied direct services on the basis of an indefensible evaluation interpretation. After dissecting Logan's report, Amy was able to defend the validity of the testing but not the accuracy of the interpreted findings. Solving the mystery of Logan's previous evaluation revealed the power—both positive and negative—of interpretation.

In another example involving defense of evaluation results, a resident-to-resident altercation at a skilled nursing facility (SNF) resulted in legal action. The legal teams for both parties carefully reviewed all available medical records pertaining to their clients, so occupational therapy documentation was part of the legal case. The occupational therapist who provided the initial evaluation for the defendant was subpoenaed for testimony. The evaluation report revealed a comprehensive review of the client, noting that they were functionally independent but required supervision for activities involving cognitive processing and safety. No further occupational therapy services were warranted as the client's discharge placement was indicated to be with significant supports. This was carefully written up in the summary section of the evaluation report, and the treatment record for occupational therapy was closed.

The subpoena occurred 5 years after the initial evaluation, during which time the occupational therapist had performed hundreds of evaluations at the SNF. The therapist could not immediately recall the resident, but after reviewing the documentation, which included the detailed evaluation report, the therapist was able to recall specifics about that client and evaluation and provide testimony. The detailed evaluation summary clearly identified that there was no need for occupational therapy since the client was discharged to a setting with significant supports. Because of this summary, the therapist was able to defend her recommendation and occupational therapy was not a part of this legal action.

DOCUMENTATION

Purpose

The primary purpose of documentation—evaluation reports, in particular—is communication. According to the *Guidelines for Documentation of Occupational Therapy*,

The purpose of documentation is to
- Communicate information about the client's occupational history and experiences, strengths and limitations, interests, values, and needs;
- Articulate the rationale for provision of occupational therapy services and the relationship of those services to client outcomes, reflecting the occupational therapy practitioner's clinical reasoning and professional judgment; and
- Provide a clear chronological record of client status, the nature of occupational therapy services provided, client response to occupational therapy intervention, and client outcomes; and
- Provide an accurate justification for skilled occupational therapy service necessity and reimbursement (American Occupational Therapy Association [AOTA], 2018, p. 1).

Evaluation and documentation occur in all service delivery settings, and it is the obligation of each occupational therapist to generate accurate and complete reports that clearly communicate the occupational therapy process for all therapeutic engagements.

Documentation is also important for educating other professionals, justifying reimbursement, research, and preserving a permanent legal record of services rendered. When occupational therapists take care in writing detailed, descriptive reports, documentation can show the value of occupational therapy services and teach people outside the profession how its distinct value can improve clients' lives. For third-party payers, documentation is the sole basis for determining whether to reimburse for occupational therapy services. Finally, documentation is a legal record of services provided and outcomes obtained. This permanent record serves as the memory of client engagements when therapists are asked to recall individual client visits after significant time has passed.

Documentation can also serve as the basis for outcome research studies, quality assurance, and other forms of program review. On a smaller scale, occupational therapists can complete an outcome study at the case report level for each client who receives services. With many reimbursement sources mandating meaningful practical improvement in clients' function, therapists are obligated to demonstrate improvement as an outcome if services are authorized (Smith, 2013).

Although some occupational therapists believe a fine line divides research and evaluation, the two are more accurately represented as a continuum with research at one end and evaluation at the other, with documentation indicative of best practices located in the middle. Documentation using empirical data can provide evidence of meaningful clinical change resulting from occupational therapy services. Like single-subject research designs, single-case reports have inherently strong internal validity but correspondingly low external validity; generalization is not possible. To improve external validity, single-case reports can be replicated and accumulated. Electronic health records (EHRs) offer an integrated way of accumulating reports. If occupational therapists collect similar information and report findings in a consistent format, the search capabilities of EHRs can enable therapists to capture information on similar people, aggregate results, analyze outcomes, and demonstrate strong evidence of the effectiveness of occupational therapy (Smith, 2013).

Types of Evaluation Documentation

Documenting evaluation results has two aspects: (1) articulating the occupational therapy process as outlined in the *Occupational Therapy Practice Framework: Domain and Process* (OTPF; AOTA, 2014) and (2) annotating the process in the context of the service delivery model. Because evaluation documentation provides a snapshot of a client's occupational performance at a particular time, evaluation results are reported in initial, progress, and discharge (sometimes called *discontinuation*) documentation.

Initial documentation includes the evaluation report; ***progress documentation*** includes reassessment, which includes progress reports and reevaluation; and ***discharge documentation*** includes the discharge summary, which is usually written after the final intervention session. Initial evaluation reports are considered ***formative evaluations,***

occurring at the beginning of treatment. The discharge summary is a *summative evaluation,* occurring once treatment is over. If the initial evaluation recommendation is that no services are needed, the evaluation report also serves as the discharge report and can be considered summative.

Evaluation report

The *evaluation report* summarizes the occupational profile, providing a detailed portrait of the client as an occupational being with "history and experiences, patterns of daily living, interests, values, and needs" (AOTA, 2014, p. S10), and the analysis of occupational performance, which identifies the client's areas of function and dysfunction within various contexts. The evaluation report summarizes and synthesizes the assessment findings, explains the therapist's clinical reasoning, and lists goals for functional outcomes. The evaluation assesses the person, the environment, and occupations in relevant contexts. This document is typically the basis for beginning therapeutic intervention and sets the stage for selection of functional measures. Although it may sound counterintuitive, a plan for reassessment and discharge is initiated during the initial evaluation.

Progress notes and reassessment reports

Progress notes and reassessment reports are integral components of the evaluation process in occupational therapy and are defined in terms of their purpose and client goals. The *OTPF* underscores the importance of data collection during intervention as a method of directing the therapy process. Documenting interim assessment data demonstrates collaboration between client and therapist and formally establishes the value of occupational therapy services to the client. As occupational therapists create the occupational profile and conduct the analysis of occupational performance, they construct the plan for intervention, the plan for determining progress, and an estimated plan for when the therapeutic intervention will meet the client's objectives.

Progress notes are generally written after each session to continuously gather data and document changes in function, participation, and progress through observations, interactions, and administration of specific assessments when necessary. As clients progress through treatment, occupational therapists continually ask themselves essential questions to guide and refine intervention, such as "Is this client making progress toward goals?" and "Are the frequency, intensity, and duration of treatment still appropriate?" Occupational therapy practitioners complete systematic documentation of the client's current state of function in the form of daily, weekly, or monthly treatment notes, as required by systems for reimbursement.

Reassessment data should influence the ongoing therapeutic process as well as the potential for discharge. The *reassessment report* often uses standardized assessment tools to documents and record progress. Many systems require *periodic reassessment*, which may be done for all aspects of intervention with the client or for one specific area of intervention. Reassessment is generally done periodically during the intervention. The *reassessment process* includes (1) data collection, (2) reflection, and (3) decision making. For example, a hand therapist might use dynamometer readings to determine whether a client's hand strength is improving and moving toward the documented goal. Additionally, the hand therapist would reassess progress by routinely collecting data from dynamometer and pinch gauge readings; client reports of pain severity, sensitivity location, and ADL performance; and goal attainment scaling scores to determine whether the client is ready for discharge from services. Like all occupational therapy documentation, a reassessment report focuses on the occupational performance of the client and the occupational value of the skills being assessed (Gillen, 2013).

Reconsidering a client's progress, providing feedback to the client, selecting next steps in treatment, and sharing information with caregivers and other professionals contribute to the establishment of progressive goals and collective decision making. A *reevaluation* that only uses assessments from the initial evaluation cannot capture the qualitative information gained through the collaborative relationship with clients and their families.

Some systems also require a full reevaluation prior to considering discharge. This would include the use of standardized and nonstandardized assessments for all aspects of treatment with the clients.

Discharge summary

Once the client has reached the previously set goals, the occupational therapist writes a *discharge summary.* In most cases, the discharge summary requires noting where the patient started with a short review of the evaluation report. This is followed by reviewing the progress made during treatment, including observations and functional performance, and discussion of the reassessment process, including where specific assessments were given to demonstrate progress. The discharge summary includes reassessment and/or reevaluation data and a statement as to whether the client has completed therapy or is going on to another facility and, if so, whether therapy should be considered at the new placement.

Style and Setting

There is no one-size-fits-all approach to writing documentation, and each facility or agency determines the style to be used in that service delivery context. This can be very disconcerting to students learning the process of note writing. Each facility (or agency) determines the appropriate documentation style that is used. Some organizations favor *narrative documentation,* which usually consists of information written in paragraph form, often with headings that show key assessment areas. This style is common in community settings, school-based practice, and home health agency settings. Narrative documentation allows occupational therapists to incorporate the context of occupation as presented by the individual client.

More typical medical-model settings favor the use of *template-based documentation,* in which practitioners record information using checklists or forms designed for efficiency. Occupational therapists using medical documentation software to complete reports or progress notes select responses from prefabricated, drop-down menus on a computer or peripheral device (e.g., tablet, smartphone). Often, when the form is completed, the documentation is done, and no further writing is required. Documentation textbooks such as those by Gateley and Borcherding (2018), Sames (2015), and Frolek Clark and Handley-More (2017) discuss the intricacies of documentation style in greater detail.

Regardless of style or setting, the content within the documentation should reflect accurately the interactions and observations that occur during the interventions. In telehealth practice, evaluation, progress documentation, and reassessment may need to take place when the occupational therapist is not in the same physical location as the client and can be provided virtually via technology interface in some states across the country. Studies of telehealth have demonstrated both feasibility and effectiveness in many areas of practice (Gately et al., 2019; Renda & Lape, 2018; Whitney & Smith, 2015; Worboys et al., 2018). Whether a client is seen in person or via electronic communication, appropriate documentation must occur. (For more information on evaluation issues in telehealth, see Chapter 14, "Evaluation in Emerging Practice Settings.")

Good descriptors for the process of client engagement, measurement of client performance, and details of the service delivery context must all be present in occupational therapy documentation. To help promote thoroughness in documentation, several systems with acronym mnemonics have emerged to help practitioners and students master the written note using acronyms. Several varieties of acronym-style documentation are used in different settings, including:

- *SOAP note—Subjective, Objective, Assessment, and Plan*
- *DAP note—Data, Assessment, and Plan* (the S and O of the SOAP note are combined into D, the Data section; Gateley & Borcherding, 2018; Sames, 2013)
- *RUMBA note—Relevant, Understandable, Measurable, Behavioral, and Achievable.*

Regardless of the style used, occupational therapists are responsible for accurate and thorough reporting based on assessment outcomes, documented observations, and clinical reasoning. When a checklist does not permit sufficient description of individual evaluation outcomes, therapists are responsible for ensuring that complete documentation is recorded in a narrative addendum to the response.

Data Gathering and Storage Formats

The data gathering and storage formats of documentation has undergone a shift in recent decades. Historically, therapists handwrote or typed evaluations and notes in a paper-based format. Now, with the advancement of technology, notations are less likely to be found in a handwritten format and more likely to be in an electronic format across the different service settings. EHRs are mandated by the **Health Insurance Portability and Accountability Act of 1996** (HIPAA; P. L. 104-191) and regulations under the **Patient Protection and Affordable Care Act of 2010** (P. L. 111-148). Many facilities are working to scan older paper-based documentation into EHRs to make it accessible electronically. In the earlier example of the subpoenaed therapist, the original handwritten documentation 5 years prior had been scanned into an electronic medical record which was viewable via computer screen.

The value of the electronic documentation format is its ease of use in entering and retrieving data. Unfortunately, the utility of medical documentation software is often limited by software designers' lack of a firm understanding of all the services for which practitioners use this documentation method. For example, checklists are often insufficiently specific to reflect the assessment areas in the occupational therapy scope of practice. In addition, digital records can become unavailable if the computer is down, the server is overloaded, the system has crashed, the router has difficulties, or the power has gone out. To provide continuity of care during electronic glitches, some therapists and departments carry printouts of their basic EHR template to record client information. Specific strengths and weaknesses of electronic documentation are outlined in Table 11.2.

TABLE 11.2. Strengths and Weaknesses of Electronic Documentation

CONSIDERATION	STRENGTHS	WEAKNESSES
Cost	- Can save employee time	- May be expensive (*see also* Integration)
Design	- Can be specified, but may not be done easily - Increases interprofessional communication - Ensures consistent language use in reporting	- May be inconsistent across different settings and medical documentation software companies
Template	- Customizable	- Prescriptive
Reliability	- Enables uniformity within facilities and across sites - Provides Internet or cloud-based access anywhere within the site	- May involve unpredictable Internet or cloud-based access
Rigidity	- Promotes consistency in data	- May entail designer-imposed rigidity - Imposes format choices that are difficult to amend
Time	- Quick - Efficient	- May create opportunities for error because of temporal demands for virtual documentation input
Integration	- Allows interface with other facility systems (e.g., payment, registration, discharge communication)	- When using external medical documentation platforms, may not easily integrate into existing facility software systems, if at all, and integration efforts may prove costly

AOTA has provided a resource occupational therapists can use to overcome many of the weaknesses in EHR software identified in Table 11.2. The **PERFORM Templates** are based on the *OTPF* and offer specific suggestions for data to be documented in an EHR (AOTA, 2017). Occupational therapists should advocate for the inclusion of these professional organization–supported template solutions in the documentation system at their facility. Professional advocacy is key for the voice of occupational therapy to be heard outside the profession. EHRs are here to stay, so practitioners must learn to navigate and improve the quality of input into electronic documentation platforms to ensure the distinct value of occupational therapy is reflected in electronic documentation.

In addition to unique storage and retrieval opportunities, electronic documentation also has data mining capabilities. Data mining allows easy comparison of a single person to norm-referenced information (a typical group) or criterion-referenced information (a standard) as well as ipsative data that allow comparison of a single person's changes over time.

Health Information Privacy and Confidentiality

Information related to people receiving health care services has had **privacy** and **confidentiality** protections for centuries, and professional codes of ethics have emphasized them as basic tenets. Privacy and confidentiality are addressed in the *Occupational Therapy Code of Ethics* as part of the principle of Autonomy: "Occupational therapy personnel shall respect the right of the individual to self-determination, privacy, confidentiality, and consent" (AOTA, 2015, p. 4). Occupational therapy practitioners have an ethical obligation to ensure the privacy and confidentiality of clients' health information, and those who fail to do so can be sanctioned, including suspended for life from AOTA membership. For additional information on ethics, see Chapter 15, "Ethical Issues in Evaluation."

In addition to the *Code of Ethics,* occupational therapy practitioners must comply with state and federal laws' that protect patient and client privacy and confidentiality. Financial information was one of the first areas to receive federal privacy protections, and educational records have been protected since 1974 by the Family Educational Rights and Privacy Act (FERPA). HIPAA extended earlier privacy legislation to health care. HIPAA's two main goals are reflected in its name: (1) health insurance portability and (2) accountability. The EHR is the key to complying with portability mandated by HIPAA. EHRs allow the capture and storage of all of a person's health-related information and permit that person to transfer it to another insurance company. HIPAA also mandates accountability: explanation of costs in an effort to decrease waste and fraud. EHRs improve the efficiency of accountability.

FERPA mandates that student records be opened to parents on written request. As a result, evaluation reports in educational settings have evolved so that they can be understood by parents and professionals with diverse backgrounds and varied education. Once the bastion of professional eyes only, medical-model facility documentation is now being accessed by patients and clients exercising their HIPAA rights to see and get copies of their personal health information.

Accessibility and Security

Increased accessibility of health information to clients and other authorized parties through new technologies has implications for privacy and confidentiality. **Accessibility** refers to who can see the records, and **security** refers to the safety of the records. Accessibility and security are inversely related; as access increases, security decreases (Strauss, 2015). Early electronic health information systems were perhaps more secure than some newer web-based systems accessed with wireless devices. Earlier systems often were closed, consisting of computers interfaced in a wired network, and security risks primarily involved the people who used the input devices. The movement to wireless devices also decreases security and, by extension, privacy and confidentiality.

More recently, some facilities and organizations have moved to open (i.e., Internet-accessible) electronic health information systems designed to allow access through secure websites. It is important to know how and where access devices are connected at all times. Because personal health information is used and stored electronically, ensuring the security of this information is of utmost importance. Newspaper accounts contain horror stories of electronic health information inadvertently released to the general public through computers or hard drives that have been stolen or donated to charitable organizations. Less public violations of confidentiality occur frequently with information available to multiple people who use a single computer station.

To protect the privacy and confidentiality of Internet-based EHRs, security needs to be ensured not only at the end points of access device and secure website, but also at the midpoints of connection, when one enters the system and transmission when one sends information. Many facilities have information technology specialists on staff to provide consultation about processes to ensure the security of documentation at each point.

Access devices containing confidential client information can be lost, stolen, or cloned. Unsecured digital information can be replicated. Privacy is becoming increasingly problematic. To improve security, users can use various types of security applications (e.g., fire walls, encryption) to help improve security of personal access devices. Be sure to consider both employer and personal devices that may contain work-related references when determining how to secure confidential information. If a computer is shared by other people, a simple way to secure electronic information is to make sure that confidential files are closed before leaving the computer station. Client information can be saved to a password-protected folder or a portable storage device (e.g., USB memory drive) that has appropriate password protection and encryption and is always kept safe.

Using a secure access device and a secure website helps improve security, but the connection between the device and website is equally important. The safer hard-wired, closed system is often not an option when accessing the Internet. Although a computer terminal may be hardwired to a facility system, the facility system at some point will "open" when connected to an outside system to access the Internet. Theoretically, if an access device is open, any file saved internally or to a memory device or linking website can be accessed and stolen. A secure wireless connection offers some safety, but many wireless hotspots are essentially radio based, which allows opportunities for stealthy electronic eavesdropping and theft. Sometimes, access devices switch from one wireless connection to another without the user being aware that a change has occurred, resulting in unintentional connection and use of network services without explicit authorization.

Working from a secured access point may offer additional security. The connection also must be secured. Occupational therapists need to ensure that every connection they use is secure. For example, if a therapist is documenting while in transit, the access device may automatically change connections many times. When therapists cannot be certain that a connection is secure, they must manually turn off the device's automatic wireless capability and work offline until they have access to a secure connection. Later, the occupational therapist can make the connection manually with full knowledge of the wireless access point. Occupational therapists working on client records need to exercise extreme caution if using unsecured wireless access sites.

Many Internet-based systems allow access from any device through any wireless hotspot, and these may be unsecured. Information from internal systems and routers is transmitted through a series of Internet hosting sites, also called *nodes,* until the information gets to the secure website. On the Internet, if something happens to one node, the network still functions. Although the website accessed is secure, many access devices may not be secure. Additionally, having a secure device, as determined by an overall computer system, does not guarantee a safe device—one free of malware or viruses. At any one time, the device, connection, transmission, and website may be infected with one or more forms of malware. Malware (a contraction of the words *malicious software*) is a reality. Started as pranks, early malware included viruses and worms that disabled system functions or shut down computers. The current generation of malware is more hostile. Newer malware applications (e.g., spyware, bots, keystroke loggers) are designed to steal data for profitable use.

Recommendations for Effective Documentation

Solving the mystery of Logan—reinterpreting the evaluation evidence to prove he qualified for direct occupational therapy services—ensured that he and his family received the early intervention services they needed. Although the original therapist might have avoided the delay in services through more effective interpretation of test results, Logan and his family were able to receive an appropriately interpreted evaluation in part because the therapist documented the original results in a way that allowed Amy to reevaluate them and resolve the mystery.

Documenting occupational therapy services is nearly as important as providing services in the first place. Long after services are provided, documentation remains as evidence of the occupational therapy services a client received. Occupational therapists display their public presence through their documentation, which reveals to other therapists their clinical reasoning skills, therapeutic abilities, and general competence. Documentation that is well written and documentation that is poorly developed and uninformative have equal longevity. The sections that follow provide general guidance for ensuring the effectiveness of occupational therapy documentation.

Treat all records as documentation

Occupational therapy practitioners should be equally cautious in creating all records pertaining to specific clients, even those that are not typically part of formal occupational therapy documentation. One poorly written note could be damaging to a professional's reputation. Records such as emails, personal notes, text messages, and voicemails are discoverable and recoverable if a lawsuit is brought, and therapists should keep in mind the legal ramifications of any communication regarding a client. With readily available technology, just about any kind of record is recoverable and discoverable and can be subpoenaed and used in court cases; digital information, which can last forever, leaves traces even after being "erased." Both client information and professional reputations can be protected by effective documentation.

Avoid the appearance of multitasking

Time, the basis of billing for occupational therapy services, can be tracked better than ever before using new technologies, and occupational therapy practitioners must avoid the appearance of nonprofessional multitasking. Today's world includes automatic record-keeping of time, date, and location. Computer systems provide a record of all actions, including signing on, making client records, using the Internet, and logging off. At home, the therapist leaves a record of phone, cable, satellite, and Internet access. Thus, overlap between professional and personal activities is increasingly discoverable. For example, if an occupational therapist uses a personal communication device during a treatment session, the client may dispute whether occupational therapy services were delivered. The third-party payer could request phone records to determine whether the communication was professional in nature and related to the person being billed for the time period. Nonprofessional multitasking could result in reimbursement being denied. Occupational therapists need to make certain there is an accurate record of service delivery during the entire session and avoid nonprofessional multitasking.

Follow AOTA's Guidelines for Documentation of Occupational Therapy

AOTA's (2018) *Guidelines for Documentation of Occupational Therapy* is an official document that provides recommendations for documentation and report writing. It also offers suggested content with examples for the various types of reports and a listing of fundamental elements that should be present in all documents—for example, including the "client's full name, date of birth, gender, and case number, if applicable, . . . on each page of documentation" (p. 2).

Request examples of best practice in documentation

Documentation varies from facility to facility, and report writing within a single facility can vary from therapist to therapist. Although some variation is purely stylistic, facilities often have specific requirements or regulations that documentation must meet. One of the best ways to become proficient in documentation at a new facility or for more than one supervisor is to request and study examples of previously written documentation that the facility or supervisor considers best practice. Before being shared, report examples need to be de-identified by removing all personal information about the client and therapist.

Respect the reader

Because the primary purpose of documentation is communication, occupational therapists must be sure their readers will understand it. The first step in respecting the reader is determining who will read the occupational therapy report, which may include the client, family members, referral sources, third-party payers, and other professionals, and then write the documentation so it can be understood by all of those readers. Therapists can make reading easier by dividing information into short paragraphs, using headings at each change in topic, and summarizing data in simple, self-explanatory tables. The report should include all the information readers need to understand the report and come to the same conclusion as the report writer. Evaluation and reevaluation reports can provide information describing delay, decline, or dysfunction in terms of percentages and justifying the need for occupational therapy services in plain language. Progress, reevaluation, and discharge reports should include all necessary preliminary information so report readers do not have to search for and read previous documentation to determine clinical change.

Demonstrate effectiveness by showing improvement

To demonstrate the effectiveness of services, occupational therapists need to document clinical change in the direction of improvement. Describing the outcome as an *improvement* in a specific outcome, rather than an *increase* or *decrease* in a score, provides clarity for readers. The discharge report should always compare initial performance with current performance and include percentage of improvement in scores, specifying the direction of improvement is key. In many cases, the direction of improvement is a higher value.

Separate facts from professional judgment and opinion

Written descriptions should describe exactly what the occupational therapist observed. By "painting a picture" that is clear, the occupational therapist will allow the reader to make a judgment or draw an appropriate conclusion. Professional judgment can be included in a consecutive sentence or phrase, an interpretation section, or a table column. Clearly label it as interpretation if including it in the same location as the corresponding description. Professional judgment and opinion should be supported by specific behavioral examples. In the following examples, the professional judgment is stated first, with the phrases beginning "as evidenced by" and "as indicated by" providing supporting evidence:

- Mr. Martin showed difficulty discriminating three-dimensional space, as evidenced by tripping on the 4-inch step at the entrance of his house.
- In the classroom, Sarah continued to disregard her central vision (looking straight at a task or object), as indicated by her viewing tasks with her head at a 45° angle and using her peripheral vision to complete activities.

Strong documentation avoids judgments; for example, rather than stating "Mr. Oberfeldt was unmotivated," the documentation should read, "Mr. Oberfeldt collected fewer nearby objects today than in the previous three sessions." Instead of, "Mrs. Martinez did a better job of walking today," the description and judgment are divided into separate sentences as follows:

> Mrs. Martinez walked 500 feet, from her room to the independent living kitchen, within 10 minutes without resting. Her functional mobility performance showed an improvement compared with a week ago, when she walked 100 feet toward the kitchen over a period of an hour and required four 5-minute rest breaks.

Additionally, instead of saying "Joey wanted to be alone during recess; given that he has ASD [autism spectrum disorder], he doesn't want to be with others" is an opinion. A more appropriate description would be, "Using the Playground Observation of Engagement, the therapist observed Joey playing the role of an onlooker during the 30-minute recess."

Explain professional jargon

Using frequent parenthetical, explanatory phrases allows occupational therapists to efficiently define professional jargon and words that readers might not understand. A combination of professional and explanatory styles helps readers at various educational levels understand the documentation. For example, in a report on Sam, a boy age 6 months, the therapist wanted to improve clarity in the report by avoiding jargon such as "ATNR has already begun to integrate." The therapist wrote the following description:

> Sam showed signs of the asymmetrical tonic neck reflex (ATNR), a primitive reflexive motor pattern, which is typical for infants of his age. He demonstrated the ATNR, primarily when supine (on his back), when he either (1) moved his head out of midline (the invisible line down the middle of his body) toward his left or right side or (2) extended (straightened) an arm to the side. The stimulus of Sam turning his head sideways or extending his arm resulted in his exhibiting the typical ATNR pattern: his arm and leg on the "face side" extended, and his arm and leg on the side opposite the nose flexed (bent). Sam was able to move out of the ATNR pattern (especially in sitting positions), a sign that the influence of this primitive reflex is disappearing. As expected, as the session progressed and he became more tired, Sam increasingly demonstrated the stimulus–response ATNR pattern.

Great examples [handwritten margin note]

By providing both professional jargon and parenthetical explanations in written documentation can also help teach readers outside the profession more about occupational therapy. Every report should include an occupational-therapy-to-English-dictionary that educates readers to be advocates of occupational therapy. In the case of Sam's ATNR, the reader learns the full name of the reflex, that the reflex is typical at his age, and the components of the reflex. Later, if another practitioner mentions ATNR without explanation, the readers of Sam's report will already have the necessary background information.

Many facilities encourage the use of approved abbreviations, acronyms, symbols, and other shortcuts in documentation, and occupational therapists must be careful to explain each one the first time they use it. In addition, therapists can consider creating a list of commonly used descriptors, qualifiers, and modifiers to refer to when writing documentation for clients with similar issues. Organizing this list by purpose (e.g., descriptors of affect, movement patterns, or pain) can improve speed and fluency in writing documentation.

Use the correct term for service recipients

Occupational therapy students often overuse the word *patient* (and especially the abbreviation "pt.") when referring to any person receiving occupational therapy services. In many settings, particularly medical-model facilities, *patient* is most appropriate, but other settings may require different terminology when referring to the person receiving services. The term *client*, for example, is used in many health care settings. In school settings, the person receiving occupational therapy services is a *student*; in industry settings, *worker* or *employee*; and in skilled nursing facilities, *resident*. Practitioners should check with their facility to determine appropriate terms and then use those terms consistently.

Use accepted conventions for good writing

Proper use of generally accepted conventions regarding grammar and punctuation promotes communication and reduces the risk for misinterpretation. Occupational therapists should write narrative reports, particularly those that will be read by the client and family, in standard English, using full sentences with all appropriate parts of speech, including articles (*a, an, the*) and individualize descriptions of the client by using personal pronouns (e.g., *she, him, her, his*)—for example, "The mother reported that her son did . . ." instead of "mom said son did . . . ." Pronouns must refer to clearly identifiable persons or objects (Whitney & Davis, 2013); Ensure it is clear who the *he* or *she* is in your sentence. For example, in the sentence "Logan's father asked Amy to reevaluate a report written by another therapist about Logan, and he appeared distressed," "he" might refer to Logan's father, the other therapist, or Logan.

Occupational therapists need to be aware of the implications of verb tense when describing what they have observed. For example, a therapist who had been working with a child to improve preschool classroom behaviors stated in the evaluation report, "Lee sits at the table with a straight back." Lee's parents maintained that their child did not have this skill. The therapist reviewed her findings and realized she had seen the behavior only once. By using present tense, the therapist implied that the behavior was ongoing or repeated over time. Use of the past tense—"Lee sat with a straight back"—indicates more accurately that the action was a one-time occurrence. Present tense should be reserved for observations of ongoing behavior, and past tense should be used for describing specific events.

The use of *can* and *is able to* (e.g., "Lee can sit with a straight back" or "Lee is able to sit with a straight back") deserves special note. Although some practitioners make liberal use of *can* and *is able to* in their notes, use of these present-tense terms leaves doubt in the reader's mind about whether the therapist actually saw the behavior during an evaluation or simply believed that the client had the potential to exhibit the behavior. If therapists wish to highlight the client's ability (rather than a specific action), the past tense—"was able to"—is appropriate; for example, "Lee was able to sit with a straight back with minimal assist and complete a 15-minute tabletop task."

Use of the active voice can significantly improve readability in documentation, but the passive voice also has uses (Whitney, 2013). Note the difference between the following two observations: "Mandy moved from prone into sitting" and "Mandy was moved from prone into sitting." The first statement uses an active verb (i.e., *moved*), indicating that Mandy accomplished the action herself. The second statement uses the passive voice (i.e., *was moved*), indicating that Mandy did not actively perform the action and that someone else manipulated her from one position to the other. In most cases, the client is an active participant, so the observation should include an active verb: "Mandy moved from prone (on her stomach) into side-sitting by pushing down with her left arm, leaning to her left side, and swinging her legs around to the right side."

Ambiguity can arise from use of passive verbs. If you observe passive action, use passive voice verbs but include the identity of the active agent in the description. For example, in the expanded statement, the actor is identified as the therapist: "Mandy was moved into sitting from prone (on her stomach) through four-point (hands and knees) by the therapist." Although this advice may remind you a bit too much of English or Language Arts class, an "active voice" in writing is clearer to the reader. Start with the subject rather than a phrase—for example, "Mandy moved from prone by leaning . . ." rather than "Leaning to her left side and swinging her legs around to the right side, Mandy moved from prone . . . ."

Occupational therapists should use precise, clear descriptions that clearly convey the events that occurred. Although some facilities allow the use of words *seem* and *appear,* other settings require professionals to avoid them in favor of more objective terms. Unlike "Mr. Oberfeldt appeared to have difficulty seeing objects nearby," the observation "Mr. Oberfeldt demonstrated difficulty seeing objects located 6 to 12 inches from his eyes when he held a newspaper at arm's length for reading" provides more definitive information about his skills. If the habit of using these two words is difficult to break, therapists can search their documentation for the terms *appear* and *seem* and rewrite the sentences in which they appear.

Other problematic words in evaluation documentation are *will*, *would*, *should*, and *could*, which imply that the client might show the behavior if given the chance or that the behavior is possible in the therapist's professional opinion, when readers need to know whether the behavior actually happened during the session. Practitioners using these four words in documentation are predicting future behaviors on the basis of their observations, but they should document only observations they specifically saw. To be useful in practice and legally defensible, documentation must accurately describe observations of behaviors that actually occurred.

In the example "Mollie would visually track an object," readers of the report have no idea whether Mollie showed visual tracking skills during the session; *would* may indicate only that this behavior was possible in the therapist's professional opinion. The observation is transformed by eliminating *would*, changing the verb to past tense, and expanding to provide additional information:

> As expected for her age, Mollie used whole-head movements (rather than moving her eyes only—as anticipated when she gets older) to track visual objects. At the starting point of Mollie looking straight forward, she tracked objects 4 inches to the left and right in the horizontal plane, 2 inches up and down in the vertical plane, and 1 inch in each direction in the diagonal planes.

Check for wordiness and possible errors

Documentation must include only concise, accurate information pertinent to the person receiving occupational therapy services. In narrative documentation, occupational therapists can check whether a phrase or sentence is really necessary by removing it and seeing how the document reads; the phrase or sentence should be deleted if the information is complete without it. Therapists should carefully proofread the document for unnecessary or inaccurate information. If the therapist stumbles on an irrelevant sentence or confusing phrase during proofreading, chances are the intended readers will also stumble. The passage should be rewritten or deleted to improve the reading rhythm (Whitney, 2013).

Typographical errors happen. But errors in documentation can make occupational therapists look careless and sloppy and, by extension, incompetent. If a spellchecker is available in the documentation system, therapists should use it. Some spellcheckers permit the addition of practice-related and technical terms to the dictionary, which can save time and increase accuracy in documentation. There are many free apps and others with modest fees; Grammarly® (www.grammarly.com) is a grammar-checking app that offers a free version and a more robust version for a small fee.

Use an appropriate reading level

For some types of documentation, reading level may be an issue. With the rise of client-centered care and clients' improved access to their own records, some documentation may need to be written at a level that matches the educational background of the client and family. Fortunately, many electronic applications have features that provide information on readability. To find out how to activate the readability statistics feature, occupational therapists can access the application help menu and search for the term *readability*. When this feature is activated, a dialog box appears after every standard spelling and grammar check that shows counts of words, characters, sentences, and paragraphs; average sentences per paragraph, words per sentence, and characters per word; and readability, which includes a passive sentences percentage, a reading ease score, and a grade level.

There are some tools that can be helpful to determining reading levels for occupational therapists. The Flesch Reading Ease tool has a 100-point scale; a document with a score of >60 is considered easy to read, whereas documents with lower scores are more difficult to read (Thomas et al., 1975). The Flesch–Kincaid Grade Level corresponds to a grade in school (Cotugna et al., 2005). For example, a Flesch–Kincaid Grade Level of 13 corresponds to the reading level of college freshmen. An occupational therapist working with a client with a Grade 7 reading level can adjust the documentation to be accessible at that client's level.

Strategies to improve reading ease and decrease grade level include decreasing word length, number of words per sentence, and number of sentences per paragraph. AOTA offers a Continuing Education course titled "Health Literacy: Effective Client Communication and Education" that can help occupational therapists learn more about health literacy considerations in documentation (Miller, 2015).

Identify ways to improve writing efficiency

Some electronic applications offer an autocorrect feature that can improve writing quality and speed. Occupational therapists can use this feature to develop codes for frequently used words or phrases. For example, a therapist who has grown weary of typing *occupational therapy* can save time by setting the autocorrect feature to expand *occther* to *occupational therapy*. Autocorrect often provides a listing of replacement items and has a removal feature. This feature can be tailored to the documentation needs of the facility, and therapists can ask the appropriate information technology personnel for more information.

Writing a description—for example, of a behavior or performance—in a professional manner sometimes takes more time than scoring a standardized assessment instrument. Rather than writing from scratch each time, occupational therapists can gather well-crafted descriptions in a central place for repeated use.

SUMMARY

The mystery of Logan illustrates the importance of interpretation in occupational therapy and the lasting power of documentation. To show the effectiveness of their services, occupational therapists solve the mystery surrounding each client by becoming lifestyle detectives who profile clients, examine clues within contexts, and synthesize multiple data points to give order to the complexities of life. Because documentation is permanent evidence of occupational therapy services, occupational therapists must always be aware that their writing is part of their public image and take care to ensure that it is ethically, legally, and stylistically sound.

QUESTIONS

1. How would you adapt your documentation for the following audiences?
   - Rehabilitation team at the facility to which the client will be transferred
   - Referring physician
   - Parent with a high school education
   - Parent with a sixth-grade education
   - Parent who speaks and understands minimal English
   - Teacher of a student with a disability
   - Older adult with mild cognitive difficulties
   - Third-party payer interested in function and functional outcomes.
2. How can you protect the security, privacy, and confidentiality of your documentation if you are using an access device that is wireless? What steps can you take to protect client information?
3. When reviewing documentation written by a fieldwork student, occupational therapy colleague, or non–occupational therapist team member, what practices discussed in this chapter would you use to ensure quality?
4. The director of rehabilitation at your skilled nursing facility informs you that the third-party payer for a client you have been treating for 6 weeks has requested additional justification for reimbursement of continued occupational therapy services.
   - What types of documentation would the payer be interested in to determine whether payment for continued therapy treatment is warranted?
   - What elements of your occupational therapy documentation would you highlight?
   - What is your responsibility in answering questions related to reimbursement in this case?
5. Regardless of the theory or style used by an occupational therapy practitioners, for the evaluation, interpretation, and documentation process, the practitioner is ultimately responsible for accurate and complete reporting. What are three critical components identified in this chapter that form the basis for meeting the directive of accurate and complete documentation?
6. Using a client you have seen on Fieldwork (either Level I or II), write a short progress note and share it with a classmate. Have the classmate determine if it is clear and concise and conveys information appropriately. If not, how can you improve it?

REFERENCES

American Occupational Therapy Association. (2014). Occupational therapy practice framework: Domain and process (3rd ed.). *American Journal of Occupational Therapy, 68*(Suppl. 1), S1–S48. https://doi.org/10.5014/ajot.2014.682006

American Occupational Therapy Association. (2015). Occupational therapy code of ethics (2015). *American Journal of Occupational Therapy, 69*(Suppl. 3), 6913410030. https://doi.org/10.5014/ajot.2015.696S03

American Occupational Therapy Association. (2017). *AOTA PERFORM documentation templates.* Retrieved from https://www.aota.org/~/media/Corporate/Files/Secure/Advocacy/Federal/Perform-Documentation-Templates.pdf

American Occupational Therapy Association. (2018). Guidelines for documentation of occupational therapy. *American Journal of Occupational Therapy, 72*(Suppl. 2), 7212410010. https://doi.org/10.5014/ajot.2018.72S203

Cotugna, N., Vickery, C. E., & Carpenter-Haefele, K. M. (2005). Evaluation of literacy level of patient education pages in health-related journals. *Journal of Community Health, 30,* 213–219. https://doi.org/10.1007/s10900-004-1959-x

Family Educational Rights and Privacy Act, 20 U.S.C. § 1232g (1974).

Folio, M., & Fewell, R. (2000). *Peabody Developmental Motor Scales–Second Edition (PDMS-2): Examiner's manual.* Austin, TX: Pro-Ed.

Frolek Clark, G., & Handley-More, D. (2017). *Best practices for documenting occupational therapy services in schools.* Bethesda, MD: AOTA Press.

Gateley, C. A., & Borcherding, S. (2018). *Documentation manual for occupational therapy: Writing SOAP notes* (4th ed.). Thorofare, NJ: Slack.

Gately, M. E., Trudeau, S. A., & Moo, L. R. (2019). Feasibility of telehealth-delivered home safety evaluations for caregivers of clients with dementia. *OTJR: Occupation, Participation and Health, 40,* 42–49. https://doi.org/10.1177/1539449219859935

Gillen, G. (2013). A fork in the road: An occupational hazard? *American Journal of Occupational Therapy, 67,* 641–652. https://doi.org/10.5014/ajot.2013.676002

Health Insurance Portability and Accountability Act of 1996, Pub. L. 104-191, 45 C.F.R. §§ 160, 164.

Miller, C. (2015). *Health literacy: Effective client communication and education* [Continuing education course]. Bethesda, MD: AOTA Press.

Patient Protection and Affordable Care Act, Pub. L. 111-148, 42 U.S.C § 18001 (2010).

Renda, M., & Lape, J. E. (2018). Feasibility and effectiveness of telehealth occupational therapy home modification interventions. *International Journal of Telerehabilitation, 10*(1), 3–14. https://doi.org/10.5195/ijt.2018.6244

Sames, K. (2013). Documentation in practice. In B. A. B. Schell, G. Gillen, & M. E. Scaffa (Eds.), *Willard and Spackman's occupational therapy* (12th ed., pp. 466–476). Baltimore, MD: Lippincott Williams & Wilkins.

Sames, K. (2015). *Documenting occupational therapy practice* (3rd ed.). Upper Saddle River, NJ: Pearson Prentice Hall.

Smith, J. (2013). Documenting occupational therapy services. In R. V. Whitney & C. A. Davis (Eds.), *A writer's toolkit for* occupational therapy and health care professionals: An insider's guide to writing and getting published (pp. 207–226). Bethesda, MD: AOTA Press.

Strauss, L. J. (2015). Electronic medical records—Benefits and liabilities. Journal of Health Care Compliance, 17(2), 57–58.

Thomas, G., Hartley, R. D., & Kincaid, J. P. (1975). Test–retest and inter-analyst reliability of the Automated Readability Index, Flesch Reading Ease Score, and the Fog Count. Journal of Literacy Research, 7, 149–154. https://doi.org/10.1080/10862967509547131

Whitney, R. V. (2013). Refreshing, renewing, and remediating your writing: Back to the basics. In R. V. Whitney & C. A. Davis (Eds.), A writer's toolkit for occupational therapy and health care professionals: An insider's guide to writing and getting published (pp. 53–64). Bethesda, MD: AOTA Press.

Whitney, R. V., & Davis, C. A. (Eds.). (2013). A writer's toolkit for occupational therapy and health care professionals: An insider's guide to writing and getting published. Bethesda, MD: AOTA Press.

Whitney, R., & Smith, G. (2015). Emotional disclosure through journal writing: Telehealth intervention for maternal stress and mother–child relationships. Journal of Autism and Developmental Disabilities, 45, 3735–3745. https://doi.org/10.1007/s10803-014-2332-2

Worboys, T., Brassington, M., Ward, E. C., & Cornwell, P. L. (2018). Delivering occupational therapy hand assessment and treatment sessions via telehealth. Journal of Telemedicine and Telecare, 24, 185–192. https://doi.org/10.1177/1357633X17691861

12

Outcomes Assessment

Andrew C. Persch, PhD, OTR/L, BCP, and Cristina C. Parsons, MOT, OTR/L

CHAPTER HIGHLIGHTS

- Frameworks for outcomes assessment
- World Health Organization's *International Classification of Functioning, Disability and Health*
- National Institutes of Health's (NIH) Patient-Reported Outcomes Measurement Information System (PROMIS)
- NIH's Common Data Element Resource Portal
- Occupational Profile
- Multiple stakeholder model of occupational therapy outcomes
- Defining the stakeholders in occupational therapy outcomes
- Consequences of misaligned outcomes
- Multiple stakeholders in transition outcomes

KEY TERMS AND CONCEPTS

- Asessment
- Common data element
- Common Data Element Resource Portal
- Core sets
- Evaluation

- *International Classification of Functioning, Disability and Health*
- Occupational profile
- Occupational therapy outcome
- Outcomes assessment
- Outcomes orientation
- Patient

- Patient-reported outcomes
- Patient-Reported Outcomes Measurement Information System
- Payors
- Policymakers
- Providers
- Stakeholders

INTRODUCTION

An **occupational therapy outcome** is "the functional consequence for the patient of the therapeutic actions implemented by an occupational therapist" (Rogers & Holm, 1994, p. 872). This definition suggests a professional focus on functional patient-level outcomes: patients' occupations. The focus has not always been on patients' occupations, nor does such a focus on patients' outcomes provide a complete view of all occupational therapy outcomes. For example, the reductionistic models of medicine and rehabilitation that were prominent in the 20th century focused on reducing impairment or improving some type of component-level skills. These types of outcomes fall at the level of body structures and functions within the *International Classification of Functioning, Disability and Health* (*ICF*; World Health Organization [WHO], 2001). They may be at the patient's level but are not functional and say little about patients' occupational performance as occupational therapy outcomes are complex and multidimensional.

This chapter uses the following terms as defined here:

- **Evaluation:** the occupational therapy process of evaluation that includes interview, occupational profile, assessment, interpretation, and treatment planning

- **Assessment:** a specific test or measure used with a client
- **Outcomes assessment:** integration of individual outcomes relevant to a stakeholder.

Occupational therapy practitioners may conduct one or more assessments as part of a comprehensive evaluation. *Outcomes assessment* refers to the process of integrating stakeholder outcomes and is distinct from a specific assessment tool or the client evaluation process. This is related to but distinct from assessment and evaluation. Unsworth (2000) has suggested that the objective of outcomes assessment is to determine positive change that is attributable to the intervention, which aligns well with Rogers and Holm's (1994) perspective. Positive changes may occur at the patient level or may be observed by other stakeholders in occupational therapy outcomes.

Occupational therapy practitioners increasingly face outside pressures from payors, employers, and clients to demonstrate the distinct value of the profession and provide quality, evidence-based therapy at a low cost (Unsworth, 2000). Payors such as the Centers for Medicare and Medicaid Services (CMS) and health care quality leaders such as the National Quality Forum are advocating for more outcomes-focused measures. Occupational therapists who integrate assessment data at multiple levels while considering the unique perspectives of multiple stakeholders are engaged in outcomes assessment at its highest level. Case Example 12.1 provides an example that integrates outcomes and stakeholders at multiple levels.

FRAMEWORKS FOR OUTCOMES ASSESSMENT

Whether therapists are conducting research, working with individual clients, or characterizing the health of a population, identifying a framework is important to ensure fidelity in measurement and a harmonious language to effectively communicate findings. Many established and acceptable frameworks can guide outcomes assessment at the person, group, and population levels. In this section, we discuss frameworks at the global, national, and professional rank; some advantages and disadvantages of these frameworks; and implications for occupational therapy practitioners.

International Classification of Functioning, Disability and Health

In 2001, the *ICF* was adopted by the 191 WHO member states "as the basis for the scientific standardization of data on health and disability world-wide" (WHO, 2002, p. 5). The *ICF*, which is part of the WHO's larger family of international classifications (WHO–ICF), categorizes the functioning and disability of a person that occurs in a given context and incorporates environmental factors (WHO, 2002). Worldwide, the *ICF* is broadly accepted by rehabilitation professionals as a framework for measuring health and disability (WHO, 2002).

Applications of the *ICF* at different client levels can be found in Exhibit 12.1. Use of the framework at the social, or population, level is valuable for epidemiological purposes, and some developed countries have begun integrating *ICF*-based reporting systems into a variety of health processes and legislation (WHO, 2019). For occupational therapists on a global scale, it is important to establish familiarity with the *ICF* as a framework because it is foreseen to be "the world standard for disability data and social policy modeling" (WHO, 2002, p. 19).

WHO (2019) has suggested that at the individual level, therapists may use the *ICF* in "functional status assessment, goal setting & treatment planning and monitoring, as well as outcome measurement" (para. 9). However, given its

---

EXHIBIT 12.1.　ICF Applications

- *Person level:* The *ICF* can be used to assess a person's level of functioning, plan treatments, evaluate outcomes of intervention for the person, and facilitate communication among health care providers.
- *Group level:* The *ICF* can be used for group education and training, resource planning and development, quality improvement initiatives, and evaluation of service provision and to better develop models of health care delivery.
- *Population level:* The *ICF* can be used to determine eligibility criteria for state entitlements, develop and change social policy, and assess needs and environmental accessibility for people with impairments, limitations, or restrictions.

---

more than 1,400 categories, the comprehensive nature of the *ICF* presents clinicians with issues related to feasibility.

Given the *ICF*'s broad language and constructs, core sets have been developed to improve its clinical practicality and utility for specific diseases such as breast cancer (Brach et al., 2004), chronic widespread pain (Cieza et al., 2004), multiple sclerosis (Coenen et al., 2011), rheumatoid arthritis (Kirchberger et al., 2007), stroke (Glässel et al., 2010), and traumatic brain injury (Laxe et al., 2013). *Core sets* are a set of *ICF* domains that are most relevant for a certain disease or condition that help make the *ICF* more accessible for use by clinicians at the individual and group levels. Researchers such as Kirchberger et al. (2007) have worked to establish content validity across core sets by comparing *ICF* measures with concepts that occupational therapists use in treating specific populations.

Although the *ICF* aims to capture the experience of disability and health (WHO, 2002), one criticism of the *ICF* is its lack of emphasis on and classification of person factors (Kirchberger et al., 2007). Haglund and Henriksson (2003) cautioned that although the *ICF* can be helpful in communicating with other health professionals, it is not sufficient for occupational therapists to use as a stand-alone language. The universal language of the *ICF* is helpful in communicating the relationship among a person, the person's environment, and the person's everyday functioning to stakeholders outside of the occupational therapy profession, but it should be paired with the clinical expertise unique to an occupational therapy perspective. Extra caution should be used to ensure occupational therapists capture clients' subjective experience.

Patient-Reported Outcomes Measurement Information System

The National Institutes of Health (NIH) established the *Patient-Reported Outcomes Measurement Information System* (PROMIS) in 2004 (HealthMeasures, 2019) as a tool to evaluate and monitor physical, mental, and social health in adults and children through person-centered measures (HealthMeasures, 2019).

PROMIS uses *patient-reported outcomes* (PROs) in the domains of global health, pain, fatigue, sleep–wake function, physical function, emotional distress, and social health (HealthMeasures, 2019). Like the *ICF*, PROMIS is a valuable tool for clinical research and practice because it allows health professionals to use the same metrics across disciplines (Bear-Lehman, 2012), which improves communication and knowledge translation. Unlike the *ICF*, using PROs helps maintain the crucial client-centered aspect of care throughout the occupational therapy process. Occupational therapists are well positioned to use PROMIS domains in their own practice to demonstrate the value of the applied science of occupational therapy in terms that other health and industry professionals can understand.

For use at the person level, PROMIS has adult, child, and short form versions available. NIH is currently developing a form for use with children ages 1–5 years as a part of the Environmental influences on Child Health Outcomes research program (NIH, 2020).

Similar to the core sets of the *ICF*, researchers have worked to close the gap in clinical utility by comparing

PROMIS measures with known, condition-specific instruments (Blackwell et al., 2019; Coster et al., 2016; Kashikar-Zuck et al., 2016; Mulcahey et al., 2018; Weinfurt et al., 2015) and establishing their content validity for use with disease-specific populations.

Common Data Element Resource Portal

NIH (2019a) published the *Common Data Element (CDE) Resource Portal,* which provides free access to information about NIH-supported CDEs. A *CDE* is defined as a data element, such as demographic information or patient-reported outcomes, that is mutual to specific populations across multiple data sets from different studies.

The CDE Resource Portal highlights intentional use of CDEs as a method to enhance and promote data quality and data sharing for fields of research funded by NIH. It provides tools and resources for investigators to develop protocols for data collection and offers a comprehensive list of data collection repositories that is updated frequently with additional instruments and measures. Table 12.1 explains the types of resources this portal provides.

Although the CDE collections and repository are primarily of use to researchers, the tools and resources available can also guide clinical outcomes assessment by practitioners. For instance, the NIH Toolbox for Assessment of Neurological and Behavioral Function is a CDE initiative that can be used by researchers and clinicians alike in a variety of settings (NIH, 2019b). The NIH Toolbox is maintained by researchers at the Feinberg School of Medicine at Northwestern University and contains easy-to-use self- and proxy-report measures of cognitive, emotional, motor, and sensory function. Paper forms are available, as well as an iPad app. Using measures that are part of a larger toolkit such as this one not only affords confidence in better data quality, but also provides practitioners with the ability to quickly assess relevant client domains to assist with necessary assessment of the whole person.

Occupational Profile

Not only is the *occupational profile* essential to the evaluation process, but it is a primary driver of effective outcomes assessment. Systematically and intentionally gathering information about a client's (person's, group's, or population's) wants and needs in relation to occupational performance serves therapists well in three ways. First, completing an occupational profile helps to establish rapport with the client. Asking questions related to why the client is seeking services and the client's life experiences (occupational history), values, and beliefs is just one example of how therapists engage clients to begin thinking from an occupational perspective. With an occupational therapist's guidance, clients may simultaneously begin to form and share their viewpoint of their own facilitators of and barriers to occupational success within a given context.

Second, the occupational profile is the basis for establishing client-centered goals. Analysis of occupational performance through the use of standardized or non-standardized tools is insufficient to capture the whole picture and often focuses on the therapist's objective perspective. It is easy to miss capturing the client's subjective experience. Although observing and measuring occupational performance is certainly a necessary part of evaluation, coming back to information discovered through use of the occupational profile frames the treatment plan in the context of the client's perspective.

Third, a previous edition of this text proposed that the occupational profile "is a legitimate occupational therapy assessment, but is also a process that may be used over time, throughout both the evaluation and treatment phases of client-centered intervention, rather than purely as an assessment" (Crist, 2014, p. 6). Not only is this notion advantageous when considering that therapists may not have sufficient time to gather a comprehensive occupational profile during the initial evaluation, it also lends itself to the idea that as therapists continue to establish rapport with the client and take on a personal occupational perspective, the information pertinent to the occupational profile is likely to become richer and more salient. These factors are essential to ensuring a meaningful outcomes assessment for all stakeholders after occupational therapy intervention.

MULTIPLE STAKEHOLDER MODEL OF OCCUPATIONAL THERAPY OUTCOMES

Human life and occupations are complex phenomena. As such, occupational therapy outcomes are rarely unidimensional and may not reflect actual individual experience. For example, consider the *ICF* participation-level outcome of

TABLE 12.1.   Resources from the NIH CDE Resource Portal

RESOURCE	DESCRIPTION
NIH CDE initiatives	Collections of CDEs that were used in NIH-supported research projects (free, although registration may be required for access)
CDE Tools and Resources	Databases of data elements and case report forms for the purpose of assisting investigators in selecting data elements that are relevant to their research; used to promote the use of existing data elements
Other CDE Resources	Other collections of CDEs that have been developed with lesser involvement from NIH but that still have potential for use in research (may require fee to access)
Relevant Standards	Clinical vocabularies, terminologies, and standards used for the purpose of improving the comparability of data

Note. CDE = Common Data Element; NIH = National Institutes of Health.
Source. Adapted from Common Data Element Resource Portal (2019a).

dining out with friends. The experience starts before you enter the restaurant. You contact your friends and set a date, look for a restaurant online, read some reviews, make a reservation, and travel to the restaurant before you ever step foot inside. By the time you enter the restaurant, your experience dining out (i.e., the outcome) is already skewed by these aspects of the experience. Next, consider these factors: Was your table ready when you arrived? Were you satisfied with the menu choices? Was your food prepared to your liking? How was the service? The list of factors that may influence an outcome is long.

When asked about a dinner date, people tend to report their experiences differently. If a friend asks how your dinner was, you may share facts about your meal or the service you received. If you wrote a review on Yelp or Google, you would enter a scaled response, contribute a short narrative report, or both. The other members of your dinner party may have different perspectives, and their experience of the same

meal might be very different. For example, your spouse may have focused on the service and be disappointed that the waiter did not keep the water glasses full. In contrast, your friends may have just experienced a death in the family, and for them, dinner out provided a much-needed distraction from the realities of everyday life. They cannot remember what they had to eat or drink but remember having a good time with you and your spouse. Which or whose outcome is primary? Of course, there is no single answer.

Similarly, occupational therapy practitioners should take a collaborative, data-based approach to evaluating complex multidimensional and multistakeholder outcomes. These stakeholders are the people, groups, and organizations that have a right to know the outcomes and a legitimate interest in the outcome (Hyland & Jackson, 2006). Case Example 12.1 illustrates the different stakeholders involved in postsecondary outcomes for children as they transition into adulthood.

CASE EXAMPLE 12.1. TRANSITION TO ADULTHOOD

The U.S. Office of Special Education Programs reported a total of 6,048,882 students with disabilities, ages 6–21 years, were served under IDEA Part B in 2016. The most prevalent disability categories were specific learning disability, speech or language impairment, other health impairment, autism spectrum disorder, intellectual disability, and emotional disturbance, respectively. *Transition age* is defined as age 14 years (or older, depending on locality) and having an individualized education program (IEP) with measurable postsecondary goals and transition services. In 2016, 69.9% of students with disabilities served under IDEA Part B graduated with a high school diploma, and 17.5% dropped out of high school (U.S. Department of Education, 2018).

What happens to these youth with disabilities when they exit the school system? Where do they go? How do they occupy their time? What services are available to them outside of the school system? The transition from adolescence to adulthood and employment has been shown to be a significant challenge for youth with disabilities. For example, although as many as 39% of youth with intellectual disability are employed in the years immediately after high school (Newman et al., 2011), only 15% of these youth maintain employment (Butterworth et al., 2015). This means that as much as 85% of youth with intellectual disability face unemployment as adults.

Students older than age 16 years with a disability and an IEP are required to receive transition services under IDEA. These transition services are designed to support a student's transition from high school to postsecondary education, competitive employment, or both (IDEA, 2004). Postsecondary education can be described as acceptance into a junior college or 4-year university. Competitive employment is work that is performed on either a full- or a part-time basis for which people are compensated. The compensation paid

FIGURE 12.1. Stakeholders involved in transition IEP meeting.

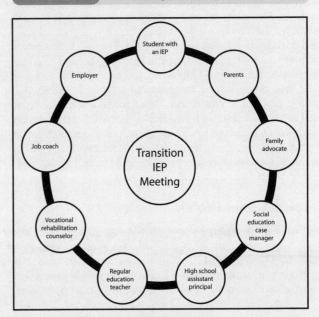

Note. IEP = individualized education program.

must be at or above the set minimum wage, but not less than the wages paid to people who are not disabled and performing work that is at the same or a similar level.

Multiple stakeholders in transition outcomes

Transition to adulthood occurs through support services that include possibly contradicting perspectives

(Continued)

CASE EXAMPLE 12.1. TRANSITION TO ADULTHOOD *(Cont.)*

of multiple stakeholders, such as the student, parents, teachers, vocational rehabilitation professionals, and other organizations (Figure 12.1). These varying perspectives can complicate the transition process. Occupational therapy practitioners who can understand and identify these perspectives can help youth and their families to prepare and plan for the complicated transition process. Figure 12.1 shows the different, and at times competing, perspectives of the stakeholders in the transition process.

Patient

Students' perspective and wishes must be primary in determining a successful transition to adulthood. Young adults with developmental disabilities seek social connections, community engagement, and employment as key factors for higher quality of life and satisfaction during and after the transition period (Blaskowitz et al., 2018). These young adults rely on teachers and vocational rehabilitation professionals to assist them in the transition process and to help them develop more autonomy to self-advocate for services they may need in the future. Parents and families are a direct influence and support for young people with developmental disabilities and can influence their goals and desired outcomes.

Current research has indicated that 88% of people with developmental disabilities live with their families or in their own households (Developmental Disabilities Assistance and Bill of Rights Act of 2000, P. L. 106-402). Parents and families prioritize competitive employment and independent living as key criteria for successful transition, just as transition specialists do. However, they view psychological well-being, health, and opportunities for social and romantic relationships as other important outcomes, suggesting a more dynamic and varied view of what successful transition means for people with developmental disabilities (Henninger & Taylor, 2014).

Providers and payors

The term *payor* refers to the health care or medical insurance that pays for the services provided. Because providers and payors often work for the same organization, it can be difficult to separate provider from payor in the context of secondary transition. For example, school districts are responsible for both providing special education services and paying for those services.

Special education teachers and related service personnel work directly with students with disabilities. They adapt lessons, teaching styles, and expectations to meet each student's capabilities and are invested in each student's success. Therefore, they are likely to view the transition to postsecondary education, competitive employment, or both as markers of a successful transition. Nevertheless, transition planning can be implemented in a way that differs from policy intention. For example, school districts may view IEPs as a mandated

obligation rather than as a benefit to the student. To increase the quality of the transition experience for students with disabilities, it is crucial to actively engage students and their family in the process (deFur, 2003; Orentlicher, 2015).

By contrast, vocational rehabilitation professionals (e.g., vocational counselors, job developers, job coaches) have emphasized the attainment of competitive employment as the primary indicator of a successful transition to adulthood. Vocational rehabilitation services are federal–state programs that provide services to help people with physical or intellectual disabilities attain and maintain employment. These agencies promote the transition of people with disabilities into postsecondary education or employment through interagency team processes, person-centered planning, and provision of essential supports. The specific services provided by vocational rehabilitation professionals can range from skills training to job coaching (Yamamoto et al., 2014). During the transition process, students may place more value on making money as a successful outcome, whereas vocational rehabilitation professionals may view working independently as a positive outcome.

Boards of developmental disabilities, which operate at the state or county level and receive federal funding, are another stakeholder group that may be involved in the transition process. Representatives from this board aim to "promote self-determination, integration, and inclusion" of people with developmental disabilities, specifically focusing on their living arrangements, health, safety, and welfare (National Association of Councils on Developmental Disabilities, 2020, para. 1). People with developmental disabilities can apply for a developmental disabilities waiver to receive various benefits and services, such as supported employment, peer mentorship, and transportation. The purpose of this waiver program is to supply home- and community-based services to assist people with intellectual and developmental disabilities. Nevertheless, the parent of a student with a developmental disability may prioritize health services, whereas the student may prioritize supported employment.

Case conclusions

Paid employment or continuation to postsecondary education supports development of social networks and self-efficacy and provides a sense of belonging and security (Schur, 2002), contributes to health and well-being (Egerter et al., 2008), and is associated with higher levels of self-reported health status (Hall et al., 2013). Therefore, identification of, and agreement on, transition outcomes for youth with disability may require discussion of outcomes among the multiple stakeholders involved in the process. Parents may envision happiness and health as a successful transition for their child, whereas vocational rehabilitation professionals may view competitive employment as a successful transition.

Defining the Stakeholders in Occupational Therapy Outcomes

A health care encounter, although very different from dinner out with friends, is similar in that the encounter begins long before a scheduled appointment, and multiple stakeholders can define the outcome. If people have a hard time navigating insurance, scheduling an appointment, or parking at the clinic, their perspective of the health care encounter has already started to be shaped. There may be additional stakeholders, depending on the patient and context. In this chapter, *stakeholders* fall into one of four categories: (1) patients, (2) providers, (3) payors, and (4) policymakers. This model of stakeholders is adapted from Ritz et al. (2014).

Patients

The Patient-Centered Outcomes Research Institute (PCORI; 2019) defines **patients** as "persons with current or past experience of illness or injury, family members or other unpaid caregivers of patients, or members of advocacy organizations that represent patients or caregivers." (See "How PCORI Defines Stakeholders.") Occupational therapists attempt to capture relevant aspects of a person's experience by completing an occupational profile and client-centered evaluation.

Despite best intentions, perceptions of client centeredness can vary between occupational therapist and patient. Maitra and Erway (2006) conducted semi-structured interviews of 11 occupational therapists and 30 clients across four facilities (i.e., long-term care, hospital outpatient, hospital inpatient, nursing homes) that revealed perceptual differences about the use of client-centered practice, particularly during goal setting. They also found that the type of facility significantly influenced clients' knowledge of certain aspects of their treatment.

It is also important to understand the patient's **outcomes orientation**, that is what the patient expects as an outcome of the intervention. If the patient is interested in reducing impairment, then measures such as range of motion, strength, and pain may provide useful endpoints. In contrast, if the patient is focused on community participation (e.g., trivia night), then these measures would be of little use. As noted in the PCORI definition, the group of patient stakeholders extends beyond the person to family members, unpaid caregivers, and advocates.

Providers

Health care **providers** include physicians, nurses, rehabilitative professionals (e.g., occupational therapists, physical therapists, speech–language pathologists), pharmacists, and a wide range of other allied health professionals. "Providers operationalize care delivery within the policy framework. They provide health services to patients and maintain health information about them. Many providers are independent businesses that must manage their own operations and finances" (Ritz et al., 2014, p. 28).

Payors

Payors are responsible for procuring health care services from providers on behalf of patients according to policy frameworks. For example, although Part B of the Individuals With Disabilities Education Improvement Act of 2004

(IDEA; P. L. 108-446) authorizes Congress to provide up to 40% of special education costs, the federal government has historically provided only 15%–20%. In this example, there are two payors: (1) the federal government and (2) the local school district, which is responsible for making up the difference. According to Ritz et al. (2014), "To be sustainable, payors endeavor to minimize the costs of funding their portfolios of care services. This incentivizes payors to encourage and even invest in the uptake of healthy-living initiatives within their beneficiary population" (p. 30).

Policymakers

Policymakers "establish the framework within which health care is provided to the country's citizens. The policymakers aggregate data from patients, providers, and payors to develop population-level metrics that inform their health and health economic policies" (Ritz et al., 2014, p. 27). These policies set the context for care. Other stakeholders must operate within these constraints. For example, providers working in a skilled nursing facility operate under Medicare Part A whereas providers working in an outpatient setting operate under Medicare Part B. These policies are set by CMS.

Consequences of Misaligned Outcomes

The literature is full of examples that illustrate the consequences of misaligned stakeholder outcomes. This section includes several examples of the real-life consequences of misaligned priorities and outcomes. We have selected examples from a variety of practice areas to provide readers with multiple contrasts.

Adolescent mental health services

Integrating evidence into practice has been slow, with serious implications for public mental health systems (Morris et al., 2011). Factors affecting the implementation of evidence-based practice were studied through multiple stakeholders' viewpoints in one of the largest counties in the United States (Aarons et al., 2009). Researchers created a focus group with 31 individuals from several organizational levels and a diverse range of mental health agencies and programs. These stakeholders included county officials, agency directors, program managers, clinical staff, administrative staff, and consumers. Their goal was to identify factors likely to facilitate or hinder the implementation of evidence-based practice in larger health systems and ascertain how these factors are perceived through importance and changeability ratings. By questioning each individual and through consolidation of the resulting data, the researchers were able to identify 14 prominent factors that affected implementation of evidence-based practice, including the impact on clinical practice, costs, and system readiness and compatibility.

Although the sample size was small, there was variability across stakeholder groups. For example, county officials rated costs as less important than agency directors or administrative staff. Consumers rated consumer values and marketing higher than did any other stakeholder group. The researchers suggested that these differences indicate the need for more communication between stakeholder groups to more effectively understand what affects implementation of evidence-based practice. These findings demonstrate that participants varied in terms of which outcomes they focused on.

Adolescent–parent–therapist triads

Garland et al. (2004) sought to identify and determine agreement on desired outcomes for adolescent mental health services according to three stakeholder groups: (1) adolescents, (2) parents, and (3) therapists. The investigators conducted interviews with 170 adolescents, their caregivers, and their psychotherapists. From these interviews, they determined 30 outcome categories across five broader outcome domains (symptoms, functioning, consumer perspectives, environment, systems).

At the aggregate level, most stakeholders report similar desired outcomes of reducing anger and aggression and improving family and peer relations. However, results also showed that individual triads (adolescent–parent–therapist) did not have high levels of agreement on desired outcomes. Parents tend to focus more on symptoms as the problem, whereas adolescents focused on family and environmental issues. This lack of consensus between key stakeholders on desired outcomes could affect engagement in mental health services and limit the effectiveness of treatment.

Hospitals

Avgar et al. (2011) sought to understand the effects of work–life balance practices in hospitals for three stakeholders: (1) hospitals, (2) employees, and (3) the patients for whom they care as measured by financial performance, employees' intentions to leave the hospital over the following year, and quality of patient care, respectively. Results indicated that work–life balance practices (e.g., family leave, flexible work time, child care support) improved outcomes for all key stakeholders by positively affecting hospital financial performance, decreasing the employee turnover rate, and decreasing errors that could harm patients. The findings reflect participants' agreement regarding what outcomes are important for the functioning of the health care system and suggest that an intervention focused on one stakeholder group (e.g., employees) may have an influence on additional stakeholder groups (e.g., patients, policymakers).

Mobile technology

Hammel et al. (2013) looked at the perspectives and priorities of multiple stakeholders related to mobility technology (MT) use and outcomes. These stakeholders included consumers (people with disabilities who use MT), caregivers, and service providers. Results indicated that service providers prioritized functional activity independence and body function and structure as a primary concern because of their relation to funding and documentation, whereas consumers emphasized participation and social outcomes. Consumers also pointed out that there are other important ways to assess impact of MT besides just activity independence. Caregivers and consumers also emphasized the importance of the person–environment fit and the dynamic MT management process to finding the best fit. These differing perspectives suggest the need for an assessment tool that allows for a wider range of valuable outcomes related to MT.

Motor skill performance

Many occupational therapists rely on performance-based measures to evaluate a child's motor skills to provide a justification for services. This approach can consequently remove the child's and parent's perspectives from the evaluation and intervention process. Kennedy et al. (2011) examined the relationships among performance-based, client-report, and parent-report measures of a child's motor skill performance. The researchers recruited 38 children and their parents to complete self-report and parent-report measures, respectively, in addition to a performance-based measure of motor skill performance. The results indicated very few significant correlations between the children's perceptions of their motor skill performance and the scores obtained from the performance-based measures and parent reports.

Based on these results, children can provide valuable insight into their motor skill performance that may not be obtained by other types of measures. It is important for the perceptions of all stakeholders to be aligned because motor skill performance can affect children's health and well-being, as well as their academic performance.

SUMMARY

The typical stakeholders in occupational therapy outcomes are patients, providers, payors, and policymakers. A thorough outcomes assessment acknowledges that these stakeholders focus on different elements of the encounter. Occupational therapy practitioners who understand the multiple stakeholder model of occupational therapy outcomes may be able to enhance the efficacy of services by aligning systems and outcomes to meet patient and other stakeholder needs. Tools such as the *ICF*, the NIH's PROMIS and CDEs, and the occupational profile described in this chapter help to provide structure for a holistic outcomes assessment.

QUESTIONS

1. What are the differences among assessment, evaluation, and outcomes assessment?
2. What frameworks support multilevel outcomes assessment?
3. Who are the key stakeholders in occupational therapy outcomes?
4. What are the consequences of misaligned outcomes?

REFERENCES

Aarons, G. A., Wells, R. S., Zagursky, K., Fettes, D. L., & Palinkas, L. A. (2009). Implementing evidence-based practice in community mental health agencies: A multiple stakeholder analysis. *American Journal of Public Health, 99,* 2087–2095. https://doi.org/10.2105/AJPH.2009.161711

Avgar, A. C., Givan, R. K., & Liu, M. (2011). A balancing act: Work–life balance and multiple stakeholder outcomes in hospitals. *British Journal of Industrial Relations, 49,* 717–741. https://doi.org/10.1111/j.1467-8543.2010.00839.x

Bear-Lehman, J. (2012). Comparison of the Occupational Therapy Research Agenda with the National Institutes of Health Roadmap for Medical Research. *American Journal of Occupational Therapy, 66,* 250–253. https://doi.org/10.5014/ajot.2012.002840

Blackwell, C. K., Elliott, A. J., Ganiban, J., Herbstman, J., Hunt, K., Forrest, C. B., & Camargo, C. A. (2019). General health and life satisfaction in children with chronic illness. *Pediatrics, 143*(6), e20182988. https://doi.org/10.1542/peds.2018-2988

Blaskowitz, M. G., Famularo, E., Lonergan, M., Mcgrady, E., Layer, L., Randall, L., & Zelenko, M. (2018). Closing the gap: Identifying quality-of-life disparities for young adults with intellectual and developmental disabilities in transition. *American Journal of Occupational Therapy, 72*(4, Suppl. 1), 7211510164. https://doi.org/10.5014/ajot.2018.72S1-PO1020

Brach, M., Cieza, A., Stucki, P. D. M. G., Füssl, M., Cole, A., Ellerin, B., . . . Melvin, J. (2004). ICF Core Sets for breast cancer. *Journal of Rehabilitation Medicine, 36,* 121–127. https://doi.org/10.1080/16501960410016811

Butterworth, J., Winsor, J., Smith, F. A., Migliore, A., Domin, D., Ciulla Timmons, J., & Hall, A. C. (2015). *StateData: The national report on employment services and outcomes.* Boston: University of Massachusetts Boston, Institute for Community Inclusion.

Cieza, A., Stucki, P. D. M. G., Weigl, M., Kullmann, L., Stoll, T., Kamen, L., . . . Walsh, N. (2004). ICF Core Sets for chronic widespread pain. *Journal of Rehabilitation Medicine, 36,* 63–68. https://doi.org/10.1080/16501960410016046

Coenen, M., Cieza, A., Freeman, J., Khan, F., Miller, D., Weise, A., & Kesselring, J. (2011). The development of ICF Core Sets for multiple sclerosis: Results of the International Consensus Conference. *Journal of Neurology, 258,* 1477–1488. https://doi.org/10.1007/s00415-011-5963-7

Coster, W. J., Ni, P., Slavin, M. D., Kisala, P. A., Nandakumar, R., Mulcahey, M. J., . . . Jette, A. M. (2016). Differential item functioning in the Patient Reported Outcomes Measurement Information System Pediatric Short Forms in a sample of children and adolescents with cerebral palsy. *Developmental Medicine and Child Neurology, 58,* 1132–1138. https://doi.org/10.1111/dmcn.13138

Crist, P. (2014). Reliability and validity: The psychometrics of standardized assessments. In J. Hinojosa & P. Kramer (Eds.), *Evaluation in occupational therapy: Obtaining and interpreting data* (4th ed.). Bethesda, MD: AOTA Press.

deFur, S. H. (2003). IEP transition planning—From compliance to quality. *Exceptionality, 11,* 115–128. https://doi.org/10.1207/s15327035ex1102_06

Developmental Disabilities Assistance and Bill of Rights Act of 2000, Pub. L. 106–402, 42 U.S.C. 15001 *et seq.*

Egerter, S., Dekker, M., An, J., Grossman-Kahn, R., & Braveman, P. (2008). *Work matters for health* (Issue Brief 4: Work and Health). Princeton, NJ: Robert Wood Johnson Foundation Commission to Build a Healthier America. Retrieved from http://www.commissiononhealth.org/PDF/0e8ca13d-6fb8-451d-bac8-7d15343aacff/Issue%20Brief%204%20Dec%2008%20-%20Work%20and%20Health.pdf

Garland, A. F., Lewczyk-Boxmeyer, C. M., Gabayan, E. N., & Hawley, K. N. (2004). Multiple stakeholder agreement on desired outcomes for adolescents' mental health services. *Psychiatric Services, 55,* 671–676. https://doi.org/10.1176/appi.ps.55.6.671

Glässel, A., Kirchberger, I., Linseisen, E., Stamm, T., Cieza, A., & Stucki, G. (2010). Content validation of the International Classification of Functioning, Disability and Health (ICF) Core Set for Stroke: The perspective of occupational therapists. *Canadian Journal of Occupational Therapy, 77,* 289–302. https://doi.org/10.2182/cjot.2010.77.5.5

Haglund, L., and Henriksson, C. (2003). Concepts in occupational therapy in relation to the ICF. *Occupational Therapy International, 10,* 253–268. https://doi.org/10.1002/oti.189

Hall, J. P., Kurth, N. K., & Hunt, S. L. (2013). Employment as a health determinant for working-age, dually-eligible people with disabilities. *Disability and Health Journal, 6,* 100–106. https://doi.org/10.1016/j.dhjo.2012.11.001

Hammel, J., Southall, K., Jutai, J., Finlayson, M., Kashindi, G., & Fok, D. (2013). Evaluating use and outcomes of mobility technology: A multiple stakeholder analysis. *Disability and Rehabilitation: Assistive Technology, 8,* 294–304. https://doi.org/10.3109/17483107.2012.735745

HealthMeasures. (2019). *PROMIS.* Retrieved from http://www.healthmeasures.net/explore-measurement-systems/promis

Henninger, N. A., & Taylor, J. L. (2014). Family perspectives on a successful transition to adulthood for individuals with disabilities. *Intellectual and Developmental Disabilities, 52,* 98–111. https://doi.org/10.1352/1934-9556-52.2.98

Hyland, M., & Jackson, S. E. (2006). A multiple stakeholder perspective: Implications for measuring work–family outcomes. In M. Pitt-Catsouphes (Ed.), E. Ernst Kossek, & S. Sweet (Series Eds.), *The work and family handbook: Multi-disciplinary perspectives and approaches* (pp. 527–549). Mahwah, NJ: Erlbaum.

Individuals With Disabilities Education Improvement Act of 2004, Pub. L. 108–446, 20 U.S.C. §§ 1400–1482.

Kashikar-Zuck, S., Carle, A., Barnett, K., Goldschneider, K. R., Sherry, D. D., Mara, C. A., . . . DeWitt, E. M. (2016). Longitudinal evaluation of Patient Reported Outcomes Measurement Information Systems (PROMIS) measures in pediatric chronic pain. *Pain, 157,* 339–347. https://doi.org/10.1097/j.pain.0000000000000378

Kennedy, J., Brown, T., & Chien, C.-W. (2011). Motor skill assessment of children: Is there an association between performance-based, child-report, and parent-report measures of childrens motor skills? *Physical and Occupational Therapy in Pediatrics, 32*(2), 196–209. https://doi.org/10.3109/01942638.2011.631101

Kirchberger, I., Stamm, T., Cieza, A., & Stucki, G. (2007). Does the Comprehensive ICF Core Set for rheumatoid arthritis capture occupational therapy practice? A content-validity study. *Canadian Journal of Occupational Therapy, 74*(3, Suppl.), 267–280. https://doi.org/10.1177/00084174070740S308

Laxe, S., Zasler, N., Selb, M., Tate, R., Tormos, J. M., & Bernabeu, M. (2013). Development of the International Classification of Functioning, Disability and Health Core Sets for traumatic brain injury: An international consensus process. *Brain Injury, 27,* 379–387. https://doi.org/10.3109/02699052.2012.750757

Maitra, K. K., & Erway, F. (2006). Perception of client-centered practice in occupational therapists and their clients. *American Journal of Occupational Therapy, 60,* 298–310. https://doi.org/10.5014/ajot.60.3.298

Morris, Z. S., Wooding, S., & Grant, J. (2011). The answer is 17 years, what is the question: Understanding time lags in translational research. *Journal of the Royal Society of Medicine, 104*(12), 510–520. https://doi.org/10.1258/jrsm.2011.110180

Mulcahey, M. J., Slavin, M. D., Pengsheng, N., Kratz, A., Kisala, P. A., Tulsky, D. S., & Jette, A. M. (2018). Examination of psychometric properties of PROMIS˚: Pediatric upper limb measures in youth with cerebral palsy. *British Journal of Occupational Therapy, 81,* 393–401. https://doi.org/10.1177/0308022618757961

National Association of Councils on Developmental Disabilities. (2020). *Home.* Retrieved from https://www.nacdd.org/

National Institutes of Health. (2019a). *Common Data Element (CDE) Resource Portal.* Retrieved from https://www.nlm.nih.gov/cde/index.html

National Institutes of Health. (2019b). *NIH Toolbox for assessment of neurological and behavioral function.* Retrieved from https://neuroscienceblueprint.nih.gov/resources-tools/nih-toolbox-assessment-neurological-and-behavioral-function

National Institutes of Health. (2020). *About the ECHO program.* Retrieved from https://www.nih.gov/research-training/environmental-influences-child-health-outcomes-echo-program

Newman, L., Wagner, M., Knokey, A.-M., Marder, C., Nagle, K., Shaver, D., . . . Schwarting, M. (2011). *The post-high school outcomes of young adults with disabilities up to 8 years after high school: A report from the National Longitudinal Transition Study–2.* Menlo Park, CA: SRI International.

Orentlicher, M. L. (2015). Transition from school to adult life. In M. L. Orentlicher, S. Schefkind, & R. W. Gibson (Eds.), *Transitions across the lifespan: An occupational therapy approach* (pp. 103–127). Bethesda, MD: AOTA Press.

Patient-Centered Outcomes Research Institute. (2019). *PCORI's stakeholders.* https://www.pcori.org/about-us/our-programs/engagement/public-and-patient-engagement/pcoris-stakeholders

Ritz, D., Althauser, C., & Wilson, K. (2014). *Connecting health information systems for better health: Leveraging interoperability standards to link patient, provider, payor, and policymaker data.* Seattle PATH and Joint Learning Network for Universal Health Coverage.

Rogers, J. C., & Holm, M. B. (1994). Nationally Speaking—Accepting the challenge of outcome research: Examining the effectiveness of occupational therapy practice. *American Journal of Occupational Therapy, 48,* 871–876. https://doi.org/10.5014/ajot.48.10.871

Schur, L. (2002) The difference a job makes: The effects of employment among people with disabilities. *Journal of Economic Issues, 36,* 339–347, https://doi.org/10.1080/00213624.2002.11506476

Unsworth, C. (2000). Measuring the outcome of occupational therapy: Tools and resources. *Australian Occupational Therapy Journal, 47,* 147–158. https://doi.org/10.1046/j.1440-1630.2000.00239.x

U.S. Department of Education. (2018, December 18). *40th Annual Report to Congress on the implementation of the Individuals with Disabilities Education Act, Parts B and C.* Retrieved from https://www2.ed.gov/about/reports/annual/osep/2018/parts-b-c/40th-arc-for-idea.pdf

Weinfurt, K. P., Lin, L., Bruner, D. W., Cyranowski, J. M., Dombeck, C. B., Hahn, E. A., . . . Reese, J. B. (2015). Development and initial validation of the PROMIS˚ Sexual Function and Satisfaction Measures Version 2.0. *Journal of Sexual Medicine, 12,* 1961–1974. https://doi.org/10.1111/jsm.12966

World Health Organization. (2001). *International classification of functioning, disability and health.* Geneva: Author.

World Health Organization. (2002). *Towards a common language for functioning, disability and health: ICF.* Geneva: World Health Organization.

World Health Organization. (2019). *Classifications.* Retrieved from https://www.who.int/classifications/icf/appareas/en/

Yamamoto, K., Stodden, R. A., & Folk, E. D. R. (2014). Inclusive postsecondary education: Reimagining the transition trajectories of vocational rehabilitation clients with intellectual disabilities. *Journal of Vocational Rehabilitation, 40,* 59–71. https://doi.org/10.3233/JVR-130662

Addressing Diversity in Occupational Therapy Assessment

Razan Hamed, PhD, OTR/L

13

CHAPTER HIGHLIGHTS

- Diversity and health outcomes
- Many facets of diversity
- Macro and micro layers of diversity
- Assessment tools in evaluation for diverse populations and needs
- Diversity and evidence-based practice
- Other issues related to diversity in occupational therapy practice

KEY TERMS AND CONCEPTS

- Access
- Choices and goals
- Community
- Core
- Culture
- Cultural effectiveness
- Cultural humility
- Cultural sensitivity
- Culturally responsive care
- Diversity
- External factors and contexts
- Health disparities
- Individual
- Intrinsicality
- Life events
- Macro
- Meaning of life
- Macro–Micro Model of Diversity
- Micro
- Social systems
- Therapeutic use of self
- Transcultural competence
- Well-being

INTRODUCTION

This chapter discusses the concept of *diversity*, how it affects clients as functional beings, the relationship of diversity to health outcomes, and diversity relevance during evaluation and assessment. This chapter introduces the Macro–Micro Model of Diversity (MMMD), which depicts how diversity, with its many layers, affects people's function and their perceptions of their own identities. The chapter aims to assist occupational therapists in addressing the different layers of diversity in their assessments.

DIVERSITY AND HEALTH OUTCOMES

Diversity is the recognition, acceptance, and inclusion of different types of people. People engage in occupations in diverse ways; diversity "extends to cultural identities, values, and histories, as well as to the lenses through which people and communities see and understand themselves and the world" (Alvarez Jaramillo et al., 2020, p. 86). Principal health care organizations recognize that health outcomes are the product of interplay among numerous health systems across countries that have varied political systems. These large organizations also recognize that health

outcomes are highly dynamic, with changing functional spheres ranging from person to community, state, nation, and continent. Some examples of these large organizations and how they recognize diversity in people and health outcomes are as follows:

- The World Health Organization (WHO; 2019) states that health care professionals should be committed to development and innovation to serve the needs of a changing world. It also recognizes the "power of diversity to achieve more" and strives to "make people feel safe, respected, empowered, fairly treated, and duly recognized."
- The U.S. Department of Health and Human Services (DHHS; 2019) specifies that culture is a key determinant of health perception and that it

defines how health care information is received, how rights and protections are exercised, what is considered to be a health problem, how symptoms and concerns about the problem are expressed, who should provide treatment for the problem, and what type of treatment should be given. (p. 4)

DHHS defines *culture* as "the integrated pattern of human behavior that includes thoughts, communications, actions, customs, beliefs, values, and institutions of a racial, ethnic, religious, or social group" (p. 4).

- The National Institutes of Health's (NIH, 2019) mission is to "seek fundamental knowledge about the nature and behavior of living systems. . . . to enhance health, lengthen life, and reduce illness and disability." NIH's National Institute on Minority Health and Health Disparities (NIMHD; 2019) envisions "an America in which all populations will have an equal opportunity to live long, healthy, and productive lives." NIMHD also raises national awareness "about the prevalence and impact of health disparities and disseminates effective individual-, community-, and population-level interventions to reduce and encourage elimination of health disparities."

- The American Occupational Therapy Association (AOTA) mirrors the visions, missions, and statements of these health institutions in describing the relationship among occupation, diversity, culture, and health. AOTA's (2015) *Occupational Therapy Code of Ethics* explicitly states that the profession values and respects all facets of people's diversity (e.g., their culture, ethnicity, race, age, religion, gender, sexual orientation, and capacities). The profession has a well-documented commitment to serve the needs of the community across different populations and practice areas. It has consistently confirmed its commitment to nondiscrimination and inclusion practices that entail treating everyone fairly and equitably (AOTA, 2014).

AOTA's (2007) *Centennial Vision* envisioned occupational therapy as having a "globally connected and diverse workforce" (p. 613). It extended this vision to *Vision 2025*, which added the pillar of equity, inclusion, and diversity to explicitly embrace diversity in all its forms (AOTA, 2017c, 2020). This pillar reflects the profession's core tenet of holistic and client-centered care; occupational therapy practitioners are urged to address diversity in their daily practice, advocacy initiatives, and professional conduct. Inherent in this statement is that practitioners should engage in culturally responsive care. *Culturally responsive care* means "actively developing a synergistic relationship grounded in mutuality and intentional respect for a person's cultures" (Muñoz, 2007 p. 256).

The concept of diversity changes over time; therefore, health care practitioners need to update their perception of what diversity means to maintain an understanding of the challenges of treating all clients. *Diversity* no longer means just the mere variation or heterogeneity of traits within a population. It is more intricate and has many dimensions, such as the association between poverty and certain races (e.g., the association of American Indian people and low financial resources) or between certain disease conditions and gender (e.g., HIV and transgender people).

In addition, it has become clear that diversity directly affects short- and long-term health outcomes (Carter et al., 2017). From a life course perspective, people who have social and physical disadvantages in childhood—who often also have socioeconomic status, racial, and ethnic disparities—have greater health problems in adulthood (Braveman & Barclay, 2009). Although health care providers believe that health care disparities result from social and economic factors, clients identify racism on the part of providers as another potential contributor to health disparities (Gollust et al., 2018).

DIVERSITY IN THE OCCUPATIONAL THERAPY LITERATURE

Occupational therapy literature on the concept of *diversity* in different contexts has been increasing. The literature has addressed diversity with respect to pedagogical curricula (Trentham et al., 2007), the occupational therapy workforce (Black, 2002; Taff & Blash, 2017), the history of the profession (Black, 2002), health promotion (Suarez-Balcazar et al., 2016), and culturally sensitive and effective practices (AOTA, 2013; Barrett et al., 2020; Iwama et al., 2009; Wells et al., 2016).

The term *diversity* is often used in the same context as or interchangeably with terms such as *cultural sensitivity, transcultural competence, cultural humility, and cultural effectiveness.* Knowing how these terms are defined is important to understanding the broad concept of diversity:

- *Cultural sensitivity* is the "ability to be appropriately responsive to the attitudes, feelings, or circumstances of groups of people that share a common and distinctive racial, national, religious, linguistic or cultural heritage" (DHHS, Office of Minority Health, 2001, p.131). It can also be conceptualized as recognizing the needs of one's culture as well as those of others (Goode et al., 2000).

- *Transcultural competence* is the "awareness of, sensitivity to, and knowledge of, the meaning of culture" (Dillard et al., 1992, p. 722).

- *Cultural humility* is "the ability to maintain an interpersonal stance that is other-oriented (or open to the other) in relation to aspects of cultural identity that are most important to the client" (Hook et al., 2013, p. 354). It also involves "redressing power imbalances in client–therapist relationships by incorporating critical self-evaluation and recognizing that cultural differences lie not within clients but within client-therapist relationships" (Hammell, 2013, p. 224).

- *Cultural effectiveness* focuses on outcomes and is "the ability to interact with people from different cultures so as to optimize the probability of mutually successful outcomes" (Stone, 2006, p. 338).

AOTA has recently increased its momentum toward accommodating diversity and cultural competence in occupational therapy practice and education through various diversity-centered committees, including recently recruiting for a new task force on diversity (AOTA, 2017b).

Occupational therapy practitioners promote engagement through occupation to achieve health, well-being, and participation in daily life (AOTA, 2014). Diversity is embedded in every facet of occupation, from the conceptualization of time to social aspects, such as language and types of interactions. Regardless of the terms associated with diversity, health care practitioners are paying more attention to diversity's impact on health outcomes (Duran & Pérez-Stable, 2019).

MACRO AND MICRO LAYERS OF DIVERSITY

Assessment is a critical part of the occupational therapy process. Conducting client-centered assessment and evaluation means addressing issues, such as diverse cultural factors, that affect clients' functional performance at all levels (Hammell, 2015). This chapter introduces the *Macro–Micro Model of Diversity (MMMD)* to show how diversity exists at different layers of the person beyond ethnicity, gender, or race and how it affects people's daily functional performance over time. Occupational therapists have to understand diversity at its deepest levels to better address and accommodate its impact on their clients' functionality.

Diversity is often perceived as variations among people in terms of gender, race, ethnicity, and heritage. Therefore, when talking about diversity in the workforce, health care, education, or community, people immediately note the obvious, or *macro,* layers of diversity (e.g., gender, race), but they rarely look at the subtle, or *micro,* layers of diversity. These micro layers may include intracultural variations, intraperson diversity, or temporal diversity (i.e., diversity that changes over time, such as identifying as transgender, converting to another faith). Both macro and micro layers affect the occupations that make up people's lives (Duran & Pérez-Stable, 2019).

Figure 13.1 displays the macro and micro layers of diversity and how they affect functioning. For example, even within a population that speaks the same language, occupational therapy practitioners have to pay attention to the interplay between this easily identifiable facet of diversity (i.e., language) and more intricate layers of diversity (e.g., socioeconomic class, generation, and geographical location). A 65-year-old Spanish-speaking client with stroke may use different terms and dialect than a 16-year-old

bilingual client with traumatic brain injury. *Therapeutic use of self* is the conscious use of an interpersonal relationship with a client to have a therapeutic effect on that client's outcomes (Solman & Clouston, 2016). Occupational therapy practitioners are urged to use therapeutic use of self to identify this micro layer of diversity and work toward a more client-centered communication style, for example, learning terms commonly used by these two distinct age groups.

This holistic look at diversity is perfectly consistent with larger models with respect to health and function (e.g., the *International Classification of Functioning, Disability and Health [ICF];* WHO, 2001) and frameworks (e.g., the *Occupational Therapy Practice Framework: Domain and Process [OTPF]* AOTA, 2014). Table 13.1 shows the macro and micro layers of diversity in relation to the *ICF* and the *OTPF*. It also shows the areas of occupation that occupational therapists should consider during assessment when using the *OTPF.*

Macro Layers

Community

A *community* is a group of people with common characteristics. This is the *macro* level. People are part of different functional communities such as a city or a family. The interplay people experience between their communities shapes how they perceive and feel about their culture, which, in turn,

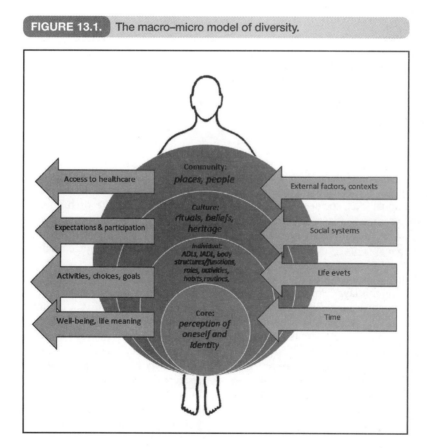

FIGURE 13.1. The macro–micro model of diversity.

Note. ADLS = activities of daily living; IADLS = instrumental activities of daily living.

TABLE 13.1.   Macro and Micro Layers of Diversity, the *OTPF*, and the *ICF*

LAYER OF DIVERSITY	MECHANISMS AFFECTING DIVERSITY	AREAS OF FUNCTIONING			
		MAY BE AFFECTED BY THE CLIENT'S DIVERSITY	AS CLASSIFIED IN THE *OTPF*	AS CLASSIFIED IN THE *ICF*	OCCUPATIONAL THERAPY AREAS OF ASSESSMENT
MACRO LEVEL					
Community	External factors and contexts may facilitate or hinder access to health care on the basis of the client (e.g., immigration status, SES)	Access to health care resources	Contexts (context and environment[a])	Environmental factors	Access that may affect health outcomes (e.g., access to rehabilitation, community-based programs, health literacy), the physical environment (e.g., wheelchair access in underserved communities)
Culture	Social systems may shape what is expected of clients on the basis of their diversity factors (e.g., gender)	Expectations, participation	Participation, performance patterns	Participation	Habits, rituals, cultural identification, attitudes, social background, social status, SES
MICRO LEVEL					
Individual	Life events, perceived in light of one's diversity (e.g., coping with loss)	Daily activities, choices, goals	Occupations, performance patterns, performance skills	Engagement in occupation	ADLs, IADLs, habits, routines, roles, rituals, life experiences, education, profession, lifestyle, motor skills, process skills, social interaction skills
Core	Time; clients' attitude toward their diversity may change over time	Well-being, meaning of life	Client factors	Personal factors, well-being	Age, sexual orientation, values, beliefs, upbringing, spirituality, body structures, body functions

Note. ADLs = activities of daily living; IADLs = instrumental activities of daily living; *ICF = International Classification of Functioning, Disability and Health; OTPF = Occupational Therapy Practice Framework;* SES = socioeconomic status.
[a]Terminology used in the *OTPF*.

shapes their overall success and functionality. People tend to be grouped within a community according to their differences (e.g., race, ethnicity, educational level, socioeconomic status, immigration status). The community macro layer is also the most extrinsic layer of people's functional being; hence, it is affected by **external factors and contexts** (e.g., change in legislative policies, availability of resources, environment).

Diversity, and how it affects (and is affected by) the community, is easily recognized at this layer. For example, occupational therapists may recognize how differences among clients (e.g., immigration status, language, economic and educational backgrounds) may affect clients' **access** to health care resources or coverage (e.g., Medicaid, home assessment coverage, access to community-based programs, health literacy). In fact, it is evident that this layer of diversity can explain a number of **health disparities** (Coulter et al., 2019) and limited access to health care interventions (Pollard & Sakellariou, 2017). For example, preliminary data on COVID-19 has shown that health disparities has led to higher numbers of cases in minority communities, particularly Black communities (Thebault et al., 2020; Yancy, 2020).

When building an occupational profile during an evaluation, occupational therapists can examine the external factors that facilitate or hinder the intervention plan, for example, by conducting an assessment of the home environment, identifying access to a social worker, or assessing a client's ability to manage medication.

Culture

People also exist within a culture that they adopt, change, and share particular behaviors, beliefs, and values. The culture layer "involves ways of being, doing, and thinking" (Coppola et al., 2020, p. 3). This layer is less visible than the community layer and is highly influenced by the pressure from or support of **social systems** (e.g., ethnicities, traditions, familial hierarchies, customs, ideologies). This macro level of diversity is unlikely to change quickly or be affected by external factors (e.g., legislation is not likely to affect wedding traditions in a Jewish community).

Occupational therapists may identify this level of diversity by working to understand how culture shapes clients' expectations and participation (e.g., attendance at family gatherings, support from one's family after an injury, relationship with parents and grandparents, gender role) regardless of their physical, mental, or psychosocial health or well-being. Occupational therapists' expectations of a certain culture may eventually lead to stereotypes and "diversity labeling" (e.g., that men outperform women in science, technology, engineering, and math jobs; Caucasian physicians provide better health care than non-Caucasian physicians), which may affect clients' daily functioning. When planning their assessments, occupational therapists should ask about the client's cultural expectations and understand them and how important they are to the client.

Micro Layers

Individual

At the *individual* level, people assume self-assigned roles and project their social and functional identities. This is the most active layer of diversity, where people define and select their roles, daily activities, routines, habits, social relationships, work dynamics, and so forth. Therefore, *life events* greatly affect the balance between diversity and function; changing jobs, getting married, losing a loved one, achieving an educational milestone, and financial status may all be affected by one's culture. Culture drives people's beliefs and traditions, as well as their behaviors and family expectations. In some cultures, the younger generation is expected to support and care for the older generation. People's *choices and goals,* made as individuals in light of their diverse cultures, may completely shift their functional activities. Occupational therapists use every facet of this layer in their assessment and intervention planning. Goals are established after the assessment and must take into account assessment data as well as clients' cultural background and preferences.

Assessment that addresses cultural diversity

Occupational therapists have to consider clients' background and culture when performing an assessment. By starting with the occupational profile, therapists gain an understanding of who the client is, the client's cultural background, and the importance of that background in the client's life.

As occupational therapists choose assessments, in particular those that are standardized, they should consider the following:

- Therapists should select assessment tools that were designed for the population with which the client identifies (e.g., Hispanic older adult).
- If no such are tools available, therapists should consider modifying existing valid and reliable assessment tools to better match the client's needs. Tools that are modified require research to reexamine their psychometric properties, and any modification of tools should be noted in the evaluation report.
- Assessment tools and evaluation methods should be suitable to address daily activities or lifestyles that match the client's needs and goals, roles, habits, preferences, and daily activities.
- The psychometric data available on the assessment should be reviewed to determine the sample demographics

and whether any study has examined the assessment's validity for the client's cultural group or groups. Normative data should include whether the standardization included people from different cultural backgrounds and areas of the country. For example, if a test was standardized only for children who live in warm climates where they can play outside throughout the year, the therapist should question whether it is relevant to children who live in the Northeastern United States, where seasonal changes prevent the same type of year-round activities. For further information, refer to Chapter 3, "Assessment Identification and Selection."

Core

The last layer of diversity lies at the person's core. This is the *micro* level. The *core* is the deepest level of the person; it is intrinsic to the person and defines who the person is and how the person views their own identity and culture. This layer is consistent with the concept of intrinsicality, as discussed by Hammell (2001). *Intrinsicality* is an active component of people's inner being and, therefore, their culture and diversity. It contributes to people's motivation, the occupations that they value and in which they participate. The core may remain constant or change over time, based on people's experiences, both past and present. The relationship among this and the other layers of diversity greatly affects people's overall *well-being* and *meaning of life*. It also affects their satisfaction with daily occupations, life roles, and outcomes.

When using the occupational profile (AOTA, 2017a) as part of an assessment, therapists should be aware of how diversity affects functioning. The following are things that occupational therapists should be thinking about while administering the occupational profile:

- Actively listen to the client's story and recognize components of gender, race, and ethnicity over time or as they relate to a life event such as an illness or disability.
- Pay attention to the verbal and nonverbal messages that may be consistent with a person's background rather than the immediate situation.
- Ask questions (if and when appropriate) about how the person feels culture and diversity may be affecting functioning.
- Document identified diversity-based challenges, and be sure to revisit them at reassessment.
- Seek resources or personnel to support themselves or their client to overcome diversity challenges so that they can better understand the experiences of those from diverse backgrounds.

Table 13.2 provides guidelines for addressing diversity in occupational therapy assessment.

DIVERSITY AND ASSESSMENT TOOLS

It is important to understand the reason for assessing a client when deciding what assessment methods should be used. Failure to do so will result in assessment data that are fragmented and not client centered (Smith, 1992). *Culture* is a live, active concept of human daily functioning (Castro et al., 2014), and it can be a determining factor in selecting

TABLE 13.2.   Guidelines for Occupational Therapy Practitioners on Addressing Issues Related to Diversity

LAYER OF DIVERSITY	MECHANISMS AFFECTING DIVERSITY	ASSESSMENT CHECKLIST FOR A CLIENT'S OCCUPATIONAL PROFILE
		MACRO LEVEL
Community	External factors and contexts	List client-identified diversity groups (e.g., race, ethnicity, gender, sexual orientation, heritage, immigration status). Identify hindering or facilitating factors for the client's diversity-related group in relation to ▪ Technology (e.g., telehealth) ▪ Natural or manmade environment (e.g., accessibility, universal design) ▪ Attitude of community members toward the client's diversity group ▪ Services, systems, policies, and legislation (e.g., health care coverage or lack of it for the client's diversity group). Explore evidence of health disparities with client-identified diversity groups (e.g., minorities, underserved populations, vulnerable populations). Discuss what literature findings your client thinks are relevant to their occupational profile. Explore (or refer the client to) supportive resources that are available to the client.
Culture	Social systems	Select assessment tools designed for the client's most relevant population. Select assessment tools and evaluation methods that are suitable to address daily activities or lifestyles or modify currently existing assessment tools to better match the client's needs. ▪ Create a list of the client's diversity-group-related habits, rituals, cultural identification, and attitudes and activities or roles unique to the family Discuss with the client how these factors affect their daily functioning. Explore and apply research evidence on the best methods and nuances of assessing health and functional outcomes in the client's population. Explore evidence from ethnographic research relevant to the client's diversity group.
		MICRO LEVEL
Individual	Life events	Create a list of the client's ▪ Impairments in body structure and body function; ▪ ADLs, IADLs, habits, routines, roles, rituals, life experiences, education, profession, lifestyle, motor skills, process skills, and social interaction skills; and ▪ Life events that may have affected the client's areas of daily functioning. Discuss with the client how these areas are affected by the client's diversity group (e.g., wedding rituals, demands in a certain culture, birthing traditions).
Core	Time	Explore the client's illness story and ▪ Actively listen to the client's story and recognize components of this layer, ▪ Pay attention to verbal and nonverbal messages, ▪ Ask questions about the client's underlying feelings, ▪ Identify challenges related to diversity, ▪ Document how the identified challenges affect daily functioning and revisit them in the reassessment, and ▪ Seek resources or personnel to support you or the client in overcoming diversity challenges.

Note. ADLs = activities of daily living; IADLs = instrumental activities of daily living.

an occupation-oriented assessment tool (e.g., assessing the ability of a client with a stroke to perform the daily prayers of the Muslim faith).

Nonstandardized Assessment Tools

Typically, culture-tailored assessment tools are nonstandardized. Therefore, in addition to using the occupational profile, therapists may opt to use a nonstandardized tool to complete a comprehensive client-centered assessment. In deciding to use a nonstandardized assessment tool, occupational therapists have to ensure the following:
▪ The nonstandardized tool is a better fit for the person, function, and context than currently available standardized tools.
▪ No adaptable standardized assessment tools are available that can be used to assess the client.

▪ The nonstandardized tool has evidence in the literature of its validity and reliability (i.e., relevant research studies for that tool's adaptability to different cultures or populations) and of expert opinion (if no research is available for the assessment area, culture, or diagnostic group) or sound clinical judgment (e.g., to ensure all test items assess the intended outcomes).

Standardized Assessment Tools

The use of standardized assessment tools (when possible) is best practice for occupational therapists because of these tools' structured nature and established validity and reliability. Standardized tools usually include a protocol that describes or provides the materials used during the assessment, the setup or context, scoring, and interpretation of findings. If normative data are used in scoring, standardized tools can help give therapists an idea of how close to or far from target outcomes the client is compared with others in the same diagnostic group or clinical population. Standardized assessments are also helpful in collecting data for reassessment, follow-up, or discharge planning. However, when using standardized tools occupational therapists have to consider the following:

- Standardized assessment tools leave little room for the invisible aspects of performance or those that indirectly affect performance, such as diversity and culture. Therefore, therapists have to decide whether using a standardized assessment tool is the best approach for a client-centered assessment.

- When using a standardized tool, therapists have to be familiar with the tool's development. For example, therapists have to be aware of the population for which the assessment was originally designed (e.g., diagnosis, age group), the context in which the tool can be most helpful (e.g., clinic vs. home), and the tool's intended purpose (e.g., screening vs. assessment). Knowledge of these aspects of a tool will later help therapists determine the appropriateness of using that tool with a client who differs from the original population—especially if the tool does not provide guidelines on how to use it in populations other than those for which it was developed. A good start for therapists is to read the assessment manual and guidelines to familiarize themselves with the tool's origins. Another helpful practice is to explore research studies that validated or standardized the tool for a new or different population than that for which it was originally developed.

Occupational therapists should also be familiar with any possible adaptations to the standardized tool of interest. For example, the authors or developers of a standardized assessment tool may allow or even recommend adapting some aspects of the tool, such as selecting different materials, grading the difficulty of the activities assessed, or changing the administration context. Therapists should therefore explore possible diversity-specific adaptations that they can apply when assessing their clients. The assessment manual, published data, research articles, or communication with the original authors (if possible) can be useful in determining the possibility of adaptation.

Occupational therapists excel at identifying differences among their clients when it comes to performance skills, performance patterns, occupations, contexts, and client factors. Cognitive function, for example, varies across clients and populations because of factors such as age, diagnosis, occupation, and environment. Occupational therapists are able to shift their perspective to the population in question when assessing or addressing cognitive function (e.g., they select assessment tools that fit the population). These considerations may lead occupational therapists to choose a nonstandardized assessment tool over a standardized one to better match the clinical outcomes expected of the population of interest. Practitioners can explore research studies that provide examples of nonstandardized assessment tools that have been found to be suitable for that population. They can also connect with other national or international occupational therapy practitioners who may have previous experience in assessing or treating that population. Physical or virtual meetings, symposiums, or networks (e.g., the World Federation of Occupational Therapists' World Occupational Therapy Day; professional groups or occupational therapy state associations on social media) can be useful resources to gain insight on this issue.

Likewise, occupational therapists may choose to use (or not use) a certain assessment tool on the basis of the client's diverse background. Hence, the decision of whether to use a standardized or a nonstandardized assessment tool is informed by the therapist's ability to complete a client-centered, culturally relevant comprehensive evaluation of the client's performance areas, skills, and patterns. Throughout the assessment process, therapists inevitably have to weigh and reevaluate which is more beneficial for the client: using a standardized assessment tool with no cultural relevance (which may lead to ineffective intervention outcomes) or using a nonstandardized assessment tool

CASE EXAMPLE 13.1. SHARIFAH: USING THE MACRO–MICRO MODEL OF DIVERSITY

Sharifah is a 37-year-old woman who was diagnosed with multiple sclerosis a year ago. She is working with the occupational therapist on energy conservation techniques, balance training, muscle strengthening, and cognitive functioning. On certain days, she uses crutches or a walker for support when moving around the house. Sharifah cares for her two children, ages 5 and 7 years, who attend public school. She also cares for her 65-year-old mother, who needs medication for several medical conditions. Sharifah works as a part-time seamstress in her home. Her husband serves in the military and is deployed overseas for a 2-year assignment.

Sharifah describes herself as a "believer" and a "caring mother, daughter, and sister." She constantly expresses her will to improve her daily functioning and maximize her time and energy to better take care of her family. When setting her therapeutic goals with the occupational therapist, she prioritizes her daily functioning activities as follows: taking care of her family and religious activities, including praying.

Sharifah has a 30-year-old sister who lives 6 hours away and who is getting married in 2 months. She shared with the occupational therapist that she is very anxious about attending her sister's wedding, where "everybody will be watching everybody," and about the travel arrangements with her two young children and her mother. She also shared that she is expected to show up for the wedding as "the big sister," regardless of her health at the time.

Sharifah lives in a rural area with limited access to transportation.

CASE EXAMPLE 13.1. SHARIFAH: USING THE MACRO–MICRO MODEL OF DIVERSITY *(Cont.)*

The occupational therapist ask Sharifah the following questions to better understand all areas of her life during the assessment and in future intervention planning:

1. What is Sharifah's racial, ethnic, and faith background and how does that affect her daily functioning? (*macro:* community, external factors)
2. What are some of the community-based factors that may support or hinder Sharifah's functional goals? (*macro:* community, external factors)
3. How does Sharifah's culture perceive her illness, and how does that affect her daily functioning? (*macro:* culture, social system)

4. How does Sharifah's family perceive Sharifah's current living conditions (e.g., illness, working at home, husband's temporary absence)? (*macro:* culture, social system, community)
5. What do Sharifah's self-described roles (e.g., "believer") entail, and how do they affect her daily functioning? (*micro:* individual)
6. How is planning to attend her sister's wedding affecting Sharifah's mental and physical functioning? (*micro:* individual, life events)
7. What does the activity analysis of praying look like? (*micro:* individual choices and goals)

---

that is client centered and culturally relevant (which may lead to effective intervention outcomes). Therapists should reconsider their choice of assessment tool as the process unfolds and on the basis of the client's feedback on its cultural relevance.

DIVERSITY AND EVIDENCE-BASED PRACTICE: HELPFUL PRACTICE HABITS

Providing client-centered, diversity-accommodating care is not a simple task. It requires a significant amount of critical thinking, reflection, clinical reasoning, and evidence seeking on the part of occupational therapists (Hammell, 2015). However, over time, providing diversity-relevant care becomes a natural and intuitive process. Note these helpful habits to accommodate diversity in occupational therapy assessment:

- Therapists should seek scientific and research evidence while constructing an occupational profile for clients of diverse backgrounds. This evidence will help therapists build experience in accommodating diversity issues in their evaluations. For example, a recent study showed that feeling connected to the activities in a treatment plan and the meaningfulness of those activities in the client's own culture is one way to accommodate clients with diverse backgrounds (du Toit & Buchanan, 2018). du Toit and Buchanan (2018) concluded that "celebrating [the] cultural diversity" (p. 7) of the client is one way to make their assessment process more relevant.
- During this continuous evidence-seeking process, therapists should make a professional habit of compiling a list of helpful research articles and assessment tools that address diversity and consult it whenever applicable.
- Therapists should make a checklist of factors to consider while conducting assessments and evaluating the macro and micro layers of diversity (Figure 13.1).
- Therapists can ask the following four questions to make sure they have addressed diversity in their assessment and evaluation:

1. Who is my client and what is available or unavailable to this client in reaching functional goals? Identify race, ethnicity, age, biological diversity factors, and living arrangements. (*macro layer:* community)
2. What does this client's culture look like, and how does it affect the client's daily functioning? (*macro layer:* culture)
3. What are the client's needs as a member of a diverse or minority group? What are my assessment options? Which option matches my client's diverse needs? Is there a better option to assess this problem, even if it is not available? (*micro layer:* individual)
4. Do my clients feel that they "belong" to their treatment plans and that care is meaningful? (*micro layer:* core)

SUMMARY

Diversity can be a determinant of health and health outcomes. It greatly affects people's daily functioning, and occupational therapists should pay close attention to its role in their assessments and interventions. The occupational therapy evaluation is a comprehensive and client-centered process that should address all aspects of the client, including diversity.

Diversity exists at macro and micro layers, and it affects how people perceive health and seek to reach their functional goals. Exploring research evidence on diverse client populations, selecting assessment tools that are relevant to clients' background, and identifying the subtleties of clients' diversity are a few examples of how occupational therapy assessment can accommodate diversity issues. Occupational therapists should always use their scientific judgment and clinical reasoning skills to select assessment tools that accommodate clients' diversity. Sharing successful practice stories, collecting diversity-friendly assessment tools, and exploring the best available evidence on diversity issues in practice are healthy practice habits for occupational therapy practitioners, students, and educators.

QUESTIONS

1. What is your perception of the relationship between diversity and health care outcomes?
2. What are the differences among the terms *cultural sensitivity, transcultural competence, cultural humility, and cultural effectiveness?* Are there similarities among these terms?
3. Considering the Macro–Micro Model of Diversity, discuss one macro and one micro level. How do they relate to each other? How do you think this model will help you as an occupational therapist?
4. How can nonstandardized assessments be helpful when working with clients from diverse backgrounds?
5. What is a standardized tool that can be used with different cultures and ethnicities? What is a standardized tool that you do not think would be appropriate for differing cultures and ethnicities? Why?
6. Think about a case that you had or saw in fieldwork. What new questions might you ask the client after having read this chapter?
7. In what ways can you ensure that you're considering aspects of a client's life that differ from your own?

REFERENCES

Alvarez Jaramillo, L., Moreno, N. A. J., Mthembu, T. G., Rivas-Quarneti, N., Tan, B. L., & Veloza, O. J. L. (2020). A journey through stories of occupational therapy around the world. In K. Barrett, S. Coppola, & L. Alvarez Jaramillo (Eds.), *International occupational therapy: Strategies for working and learning abroad* (pp. 85–98). North Bethesda, MD: AOTA Press.

American Occupational Therapy Association. (2007). AOTA's *Centennial Vision* and executive summary. *American Journal of Occupational Therapy, 61,* 613–613. https://doi.org/10.5014/ajot.61.6.613

American Occupational Therapy Association. (2013). *Frequently asked questions: How can occupational therapy strive towards culturally sensitive practices?* Retrieved from https://www.aota.org/~/media/Corporate/Files/Secure/Practice/Multicultural/FAQCulturalSensitivity.pdf

American Occupational Therapy Association. (2014). Occupational therapy practice framework: Domain and process (3rd ed.). *American Journal of Occupational Therapy, 68*(Suppl. 1), S1–S48. http://dx.doi.org/10.5014/ajot.2014.682006

American Occupational Therapy Association. (2015). Occupational therapy code of ethics and ethics standards (2015). *American Journal of Occupational Therapy, 69*(Suppl. 3), 6913410030. http://dx.doi.org/10.5014/ajot.696S03

American Occupational Therapy Association. (2017a). AOTA occupational profile template. *American Journal of Occupational Therapy, 71*(Suppl. 2), 7112420030. https://doi.org/10.5014/ajot.2017.716S12

American Occupational Therapy Association. (2017b). *Representative Assembly motion submission form: Diverse workforce: Education, competence, and ethics.* Retrieved from https://www.aota.org/~/media/Corporate/Files/Secure/Governance/RA/RA-Spring-2017/Diverse-Workforce-EC-COP-COE-final%20to-post.pdf

American Occupational Therapy Association. (2017c). Vision 2025. *American Journal of Occupational Therapy, 71,* 7103420010. https://doi.org/10.5014/ajot.2017.713002

American Occupational Therapy Association. (2020). *AOTA unveils Vision 2025.* Retrieved from https://www.aota.org/AboutAOTA/vision-2025.aspx

Barrett, K., Coppola, S., & Alvarez Jaramillo, L. (Eds.). (2020). *International occupational therapy: Strategies for working and learning abroad.* North Bethesda, MD: AOTA Press.

Black, R. M. (2002). Occupational therapy's dance with diversity. *American Journal of Occupational Therapy, 56,* 140–148. https://doi.org/10.5014/ajot.56.2.140

Braveman, P., & Barclay, C. (2009). Health disparities beginning in childhood: A life-course perspective. *Pediatrics, 124*(Suppl. 3), S163–S175. https://doi.org/10.1542/peds.2009-1100D

Carter, R., Lau, M., Johnson, V., & Kirkinis, K. (2017). Racial discrimination and health outcomes among racial/ethnic minorities: A meta-analytic review. *Journal of Multicultural Counseling and Development, 45,* 232–259. https://doi.org/10.1002/jmcd.12076

Castro, D, Dahlin-Ivanoff, S., & Mårtensson, L. (2014). Occupational therapy and culture: A literature review. *Scandinavian Journal of Occupational Therapy, 21,* 401–414. https://doi.org/10.3109/11038128.2014.898086

Coppola, S., Alvarez Jaramillo, L., Tupe, D., & Barrett, K. (2020). Occupation and intercultural practice. In K. Barrett, S. Coppola, & L. Alvarez Jaramillo (Eds.), *International occupational therapy: Strategies for working and learning abroad* (pp. 1–12). North Bethesda, MD: AOTA Press.

Coulter, R. W. S., Egan, J. E., Kinsky, S., Friedman, M. R., Eckstrand, K. L., Frankeberger, J., . . . Miller, E. (2019). *Mental health, drug, and violence interventions for sexual/gender minorities: A systematic review. Pediatrics, 144,* e20183367. https://doi.org/10.1542/peds.2018-3367

Dillard, M., Andonian, L., Flores, O., Lai, L., MacRae, A., & Shakir, M. (1992). Culturally competent occupational therapy in a diversely populated mental health setting. *American Journal of Occupational Therapy, 46,* 721–726. https://doi.org/10.5014/ajot.46.8.721

Duran, D., & Pérez-Stable, E. (2019). Novel approaches to advance minority health and health disparities research. *American Journal of Public Health, 109*(Suppl. 1), S8–S10. https://doi.org/10.2105/AJPH.2018.304931

du Toit, S. H. J., & Buchanan, H. (2018). Embracing cultural diversity: Meaningful engagement for older adults with advanced dementia in a residential care setting. *American Journal of Occupational Therapy, 72,* 7206205090. https://doi.org/10.5014/ajot.2018.027292

Gollust, S. E., Cunningham, B. A., Bokhour, B. G., Gordon, H.S., Pope, C., Saha, S. S., . . . Burgess, D. J. (2018). What causes racial health care disparities? A mixed-methods study reveals variability in how health care providers perceive causal attributions. *Inquiry, 55,* 46958018762840. https://doi.org/10.1177/0046958018762840

Goode, T., Sockalingam, S., Bronheim, S., Brown, M., & Jones, W. (2000). *A planner's guide . . . Infusing principles, content and themes related to cultural and linguistic competence into meetings and conferences.* Retrieved from https://nccc.georgetown.edu/documents/Planners_Guide.pdf

Hammell, K. W. (2001). Intrinsicality: Reconsidering spirituality, meaning(s) and mandates. *Canadian Journal of Occupational Therapy, 68*(3), 186–94. https://doi.org/10.1177/000841740106800307

Hammell, K. W. (2013). Occupation, well-being, and culture: Theory and cultural humility. *Canadian Journal of Occupational Therapy, 80,* 224–234. https://doi.org/10.1177/0008417413500465

Hammell, K. W. (2015). Client-centred occupational therapy: The importance of critical perspectives. *Scandinavian Journal of Occupational Therapy, 22,* 237–243. https://doi.org/10.3109/11038128.2015.1004103

Hook, J. N., Davis, D. E., Owen, J., Worthington, E. L., Jr., & Utsey, S. O. (2013). Cultural humility: Measuring openness to culturally diverse clients. *Journal of Counseling Psychology, 60,* 353–366. https://doi.org/10.1037/a0032595

Iwama, M., Thomson, N., & Macdonald, R. (2009). The Kawa model: The power of culturally responsive occupational therapy. *Disability and Rehabilitation, 31,* 1125–1135. https://doi.org/10.1080/09638280902773711

Muñoz, J. (2007). Culturally responsive caring in occupational therapy. *Occupational Therapy International, 14,* 256–280. https://doi.org/10.1002/oti.238

National Institutes of Health. (2019). *Mission and goals.* Retrieved from https://www.nih.gov/about-nih/what-we-do/mission-goals

National Institute on Minority Health and Health Disparities. (2019). *Mission and vision.* Retrieved from https://www.nimhd.nih.gov/about/overview/mission-vision.html

Pollard, N., & Sakellariou, D. (2017). Occupational therapy on the margins. *World Federation of Occupational Therapists Bulletin, 73,* 71–75. https://doi.org/10.1080/14473828.2017.1361698

Solman, B., & Clouston, T. (2016). Occupational therapy and the therapeutic use of self. *British Journal of Occupational Therapy, 79*(8), 514–516. https://doi.org/10.1177/0308022616638675

Stone, N. (2006). Conceptualising intercultural effectiveness for university teaching. *Journal of Studies in International Education, 10,* 334–356. https://doi.org/10.1177/1028315306287634

Smith, R. O. (1992). The science of occupational therapy assessment. *Occupational Therapy Journal of Research, 12,* 3–15. https://doi.org/10.1177/153944929201200101

Suarez-Balcazar, Y., Hoisington, M., Orozco, A. A., Arias, D., Garcia, C., Smith, K., & Bonner, B. (2016). Benefits of a culturally tailored health promotion program for Latino youth with disabilities and their families. *American Journal of Occupational Therapy, 70,* 7005180080. https://doi.org/10.5014/ajot.2016.021949

Taff, S. D., & Blash, D. (2017). Diversity and inclusion in occupational therapy: Where we are, where we must go. *Occupational Therapy in Health Care, 31,* 72–83. https://doi.org/10.1080/07380577.2016.1270479

Thebault R., Ba Tran, A., & Williams, V. (2020, April 7). The coronavirus is infecting and killing black Americans at an alarmingly high rate. *Washington Post.* Retrieved from https://www.washingtonpost.com/nation/2020/04/07/coronavirus-is-infecting-killing-black-americans-an-alarmingly-high-rate-post-analysis-shows/

Trentham, B., Cockburn, L., Cameron, D., & Iwama, M. (2007). Diversity and inclusion within an occupational therapy curriculum. *Australian Journal of Occupational Therapy, 54*(1), S49–S57. https://doi.org/10.1111/j.1440-1630.2006.00605.x

U.S. Department of Health and Human Services. (2019). *About HHS.* Retrieved from https://www.hhs.gov/about/index.html

U.S. Department of Health and Human Services, Office of Minority Health. (2001). *National standards for culturally and linguistically appropriate services in health care: Final report* (Contract No. 282-99-0039). Retrieved from https://minorityhealth.hhs.gov/assets/pdf/checked/finalreport.pdf

Wells, S. A., Black, R. M., & Gupta, J. (Eds.). (2016). *Culture and occupation: Effectiveness for occupational therapy practice, education, and research* (3rd ed.). Bethesda, MD: AOTA Press.

World Health Organization. (2001). *International classification of functioning, disability and health.* Geneva: Author.

World Health Organization. (2019). *Our values, our DNA.* Retrieved from https://www.who.int/about/who-we-are/our-values

Yancy, C. W. (2020). COVID-19 and African Americans. *Journal of the American Medical Association, 323,* 1891–1892. https://doi.org/10.1001/jama.2020.6548

Evaluation in Emerging Practice Settings: Primary Care, Telehealth, and Group- and Population-Based Evaluation

14

Lydia Royeen, PhD, OTR/L; Lauren Little, PhD, OTR/L; Laurette Olson, PhD, OTR/L, FAOTA; and Paula Kramer, PhD, OTR, FAOTA

CHAPTER HIGHLIGHTS

- Occupational therapy in the primary care setting
- *Standards of Practice for Occupational Therapy* and primary care
- *Occupational Therapy Practice Framework* and primary care
- Telehealth similarities to and differences from traditional settings
- Telehealth assessment methods
- Beginning the evaluation process for groups and populations
- Developing group or population occupational profiles
- Occupational performance analysis for groups and populations

KEY TERMS AND CONCEPTS

- Advocacy
- Context and environment
- Ecological models of practice
- Effective communication
- Evaluation report
- Focus group
- Groups
- Health disparity

- Holistic evaluation
- Interviewing
- Literature review
- Motivational interviewing
- Occupational performance analyses
- Occupational profile
- Occupational therapy–directed health promotion

- Primary care
- Store and forward
- Surveys
- Telehealth
- Videoconferencing
- Virtual rapport
- Webside manner

INTRODUCTION

For the profession to continue being relevant, occupational therapy needs to be responsive to changes in society. If a profession does not change, it runs the risk of becoming irrelevant and disappearing. Occupational therapy has continually evolved since its inception in the early 20th century, with its domain of concern growing and adjusting in response to the needs of individuals. Although evaluation will continue to identify clients' strengths and weaknesses as new settings emerge, the setting may affect how the evaluation is conducted or what is part of the evaluation. For example, in school-based practice, evaluation cannot focus on all areas of the domain of concern but by law must focus on the areas that have relevance to the child's performance in the school setting.

In the past decade, evaluations and setting for practice have changed. Many evaluations use computers for scoring, rather than relying solely on computation or the therapist's judgment. For example, the Sensory Integration and Praxis Tests (Ayres, 1989) use computerized scoring. Other evaluations are also now computer based, such as driving evaluations (Dickerson et al., 2014; Ratzon et al., 2017;

Stephenson et al., 2019). This chapter focuses on evaluation in three emerging areas of practice: (1) primary care, (2) telehealth, and (3) evaluating groups and populations.

OVERVIEW OF OCCUPATIONAL THERAPY IN THE PRIMARY CARE SETTING

Occupational therapy in the primary care setting is an emerging field (Roberts et al., 2014). This section reviews considerations regarding evaluation and assessment as it relates to the American Occupational Therapy Association's (AOTA, 2014a) *Occupational Therapy Practice Framework: Domain and Process (OTPF)*, traditional settings, and *Standards of Practice for Occupational Therapy* (AOTA, 2015b). In addition, specific evaluation tools that have been implemented in primary care settings are described throughout the section, with case examples.

Occupational therapists use different practice models in primary care settings. For this section of the chapter, *primary care* is a broad term that also includes primary care settings, specialty care offices, and telehealth (Roberts et al.,

2014). A widely used definition of *primary care* is from the Institute of Medicine (1994):

> the provision of integrated health care services provided by clinicians who are accountable for addressing a large majority of personal health care needs, developing a sustained partnership with patients and practicing in the context of family and community. (p. 1)

Occupational therapists strive to include occupational therapy as part of integrated health care by establishing occupational therapy's role in the primary care setting (AOTA, 2014b; Halle et al., 2018). Occupational therapists have the potential to be contributing and valuable members of the primary care team (AOTA, 2014b).

Traditional Practice Settings and Primary Care

Assessment tools used during evaluations in primary care settings are similar to those used in traditional practice settings, such as inpatient rehabilitation, acute care, or outpatient settings. During the evaluation, an *occupational profile* is obtained, and an analysis of occupational performance is conducted (AOTA, 2014a, 2017).

Primary care providers must place a referral for occupational therapy to evaluate and treat the patient, just as in traditional practice settings. Primary care providers can include medical doctors, doctors of osteopathic medicine, nurse practitioners, and physician assistants, but this may vary depending on the practice act in a specific state. In some primary care practice models, the provider communicates the referral request in person to the occupational therapist in addition to giving a written referral, which is required by most state practice acts. This interaction can provide valuable information to the occupational therapist and help them complete the occupational profile and understand the client's occupational performance before the start of the occupational therapy evaluation.

The interactive component, during which the members of the primary care team prioritize discussion and work together to refine communication over time, is an example of *effective communication* (Mitchell et al., 2012). Effective communication in primary care differs from traditional practice models, because in a traditional practice setting, the occupational therapist may only see the referral and have minimal other interaction with the provider. An occupational therapist working in a primary care setting may have direct communication about a patient, with the provider giving a verbal rationale as to why occupational therapy services are warranted. The collaborative relationship between the occupational therapist and primary care provider is strengthened the longer the occupational therapist works in the primary care setting. In addition, occupational therapists may work closely with other members of the primary care team, including social workers, medical assistants, pharmacists, psychologists, or physical therapists.

Once an evaluation is complete and the occupational therapist has identified the patient's pertinent barriers or concerns, they can follow up directly with the provider and other relevant primary care team members in the primary care setting. Collaboration and effective communication among the occupational therapist and primary care team members help the team work toward the mutual goal of providing the best care for the patient.

In traditional occupational therapy settings, occupational therapists' roles are usually clearly defined. In primary care settings, occupational therapists can have various roles, and it is important that occupational therapists educate team members about occupational therapy's role for future referrals (Koverman et al., 2017). Literature identifies the role of the occupational therapist as a generalist when working in the primary care setting, because occupational therapists may implement various interventions across the life course (Donnelly et al., 2014). The generalist approach is different from a traditional practice setting, such as an outpatient setting that specializes solely in orthopedic clients. In the primary care setting, occupational therapists' role could be to help manage client's chronic conditions by using health prevention and promotion interventions (AOTA, 2014b; Donnelly et al., 2014; Royeen, 2020), which may differ from traditional rehabilitation settings, where remediation and modification interventions may be the primary interventions used.

Occupational therapists perform evaluations using a holistic approach in both traditional practice settings and primary care settings (Jordan, 2019). During a *holistic evaluation,* the occupational therapist looks at the whole person rather than focusing on one specific area (e.g., orthopedics, ADLs, cognitive performance). When therapists perform such evaluations in the primary care setting, they may identify barriers or concerns that other members of the primary care team have not identified. Therapists bring these concerns or barriers to the primary care team and have the opportunity to educate the team on occupational therapy services.

Occupational therapists evaluate and address patients who have chronic conditions in primary care settings; this may differ from traditional practice settings in that chronic conditions can be the first priority for the therapist when working in a primary care setting, but just the start of the evaluation rather than the sole focus (Donnelly et al., 2014; Roberts et al., 2014). For the evaluation process to be successful, it is important to focus on a person holistically and address concerns related to environmental, physical, mental, and psychosocial aspects of health (Dahl-Popilizio et al., 2017). Currently, 6 in 10 adults in the United States have a chronic condition, and 4 in 10 adults have two or more chronic conditions (Centers for Disease Control and Prevention, 2019). Health prevention– and health promotion–focused evaluations are important in primary care settings to help address habits, routines, and education geared toward managing chronic conditions (see Case Example 14.1).

In traditional occupational therapy practice settings, a referral is initiated, and the occupational therapist evaluates the patient in either an inpatient or an outpatient setting. The primary care setting can be different. The providers may not be aware of the broad scope of services an occupational therapist can provide and may not place a referral for all appropriate clients. Furthermore, the therapist may need to initiate the referral by suggesting potential occupational therapy services for a client.

Occupational therapists can screen potential clients in different ways depending on the model of practice. They

CASE EXAMPLE 14.1. STEVE: HOLISTIC EVALUATION FOR A CHRONIC CONDITION

Dr. London asked the occupational therapist working in a geriatric primary care clinic to evaluate **Steve,** a 66-year-old man who has lateral epicondylitis. During the holistic evaluation, the occupational therapist identifies that Steve is having difficulty opening his medication bottles for diabetes and monitoring his glucose levels. The occupational therapist administers the Diabetes Self-Efficacy Scale (Allen et al., 2018), which is an eight-item self-assessment that identifies

Steve's confidence level in performing tasks related to self-management of diabetes (Loring et al., 2009). Steve has poor self-efficacy for managing his diabetes, and the occupational therapist schedules him for follow-up visits to address self-care management of his chronic condition, which Steve identified as a higher priority than the pain in his elbow at this time. The occupational therapist followed up with Dr. London about this plan of care.

CASE EXAMPLE 14.2. TEAM MEETINGS AND ASKING FOR REFERRAL

During the morning team meeting before a muscular dystrophy clinic, Dr. Rowan was reviewing information on a 38-year-old patient who was having increased difficulty swallowing and holding onto objects and was having frequent falls. Physical therapy and speech therapy services were scheduled for the client. The occupational therapist asked Dr. Rowan during the team meeting whether she could evaluate

the client, and Dr. Rowan agreed, placing the order. The occupational therapist performed an evaluation, which included dynamometer testing and an evaluation of ADLs. The therapist recommended therapeutic exercises, identified contraindications to specific exercise because of the patient's muscular dystrophy, and modified equipment during the visit to improve participation in ADLs.

can screen patients for potential services in the primary care setting through electronic medical records (EMR) or verbal communication with primary care team members. In addition, occupational therapists may serve on team meetings to identify potential clients who may benefit from occupational therapy services (see Case Example 14.2).

Specific screening tools are another option; however, there are few available at this time, and often they are self-made and specific to a particular type of clinic. Occupational therapists can use a screening questionnaire before the client's first visit to determine the need for occupational therapy. However, such a questionnaire may not be sensitive enough to identify the specific problems that the therapist might pick up in an interview in person or when completing an occupational profile with the client.

OTPF and Primary Care

Occupational therapists follow the *OTPF* (AOTA, 2014a) when performing evaluations in primary care settings. This includes obtaining an occupational profile, which is heavily based on the client history or family member history, and performing an analysis of occupational performance, which includes evaluation and assessments of identified areas of concern (AOTA, 2014a).

Evaluation: Focus on function

Occupational therapists' unique value in the primary care team is their focus on function (Donnelly et al., 2014; Roberts et al., 2014). During the evaluation, occupational

therapists may address different domains of occupational therapy, including occupations, client factors, performance skills, performance patterns, and contexts and environments (AOTA, 2014a). Occupational therapists are uniquely skilled in obtaining information related to these domains during the evaluation and identifying potential barriers to function. Table 14.1 describes different assessment tools that can be used in primary care settings for each domain.

Advocacy

Advocating for occupational therapy services is important and is discussed in the *OTPF* as it relates to interventions and outcomes (AOTA, 2014a). Advocacy is also important to therapists because they can help with legislature affecting practice through becoming part of a state or national organization. Advocacy is imperative when considering evaluation and assessment in primary care settings. In the context of primary care, ***advocacy*** can also be about educating and encouraging patients to advocate for themselves.

At this time, the roles of occupational therapy in primary care have not been clearly defined and are still evolving; these roles span many areas such as ADLs, IADLs, psychosocial issues, and other issues that may interfere with function and occupational performance. It is important for occupational therapists to advocate their role to the provider and primary care team so they can work to the top of their license (i.e., to the full extent of their scope of practice; Russell-Babin & Wurmser, 2016) and provide evaluation and assessments to a wide variety of clients. Scope of practice gives occupational therapists the autonomy to

TABLE 14.1.   Assessments for Domains of Occupational Therapy in Primary Care

DOMAIN	ASSESSMENT TOOL	DESCRIPTION	SOURCE
Occupation: IADLS	Lawton Instrumental Activities of Daily Living Scale	Assesses independent living skills; measures 8 domains of function	Graf (2008)
Occupation: rest and sleep	Pittsburgh Sleep Quality Index	Subjective Likert scale that measures sleep pattern and quality	Buysse et al. (1989)
Client factors	Disabilities of the Arm, Shoulder, and Hand Outcome Questionnaire	Subjective 30-item Likert scale that measures musculoskeletal disorder and disability of the upper extremity	Gummesson et al. (2003)
Client factors	Timed Up and Go	Observational test that measures a client's balance and fall risk	Bischoff et al. (2003)
Performance skills	Generalized Anxiety Scale	Subjective Likert scale that measures severity of anxiety	Spitzer et al. (2006)
Performance patterns	Canadian Occupational Performance Measure	Subjective rating of performance on everyday activities	Law et al. (2019)
Context and environment	Occupational profile	Verbal interview obtaining history on "clients' experiences, patterns of daily living, interests, values, and needs" (AOTA, 2017, p. S10)	AOTA (2017)

Note. AOTA = American Occupational Therapy Association; IADLs = instrumental activities of daily living.

perform evaluations they think are most relevant in the primary care setting (see Case Example 14.3).

Providers may ask occupational therapists to evaluate a patient through one-on-one communication or in a team meeting in the primary care setting, although written referrals are often required by state practice acts. Providers may state information that contributes to the occupational profile and analysis of occupation, and they may ask therapists to evaluate because of a specific diagnosis or area of concern. Either through chart review or by performing a holistic evaluation, therapists may identify other barriers of which the provider was not aware. When this happens, the therapist can advocate and educate the provider on areas of evaluation the therapist can address so they can practice at the top of their license. It is important to note that this advocates for clients to receive occupational therapy services to best serve the clients' needs.

Context and environment: Health disparities

Context and environment are important considerations when occupational therapists are performing evaluations and assessments in the primary care setting. The *OTPF* describes **context and environment** as "reflecting the importance of considering the wide array of interrelated variables that influence performance" (AOTA, 2014a, p. S8). Context and environment are important to evaluate and understand because they affect clients' performance patterns, which relate to their function. In addition, evaluating context and environment contributes to a holistic evaluation.

CASE EXAMPLE 14.3. JERRY: ADVOCATING FOR THE PATIENT'S NEEDS

Dr. Ramirez asks the occupational therapist to see **Jerry,** a 67-year-old man presenting with back pain, to evaluate his ADLs. The occupational therapist performs a holistic evaluation and identifies that Jerry is not taking all his medication doses, which is contributing to his high blood pressure. While obtaining information for the occupational profile, the therapist sees that Jerry's information is inconsistent; his answers do not always make sense or reflect the information received from his physician. The therapist uses clinical reasoning and completes the Montreal Cognitive Assessment (Nasreddine et al., 2005), a cognitive assessment that screens for mild cognitive impairment. Jerry scores a 21/30 and the therapist identifies that Jerry is having difficulty with short term-memory, specifically recall. Although Jerry's initial area of concern was back pain, through a holistic evaluation the therapist finds that cognitive areas are also a large area of concern, possibly more important at this time than the back pain. The therapist brings this information to Dr. Ramirez, and they collaborate to create a plan of care to best serve Jerry's needs.

CASE EXAMPLE 14.4. MARIA: HEALTH DISPARITY

Dr. Patel, a palliative care provider, asked the occupational therapist to perform an evaluation on **Maria** to address the chronic pain she has had for the past 5 years. The therapist planned on using the Pain Self-Efficacy Questionnaire (PSEQ), which is a 10-item patient self-report that measures the confidence level an individual has to perform activities while in pain (Nicholas, 2007). Instead, while obtaining the occupational profile and analysis of occupational performance, the occupational therapist identifies that Maria has recently fallen and has trouble getting into and out of her tub–shower combination at home. Maria does not have the finances to pay for a tub–shower bench. Instead of continuing the evaluations with the PSEQ, the occupational therapist brought this information to the social worker, and the social worker connected the patient with lending closet resources.

In this example, Dr. Patel asked the occupational therapist to address Maria's chronic pain. During the evaluation, the occupational therapist identified a recent fall and acknowledged Maria's health disparity of low socioeconomic status because she was not able purchase a tub bench. The occupational therapist identified an appropriate resource to connect Maria with to help overcome this barrier. Time can be a barrier to performance of evaluations in the primary care setting; therefore the occupational therapist prioritized Maria's concerns and addressed the most pertinent need. Through an evaluation that considered contexts and environments, a higher priority barrier was identified by the patient and addressed by the occupational therapist and primary care team.

Context and environment do not explicitly address health disparities, but they are an important area to consider. A *health disparity* is a difference in health between the general population and disadvantaged social groups, such as people with low socioeconomic status, racial and ethnic minorities, or women. Such differences may exist because of systematic influences, such as health care policy (Braveman, 2006). It is important for occupational therapists to understand the contextual nature and environment a client lives in and interacts with daily; this includes examination of the client's priorities, barriers, and values, because this provides a scanning assessment of health disparities during the evaluation. During the evaluation there may be many barriers to address, but the occupational therapist's consideration for health disparities will help prioritize what should be initially evaluated (see Case Example 14.4).

Standards of Practice for Occupational Therapy and Primary Care

Occupational therapists should consider the guiding principles in the *Standards of Practice for Occupational Therapy* when implementing evaluation and assessments in primary care settings (AOTA, 2015b). Logistically, the principles are important to evaluations for all occupational therapy practice models in primary care. Referrals must be placed before the occupational therapist performs the evaluation, and once the order is placed the occupational therapy can respond appropriately and evaluate the client according to regulatory agencies (AOTA, 2015b). The occupational therapists or the leadership managing the occupational therapists need to establish this expectation while the occupational therapy team is creating their programming in a primary care setting.

The *Standards of Practice for Occupational Therapy* emphasize client-centered care, which includes collaboration with the patient. To successfully collaborate with the client and identify appropriate activities on the basis of the client's abilities in appropriate environments (AOTA, 2015b), occupational therapists can use motivational interviewing as part of an evaluation. *Motivational interviewing* is a type of interpersonal interaction that promotes behavior change by identifying barriers and addressing them appropriately (Rollnick & Miller, 1995). For example, in an evaluation, occupational therapists help guide clients to identify their barriers to functioning or foster clients in achieving a goal by engaging in problem solving.

Standardized and nonstandardized evaluation tools can be used; it is important that the occupational therapist abide by the administration protocol when using a standardized evaluation tool. It is essential that the therapist communicate to the team the information obtained during the evaluation. If the therapist obtains information that they do not communicate or share, the primary care team members may not understand the full contribution that occupational therapy can make to the primary care team. Information from the evaluation can be shared verbally with the primary care team members, which is essential for the advocacy described earlier. Therapists should document evaluation notes in the EMR so primary care team members and other relevant health care providers can access this information.

It is also important to document evaluations for external stakeholders, such as regulatory agencies or insurance agencies. Occupational therapy in primary care is an emerging field, and insurance agencies may be reluctant to reimburse for occupational therapy services in this setting, so thorough and detailed evaluation notes are essential to establish practice. Exhibit 14.1 shows an example of an occupational therapy evaluation performed by an occupational therapist working in a primary care setting.

The end result of the occupational therapy evaluation is to create a treatment plan based on the results of the evaluation. In some practice models, occupational therapists may implement a treatment plan immediately after the provider visit. The client may only have a one-time occupational therapy visit for a variety of reasons, such as a lack of transportation for follow-up. In addition to creating a treatment plan, the therapist may identify other appropriate team members with whom the patient may need to connect (Dahl-Popolizio et al., 2017)—for example, social work to

EXHIBIT 14.1.   Sample Evaluation Note

SMITH MEDICAL CENTER
Occupational Therapy: Geriatric Primary Care

Initial Evaluation

Name: Maria Lopez
MRN: 0123456
Date: 01/01/2020

Referring body: Dr. Smith
Insurance: Medicare Part B

Diagnosis/Diagnostic Code: ICD-10-CM--W19.XXA

1. Unspecified Fall, Initial Encounter

Pain Assessment Status: Vitals: 2/10 pain, lower back

Subjective: "I fell while I was getting out of the shower."

Occupational Profile

Prior roles, Interests, Daily Routine & Level of Function:
Per patient report, patient lives alone with her cat. She lives in a one-story house with 2 stairs to enter. She reports a recent fall while getting out of the shower; she has a walk-in shower. She also endorsed losing balance while cooking, specifically while carrying a heavy pot. She has a son in the area who assists with IADLs, such as changing lightbulbs, and has a housekeeper x1 month. She is currently driving. She reports she is sleeping 7 hours a night and endorses no difficulties with sleep. She enjoys taking daily walks, when weather permits, at a nearby park. Maria enjoys going to church on Sunday and has social support with friends from church.

Analysis of Occupational Performance

Areas of Occupation:
ADLs
Safety and Quality Performance measure: 06. Jane is independent in all ADLs.

Functional Transfers
Safety and Quality Performance measure: 06. Jane is independent; when her back pain flares she uses a cane.

Lawton–Brody Instrumental Activities of Daily Living Scale
Ability to Use Telephone: 1—operates telephone on own
Shopping: 1—takes care of all shopping needs independently
Food Preparation: 1—plans, prepares, and serves adequate meals
Housekeeping: 1—maintains house with occasional assistance
Laundry: 1—does personal laundry completely
Mode of Transportation: 1—drives own car
Responsibility for Own Medications: 1—responsible for taking medication in correct dosage
Ability to Handle Finances: 1—manages financial matters independently
Total Score: 8/8 (8 = high function, independent woman)

Client Factors

Neuromusculoskeletal and Movement Skills:

	Left ROM	**Right ROM**	**Left Strength**	**Right Strength**
Shoulder	Within normal limits	Within normal limits	Within normal limits	Within normal limits
Elbow	Within normal limits	Within normal limits	Within normal limits	Within normal limits
Hand	Within normal limits	Within normal limits	Within normal limits	Within normal limits

(Continued)

EXHIBIT 14.1.   Sample Evaluation Note *(Cont.)*

Other Standardized Assessments:

When administered the Timed Up and Go to assess the pt's fall risk while completing a functional task (with walker or cane), pt completed task in 16 seconds indicating pt is at increased risk of falls (14 seconds or more indicates risk of falls).

When administered the **FES–I** to assess self-confidence as it relates to avoiding or preventing falls during everyday activities, pt scored 35, with responses indicating the pt has concern (*high concern* = 28–64) of falling during functional activities.

Summary

Assessment:

Patient was seen for skilled OT services by the request of the provider to address recent falls. Patient completed standardized assessments indicating she is a fall risk, as well high fear of falling, which has negative consequences such as decreased social and physical engagement activities. Pt also states that she completes all IADLs, however has concerns with falling when reaching outside base of support; pt also with high concerns of falling again in the bathroom. Patient educated on bathroom safety fall prevention techniques, including shower chair. Patient was connected with social worker to explore potential financial coverage options. Also discussed potential PT referral with provider. Pt would benefit from continued OT to address areas of deficits and improve functional participation in ADLs and IADLS, as well as decreasing fall risk and fear of falling.

Plan of care: Will follow up in outpatient x1 times per week for 4 weeks.

Janet Stevens, MOT, OTR/L

Goals:

1. Pt will identify 3 fall prevention intervention techniques to incorporate into her daily routine in 4 weeks to decrease risk of falls.
2. Pt will complete a complex cooking activity, including high reaching and carrying items, with no difficulty in 4 weeks.
3. Pt will improve FES–I score by 5 points to improve confidence with participation in social activities and IADLs in 4 weeks.

Note. ADLs = activities of daily living; FES–I = Falls Efficacy Scale–International; IADLs = instrumental activities of daily living; OT = occupational therapy; pt = patient; PT = physical therapy; ROM = range of motion.

connect with community resources, or physical therapy if the patient has gait difficulty.

The *Standards of Practice* identify the importance of occupational therapists following the *Occupational Therapy Code of Ethics* (AOTA, 2015a). Ethical considerations are important in evaluations and assessments in primary care settings, because it is the therapist's responsibility to abide by the *Code of Ethics*. Two ethical considerations are described in greater detail as they relate to occupational therapy evaluation in primary care. First, it is important that therapists practice and evaluate clients to their level of competence (Roberts et al., 2014). It is important for therapists to practice at the top of their license but also to be aware of and identify their limitations. For example, a therapist may require external training for a specific diagnosis or condition, such as lymphedema. If the therapist is not experienced with lymphedema, they should recommend that the client be evaluated by a therapist who is certified in the treatment of lymphedema in a nearby outpatient clinic.

Issues related to reimbursement are another ethical consideration. Reimbursement for services, including evaluations, varies depending on each clinic and must be established in a way that complies with the *Code of Ethics* (AOTA, 2015a), regulatory agencies, and the institution's billing department and protocol. The occupational therapist must be ethical when charging for an evaluation; they must complete and document a full evaluation. There may be pressures of productivity, but this must not influence billing decisions.

In addition, the occupational therapist must identify whether the client is receiving occupational therapy services elsewhere to avoid duplicating services. Depending on the model of practice and how the occupational therapy is reimbursed, therapists may need to identify whether the patient is also receiving home health services because outpatient services cannot be billed if the patient is receiving home health. Chapter 15, "Ethical Issues in Evaluation," provides a more in-depth discussion of ethical issues.

OVERVIEW OF TELEHEALTH AND OCCUPATIONAL THERAPY

The use of telehealth to deliver occupational therapy interventions is expanding. *Telehealth* refers to the use of information and communication technology, such as live videoconferencing, to deliver services to individuals at a location that is different from the provider. Telehealth addresses issues related to service accessibility, such as provider shortages, travel time, transportation challenges, and access to specialists (AOTA, 2018). Increased use of telehealth was evidenced during the COVID-19 pandemic.

Research suggests that various occupational therapy interventions delivered through telehealth are efficacious (Nobakht et al., 2017) and cost-effective (e.g., Little et al., 2018). As occupational therapists continue to use telehealth to deliver interventions, they must consider how to conduct evaluations using this delivery mechanism. The purpose of this section is to provide an overview of evaluation and assessment considerations in the context of telehealth. This section also outlines specific evaluations methods that fit most effectively within telehealth, including observation, self-report, and caregiver and parent report.

Similarities and Differences From Traditional Settings

When occupational therapists use telehealth, the focus of their evaluation remains on clients' performance skills, performance patterns, and overall participation. Therapists who conduct evaluations using telehealth may use similar measures as they would in traditional, in-person settings. They can use observations, interviews, and questionnaires to understand a client's current functioning and goals for therapy. When therapists use live videoconferencing, they can easily administer a routines-based interview or complete an occupational profile. *Videoconferencing* refers to use of online applications that allow video-based calling features. The videoconferencing software used with health data needs to have privacy protection capability. *Store and forward* techniques refer to video or audio recordings or typed data stored in a computer or on a website that can be forwarded to therapists at a later time. This can be used when clients are not amenable to an interview.

Through telehealth, occupational therapists can use skilled questioning to ask a client to fully describe what everyday activities look like for them. By using videoconferencing, clients can feel like they have valuable face-to-face time with a therapist, and the only way for the therapist to learn more is to listen. Qualitative studies on the client–therapist relationship over telehealth show that clients feel empowered by the use of telehealth because it demands that they be true partners in the evaluation and intervention process (Serwe et al., 2017; Wallisch et al., 2019).

Although there are similarities with traditional practice in completing an evaluation over telehealth, occupational therapists must also consider some differences. There are legal and regulatory considerations to using telehealth with clients (Cason & Richmond, 2018). Many state practice acts dictate how occupational therapists may or may not use telehealth, although some state practice acts do not directly address the use of telehealth (Bierman et al., 2018). Therapists are advised to consult their own state's practice act to understand the guidelines that may pertain to their services.

Currently, to provide services by telehealth, occupational therapists must be licensed in the state in which they reside as well as the state in which the client resides. For example, if an occupational therapist living in Illinois is providing services to a client residing in Indiana, the occupational therapist must be licensed in both Illinois and Indiana. To resolve issues associated with having to obtain licensure in multiple states, AOTA implemented an initiative aimed at advancing an interstate licensure compact by 2025, which would allow occupational therapists to practice across state lines. Additionally, the videoconferencing technology that is used to conduct evaluations must be compliant with the Health Insurance Portability and Accountability Act of 1996 (HIPAA; P. L. 104-191), and occupational therapists must ensure that the interview occurs in a setting that adheres to all privacy and confidentiality considerations.

There is the additional benefit that evaluations may be recorded through the videoconferencing technology for either party (client or therapist) to refer to at a later time; however, occupational therapists must consider whether the recording of an evaluation fits their organization's guidelines for privacy and confidentiality as well as where the recordings are stored. Many states have implemented an informed consent requirement before services can be provided over telehealth; occupational therapists and their organizations should ensure they are following state laws and regulations with this requirement (see Bierman et al., 2018).

All occupational therapists using telehealth must consider current reimbursement models. Currently, reimbursement of occupational therapy services delivered by telehealth is complex and differs by state, practice setting, and insurance type. Although it is beyond the scope of this chapter to outline the complexities of reimbursement for occupational therapy delivered using telehealth, therapists may consult the Telehealth Resources section of AOTA's website (https://www.aota.org/Practice/Manage/telehealth.aspx). Another helpful resource is the Center for Connected Health Policy (https://www.cchpca.org), a nonprofit organization that provides information about current policy related to health professionals, including occupational therapy.

Telehealth Assessment Methods

Occupational therapists may use various assessment methods over telehealth to evaluate occupations, client factors, performance skills, and performance patter[...] contexts and environments (AOTA, 2014a). S[...] ods of evaluation that may be administered o[...] include interview, standardized behavioral [...] observation, and standardized parent and car[...]

Interview

Occupational therapists conducting evaluati[...] health must consider the establishment and [...] of rapport. The process of establishing rapport over videoconferencing or other information technology has been referred to as *webside manner* or *virtual rapport* (Hollander et al., 2018). The ways communication occurs during an interview over telehealth require slightly different considerations than in-person interviews. The provider must look directly at their device's camera (not the screen) to make it appear as if they are making eye contact. Additionally, the provider must be mindful of the environment in which they are located to conduct the interview. The provider's backdrop (i.e., the background of the videoconference) must be considered. Clients may feel more at ease with the therapist if the therapist's background seems professional (e.g., bookcase, neutral wall) rather than a messy office or busy space.

Occupational therapists may use an interview format over videoconferencing to complete an occupational profile or learn more about a client's performance patterns (i.e., habits, routines, rituals, and roles). Therapists conducting evaluations by telehealth must use similar approaches as used during in-person services to establish and maintain rapport. Although research has not yet systematically investigated how therapeutic use of self may be different for therapists over telehealth versus in person, some studies suggest that clients feel a similar therapeutic relationship

CASE EXAMPLE 14.5. JEREMIAH: AUTISM SPECTRUM DISORDER AND TELEHEALTH

Jeremiah is a 33-month-old boy who lives with his mother, father, and two older sisters. Jeremiah has a diagnosis of autism spectrum disorder and is receiving occupational therapy delivered by telehealth through his state's early intervention system. Given Jeremiah's parents' concerns about his extreme picky eating, his occupational therapist begins the evaluation to ensure that Jeremiah does not have any swallowing difficulties or aspiration concerns.

Jeremiah's mother shares a report from an interdisciplinary feeding team evaluation, which noted that Jeremiah did not show swallowing or aspiration concerns; the team's findings concluded that his picky eating was sensory and behavioral in origin. Because initial safety concerns were addressed, the occupational therapist then used interview, standardized parent report, and observation as her evaluation methods. Table 14.2 shows specific evaluation methods and findings for Jeremiah.

The occupational therapist considers that Jeremiah has low sensory thresholds; that is, he prefers environments and activities in which there are few sensory stimuli as well as sensory stimuli he can control. His sensory processing preferences related to food are also reflected in his Let's Eat! scores (Little & Wallisch, 2018) as well as factors related to his oral–motor development and decreased ability to use utensils.

The occupational therapist gleans that Jeremiah accepts different textures during breakfast and that this time of day is the most quiet, slow paced, and self-directed. Therefore, the occupational therapist designs an intervention plan based on Jeremiah's sensory processing preferences, which includes trying to introduce new foods in the morning, during his quiet meal, rather than when environmental demands are high, such as during busy and noisy dinnertimes. The therapist recommended allowing Jeremiah to use his own utensils and eat familiar foods during dinnertime.

TABLE 14.2. Jeremiah's Evaluation Methods and Findings Through Telehealth

TYPE OF EVALUATION	CONTENT	FINDINGS
Interview	In the first session, the occupational therapist interviewed Jeremiah's mother over HIPAA-compliant videoconferencing software to understand the family's daily routine, with a focus on mealtimes. The occupational therapist led the mother through an interview of what Jeremiah's eating and mealtime behavior looked like, the details of the contexts and environments in which all behavior occurred, and the behaviors of the family members during mealtimes.	Jeremiah's mother reported that the morning routine went smoothly; Jeremiah was typically very hungry at breakfast and would accept different textures of foods then (e.g., bagel with cream cheese, oatmeal, or scrambled eggs). During dinnertime, Jeremiah would accept very few foods; he showed difficult behaviors, such as throwing food and tantruming when a new food was introduced.
Standardized parent report	The occupational therapist sent Jeremiah's mother the following questionnaires and asked her to return them before the first session: ■ *Sensory Profile–2 (Dunn, 2014)*: An 86-item measure of children's sensory processing patterns in everyday activities ■ *Let's Eat! (Little & Wallisch, 2018)*: A 29-item measure of sensory–motor contributions to children's eating habits ■ *3-Day Food Diary (unpublished)*: Parents completed this measure to understand the types of foods that Jeremiah would accept	Jeremiah's Sensory Profile–2 scores showed that he showed "much more than others" in sensitivity and avoidance. His scores in registration and seeking were "just like others." Jeremiah's Let's Eat! results showed increased scores on the Vigilance and Development subscales, which indicate that he had highly specific food preferences as well as some difficulties in oral–motor manipulation and utensil use. The 3-Day Food Diary showed that Jeremiah would accept both smooth and crunchy textures; however, he was consuming much more food in the morning and afternoon than during the evening meal.

(Continued)

(Continued)

CASE EXAMPLE 14.5. JEREMIAH: AUTISM SPECTRUM DISORDER AND TELEHEALTH *(Cont.)*

TABLE 14.2.   Jeremiah's Evaluation Methods and Findings Through Telehealth *(Cont.)*

TYPE OF EVALUATION	CONTENT	FINDINGS
Observation	The occupational therapist scheduled Jeremiah's second session during a mealtime. Jeremiah's mother explained that breakfast time was different from dinnertime, so she sent the occupational therapist a recording of breakfast time; then the therapist observed dinner time. She asked Jeremiah's mother to place her laptop on the table so that the occupational therapist could "see" each mealtime and better understand what person and environmental factors were influencing Jeremiah's eating and mealtime behaviors.	*Breakfast* The therapist observed, from video, that Jeremiah ate breakfast alone with his mother, after his siblings boarded the bus to attend school and his father left for work. At breakfast time, Jeremiah was eating his breakfast with his hands, carefully inspecting each bite carefully before bringing it to his mouth. *Dinner* At dinnertime, all of Jeremiah's family was present around the table. His sisters were talking loudly and arguing about a television show while his father was holding a spoon to Jeremiah's face to try to get him to eat a bite of turkey. Jeremiah's mother was bustling around the kitchen, trying to get everyone settled at the table. The dog was barking in the background. Jeremiah was crying and pushing the spoon away.

Note. HIPAA = Health Insurance Portability and Accountability Act of 1996.

CASE EXAMPLE 14.6. BETH: TELEHEALTH AFTER STROKE

Beth is a 76-year-old woman who had a stroke 2 years ago. Beth shows left side hemiparesis and difficulties with cognitive function, in particular executive functioning skills. Beth lives in a ranch-style home with her sister, Barb, who is also her full-time caregiver. Beth and Barb live in a rural area, and although Beth used to receive home-based services, there is no longer an occupational therapist available to serve her county. Therefore, Beth and Barb decided to consult with an occupational therapist to receive services by telehealth.

The occupational therapist had an initial phone call with Beth and Barb to ensure that Barb could use her smartphone to videoconference during their first session and to ensure that Barb did not have any safety concerns about Beth that could not be addressed through telehealth. During the first online session the occupational therapist completed a variety of assessment methods (see Table 14.3).

The occupational therapist considers that Beth has sleep difficulties and notes the absence of a sleep preparation routine. The occupational therapist also determines that Beth has decreased occupational engagement in meaningful activities throughout the day. The occupational therapist also concludes that Barb needs support in her role as a caregiver, such as learning additional strategies to engage Beth during the day and to support a meaningful sleep preparation routine in the evening. Therefore, the occupational therapist designs an intervention plan based on working with both Beth and Barb to create a sleep preparation routine, support Beth's participation in activities during the day to keep her awake and active, and find additional community supports for Barb to relieve some of her caregiving demands.

(Continued)

CASE EXAMPLE 14.6. BETH: TELEHEALTH AFTER STROKE *(Cont.)*

TABLE 14.3. Beth's Evaluation Methods and Findings Through Telehealth

TYPE OF EVALUATION	CONTENT	FINDINGS
Interview	In the first session, the occupational therapist interviewed Beth and Barb over HIPAA-compliant videoconferencing software. The therapist completed an occupational profile on Beth and then interviewed Beth and her caregiver, Barb, about the daily routine. Beth reported that she was having difficulty during the day because she was very tired. She had the support she needed from Barb for most ADLs and IADLS; however, Beth was struggling to fall and stay asleep at night. The occupational therapist asked skilled questions about what Beth's bedtime routine looked like.	Interview findings showed that Beth used to spend her time needlepointing. After her stroke, she was no longer able to needlepoint and instead spent most of the day watching television, often falling asleep in her chair. At night, Beth was restless and would often turn on the television in her bedroom (which is next to Barb's bedroom) through the night. Barb reported that she was very frustrated because she could not rest when Beth was up through the night.
Standardized self-report	The occupational therapist sent Beth and Barb the following questionnaires and asked them to return them before the first session: • PSQI (Buysse et al., 1989): A 14-item measure of sleep quality and patterns administered to Beth and Barb • CSI (Robinson, 1983): A 13-item measure administered to Barb	The PSQI showed that both Beth and Barb fell within the range of "poor sleepers," with Beth's scores showing that she had more difficulty falling and staying asleep, whereas Barb's scores were related to sleeping through the night and enthusiasm about getting things done during the day. Barb's CSI score was high (7).
Observation	The occupational therapist asked Barb to hold the smartphone to "walk through" the bedroom in which Beth sleeps. The occupational therapist then asked Beth to demonstrate her bedtime routine, such as showing where the bathroom is in relation to the bedroom, how she takes her medications, whether she leaves any lights on, and whether she drinks any beverages before bed.	*Sleeping environment* As Beth shows the occupational therapist the bedroom, the occupational therapist notices that the television is quite large and directly next to Beth's bed. She also notices that there are no window coverings and the light from outside pours into the room. *Routine* Beth reports that whenever she feels tired, she walks to her bedroom, sometimes too exhausted to change into pajamas, and falls asleep. She reports that it is frustrating, however, because 1 hour later she is "wide awake."

Note. CSI = Caregiver Strain Index; HIPAA = Health Insurance Portability and Accountability Act of 1996; PSQI = Pittsburgh Sleep Quality Index.

with providers over telehealth (Kairy et al., 2013; Little et al., 2018; Liu et al., 2007; Serwe & Bowman, 2018; Serwe et al., 2017).

Standardized behavioral assessments

Occupational therapists use standardized behavioral assessments to evaluate performance skills; however, many standardized behavioral assessments are material intensive and require specific elements of environmental set-up. Therefore, the process of administering standardized behavioral assessments over telehealth may differ from traditional settings. For example, therapists working with pediatric populations often administer global developmental measures, such as the Peabody Development Motor Scales (Folio & Fewell, 2000) or the Bruininks–Oseretsky Test of Motor Proficiency (Bruininks & Bruininks, 2005).

Both of these assessments require many materials and supplies, and the occupational therapist must administer each item in a standardized manner. Therefore, some

therapists may opt to have a certified occupational therapy assistant (COTA) or paraprofessional administer each item in person while the occupational therapist watches the standardized administration and scores over a videoconference. The occupational therapist must train the individual on the other end of the videoconference to administer the items in a standardized fashion that is visible to the camera.

Another approach to administering standardized behavioral assessments is for the occupational therapist to instruct nonprofessionals, such as parents or caregivers, on how to set up an environment and administer specific items. Studies have shown that parents can reliably administer such standardized items (Reese et al., 2013), but more research is needed to better understand what type of training parents may require to administer standardized behavioral assessments over telehealth so therapists can reliably and accurately provide scores and interpretation.

Research has established that certain standardized assessments may be reliably administered by telehealth for adults, including the Montreal Cognitive Assessment (MOCA; Nasreddine et al., 2005; Stillerova et al., 2016), the Kohlman Evaluation of Living Skills (KELS; Dreyer et al., 2001; Thomson & Robnett, 2016), the Timed Up and Go Test (TUG; Hwang et al., 2017; Podsiadlo & Richardson, 1991), and the Functional Independence Measure (FIM; Hoffmann et al., 2008; Uniform Data System for Medical Rehabilitation, 2012). Although these studies show that a distant assessor is able to administer the standardized assessments and the occupational therapist who observes over telehealth can reliably score, research must continue to investigate how COTAs or caregivers may reliably and safely administer items to glean similar information from such assessments.

Observation

One of the primary advantages of telehealth, if the client is connecting from home or another primary context, is that an occupational therapist can "see" the client in their natural environment. Through observation in the client's natural environment, the therapist can assess specific performance skills that occur while the client performs an occupation. As with more traditional practice settings, therapists must consider any safety concerns that may arise from observing a client perform an occupation. Observing a client's engagement in an occupation may differ with telehealth, however, because the therapist may need a second person at the same site as the client to ensure safety and assist in any necessary accommodations.

For example, if an occupational therapist is using telehealth to evaluate the need for home modifications, they should have a caregiver or other second person present to navigate the physical space while holding the telehealth device. If it has been determined that the client requires home modifications to safely navigate the home, the client should not then be navigating the home while holding a device. Research on home modification evaluations, however, guides therapists in creating adjustments to ensure safety considerations. Studies have investigated various ways to conduct an evaluation of home modifications over telehealth, including sending a technician to the home, with the occupational therapist instructing and assessing remotely, and using software programs that allow caregivers to upload digital photos (Ninnis et al., 2019). Overall, structured methods of home modification evaluation have been found effective when implemented with proper safety considerations.

Standardized caregiver, parent, and self-report

Standardized caregiver or parent reports are commonly used in traditional practice settings to gain an understanding of individuals' characteristics across contexts and in everyday settings. Telehealth occupational therapy interventions are gaining traction with providing services to caregivers of children with developmental conditions in early intervention as well as caregivers of individuals with chronic conditions. Therefore, occupational therapists may use standardized parent reports of child behavior (e.g., Sensory Profile–2, Adaptive Behavior Assessment System;

Dunn, 2014; Harrison & Oakland, 2015) or caregiver strain (e.g., Caregiver Strain Questionnaire; Brannan et al., 1997) to characterize and quantify what they are gleaning from interview and observation. Many such standardized reports may also be used to show change over time as a result of occupational therapy intervention (see Case Examples 14.5 and 14.6).

OVERVIEW OF GROUP- AND POPULATION-BASED EVALUATION

Occupational therapy leaders and scholars have been advocating for the profession to more specifically develop its role within population health (Braveman, 2016; Lamb, 2017; Mallinson et al., 2009). In the *2018 Accreditation Council for Occupational Therapy Education (ACOTE®) Standards and Interpretive Guide* (ACOTE, 2018), groups and populations are included with individuals in the definition of *client*. *Groups* are defined as "collectives of individuals" and populations as "collectives of groups or individuals living in the same locale or sharing the same or like concerns" (ACOTE, 2018, p. 48). The evaluation or assessment of populations or groups is not specifically identified in the standards related to evaluation, because they are identified in the specific sections on theories, basic tenets of occupational therapy, and intervention. It should be noted that the word *client*, not *groups* or *populations*, is used in the evaluation-related standards.

Occupational therapy has a recognized, discipline-specific evaluation process that includes developing occupational profiles, followed by completing occupational performance analyses related to those occupations that are of concern and meaningful to the client (Chisholm & Schell, 2019). This process is most commonly applied to individual clients. Scaffa (2019) recommended applying this occupation-based evaluation process to groups and populations as well.

In this section, the evaluation of groups and populations is discussed relative to this accepted occupational therapy evaluation process. In addition, recommended evaluation processes for identifying group- or population-based needs are integrated into this process and how it can be expanded (Clark et al., 2015; Cole, 2018; Fazio, 2017; Gewurtz & Kirsh, 2016; Reitz & Graham, 2019). Kramer and Grampurohit's framework in Chapter 1, "Evaluation: Where Do We Begin?" identifies the importance of theoretically based, evidence-based, and outcome-focused evaluations in influencing comprehensive intervention plans, and this is applied in this chapter to population and group evaluation. Examples are used to support the reader's understanding and application of the occupational therapy evaluation process to groups and population.

Beginning the Evaluation Process: Groups and Populations

The evaluation of a group or population begins when an occupational therapist or a referral source, such as school, community organization, or group setting, identifies a critical need that is not currently being addressed and that an occupational therapy perspective might be instrumental in addressing for a population or group. An occupational therapist then works to understand the need identified from the perspective of the client—the group or population.

Ecological models of occupational therapy applied within a theory of health promotion are considered best practice for populations and groups (Scaffa, 2019). *Occupational therapy–directed health promotion* is "the client-centered use of occupations, adaptations to context or alterations of context to maximize individuals', families, and groups' pursuit of health and quality of life" (Reitz & Graham, 2019, p. 676). *Ecological models of practice* recognize that physical, social, cultural, and temporal environments predict the occupational participation and performance of individuals, groups, or populations and that aspects of environments can inhibit or facilitate function (Brown, 2019).

Some groups are developed within organizations and institutions to use the power of a group to facilitate individual clients working toward their individual goals. In these cases, other occupational therapy frames of reference and models may be best practice for framing and guiding the evaluation process (Cole, 2018; Krupa et al., 2016).

Occupational Profile of a Group or Population

Developing an occupational profile is the first step of the occupational therapy process. Key components of this step are identifying the clients' needs, occupations, contexts, interests, occupational history, and resources from the clients' point of view (AOTA, 2017). For a group or population, that means aggregating or synthesizing data across individuals who are members of a group or population.

Various professional groups commonly use a needs assessment process to systematically investigate the concerns of an organization, community, population, or group and potential service needs. Assessment strategies used for this purpose are focus groups, client or stakeholder interviews, surveys, and literature reviews. Members of a profession direct their needs assessment toward their profession's domain of concern. In the case of occupational therapy, its practitioners design need assessments for learning about and uncovering patterns about a group or population's occupation-based needs, desires, and goals as perceived by its members (Clark et al., 2015; Finlayson, 2017; Scaffa & Brownson, 2014).

Focus groups

A *focus group* is a method of systematically listening and learning from discussions by a group of people. It is essentially a group interview and makes use of the power of group process for facilitating participant engagement. It allows participants to share their own ideas on a topic, as well as extend or build on what their fellow group members share. A focus group process supports the investigation and understanding of complex behaviors and concerns that might not be understood through other methods. It may also uncover facets of topics that a potential service, program, or group developer might not have considered (Krueger & Casey, 2015).

To use a focus group as an accountable and evidence-based assessment method, occupational therapists must also carefully develop a logical sequence of questions to facilitate focus group members' sharing their viewpoints and experiences related to the group's or population's occupational profile. Therapists also must develop the skills for focus group data collection, data management, and analysis. Such data analysis is similar to the techniques used in qualitative research. Clark et al. (2015) provided excellent examples of the use of focus groups for developing the University of Southern California's Well Elderly Studies and for related community project development serving older adult populations in other communities.

Interviewing

Interviewing representative members of a group or population or interviewing other stakeholders of an organization that serves the targeted population, such as administrative leadership or service providers, is an important way to get in-depth information and perceptions of the needs and profile of a population or group. Clark et al. (2015) described their application of qualitative research methods for interviewing to understand the viewpoints and needs of an older adult population in Southern California. Such an interview process is open ended to support the interviewer learning what interviewees believe is most relevant and important to share. Interviewers develop a tentative interview guide so that they have a map of key questions and topics and can refocus the conversation as needed, but they generally work to follow the lead of the interviewee to promote the interviewee elaborating on topics shared.

It is critical that occupational therapists develop their skills for interviewing as well as for managing and analyzing interview data across interviewees, to use interviewing as an assessment for population and groups. Stake (2014) and Taylor (2017) provided guidance for occupational therapists interested in developing beginning skills for applying qualitative research interview methods as an assessment tool for populations and groups. To efficiently manage, analyze, and develop visualizations for sharing results of themes across interviewees, qualitative research software can be an indispensable tool. Atlas.ti (www.Atlasti.com) and NVivo (www.qsrinternational.com) are user-friendly tools for managing and analyzing data across interviews.

Surveys

Surveys are also a helpful assessment tool for learning about population-based needs and developing a group- or population-based occupational profile. Surveys are systematically designed questionnaires that can be completed by a client without a professional present. Developing a survey to explore a population's needs, perspectives, or interests requires basic knowledge about survey construction, and is relatively easy to administer. If an online survey is feasible for engaging the target population, there are time- and resource-efficient ways to collect and analyze data. Survey Monkey® and Qualtrics™ are two online survey platforms that are user friendly and include prompts to support actual survey construction. The basics of survey research and construction were addressed by Forsyth and Kviz (2017); Dillman et al. (2014) provided in-depth guidance on the design of different types of surveys.

Literature review

When occupational therapists are developing an occupational profile of a group or population, carrying out a **literature review** can be an invaluable tool. *Literature review* refers to a comprehensive summary of results from prior literature on a topic. The literature can support understanding of the specific population or group and can help the therapist learn more about specific needs that may come up in interviews, focus groups, or surveys. Brown (2017) provided an occupational therapy–specific guide to learning skills for pursuing and organizing an evidence-based literature review. Case Examples 14.7–14.9 demonstrate developing occupational profiles for groups and populations.

Occupational Performance Analysis

Occupational performance analyses are necessary for examining objective factors that facilitate or are barriers to the occupational performance of the target group or the population (Scaffa, 2019). This includes exploring population and group data related to health indicators, lifestyles, trends in impairments, conditions, and risk behaviors, as well as a population's or group's commitment to and preparedness for change.

Any relevant secondary data collected by an organization or municipalities about the population or group being evaluated should be reviewed. Data about health indicators and goals of different populations of the United States can be found at HealthyPeople.gov and at cdc.gov.

CASE EXAMPLE 14.7. COMMUNITY MENTAL HEALTH CLINIC: OCCUPATIONAL PROFILE

An occupational therapist noticed a pattern in the occupational profiles of the female clients she serves at a **community mental health clinic.** This pattern was related to the clients' concerns about parenting their young children. The practitioner created a draft of a group occupational profile that articulated commonalities across individual occupational profiles. She then identified gaps in the group occupational profile that required more information from members of this population. She decided that she would develop a focus group of clients who are mothers of young children to explore their parenting experiences, concerns, and self-identified needs.

CASE EXAMPLE 14.8. COMMUNITY-BASED PRACTICE AND OLDER ADULTS: OCCUPATIONAL PROFILE

An occupational therapist has a **community-based private practice** in an area with a large population of older adults. The therapist has beginning relationships with organizations that provide services for this population and that have expressed interest in learning more about developing a partnership with him for providing health promotion occupation-based groups for older adults.

One organization is member run and focuses on offering cultural and educational activities for its members. Its members are retired, are generally healthy, fall in the middle- to upper-middle class income levels, are college educated, and range in ages from 60 to 95 years. Another organization interested in partnering with the occupational therapist is a vibrant senior center supported by the local municipality. It offers a range of classes and activities for a diverse group of older adults within the same age range as the other organization, but its member population is ethnically and racially diverse. This group has limited English proficiency, low income levels, and more health concerns than the other older adult community organization.

Because of the demands of evaluating the population of each center, the occupational therapist decides to meet with a local graduate occupational therapy program. Together, the faculty and community-based occupational therapist plan meetings with the leadership of each program to learn about the organizational leaders' views of their overall population and any subpopulations for whom they identify needs or concerns. After gathering this information, the occupational therapy team decides to interview a cluster of center members who are representative of the different groups. The members interviewed are of different age groups and genders.

The occupational therapy team seeks to learn about groups within the larger population and focus on their views, needs, interests, occupations, and occupational history. After getting to know these members, they decide to develop a focus group of participants at each center so they can deepen their understanding of the populations and the groups within the population relative to needs, interests, and occupational perspectives on lifestyle and health.

Besides creating occupational profiles of the populations, the occupational therapy team creates organizational profiles of both centers to focus their thinking about their mission, philosophy, goals, programs, and outcomes of the program. As the team goes about the project, they can also search for articles to help them understand each population of older adults.

CASE EXAMPLE 14.9. ELEMENTARY SCHOOL COMMUNITY: OCCUPATIONAL PROFILES

The superintendent of a **suburban school district** requested that one of the district's occupational therapists develop a program to address the fine motor skill development of all kindergartners in its four elementary schools. Although she has worked for the school district for several years and understands the rationale for developing such a program, the occupational therapist chooses to get more information. She decides to develop a population-based occupational profile of kindergarteners, kindergarten teachers, and parents of kindergarteners of the school district as a whole. Additionally, she develops a community profile of each elementary school to focus the occupational therapy department on similarities and differences of each school.

She decides that the most efficient way to proceed is to set up a series of focus groups to learn about the views of each group of stakeholders who would need to collaborate and value such a districtwide program. She first plans a series of meetings with the occupational therapy practitioners to learn about their views and experiences with kindergarteners, teachers, and the culture of kindergarten classes and the school district at large. In addition, she plans focus groups with kindergarten teachers and individual interviews of elementary school principals. Her plan is to discuss their views about kindergarteners' fine motor skill development, curricular needs, and how the principals understand teacher and parent concerns related to the project. As she goes about these tasks, she searches the literature to learn what has been written about kindergarteners' development of skills for drawing, writing, and cutting with scissors.

After completing these interviews and focus groups, the occupational therapist creates a districtwide profile of the perceived needs for fine motor skill development of kindergarteners. She also has gained an understanding of the priorities of the parents, teachers, and leadership related to the topic, as well as overall kindergarten curricular and classroom routines.

To better understand trends in impairments, conditions, or risk behaviors for similar groups or populations, an evaluator should also search other databases for population or group data, as well as systematic reviews and epidemiological research literature.

In addition, occupational therapists should use opportunities to directly assess concerns. There are only a few reliable and valid assessment tools available to guide an occupation-based group or population assessment. Morgan-Brown and Chard (2014) described the Assessment Tool for Occupation and Social Engagement, which measures the interaction and engagement of all people in communal areas of long-term care facilities. A therapist may use the Social Profile (Donohue, 2013) to understand the interaction and effectiveness of the overall level of group member participation for intended occupations of that group.

Gewurtz and Kirsh (2016) described the use of publicly available interdisciplinary workplace assessments that examine an organization's culture for workers. The intent of these assessments is to prevent mental health problems and to improve the mental health of all workers. There are also interdisciplinary guidelines for conducting ecological and situational assessments within frameworks for planning health promotion programs (Public Health Ontario, 2015; Reitz & Graham, 2019). Case Examples 14.10–14.12 illustrate the use of the occupational performance analysis in group settings.

Evaluation Report for Groups and Populations

An evaluation report for a group or population is consistent with the tenets described for a traditional occupational therapy report (Chisholm & Schell, 2019); however, the data collection, analyses, and synthesis are more in depth. For a group the *evaluation report* includes what methods the therapist used to collect the data, how the therapist analyzed the data, and any specific methods used for synthesizing the information.

The report's audience is also different than that of traditional occupational therapy reports. It is important to share the report with an organization's administration and potential funders as well as the client. The report may have implications for or recommend policy and program changes for the organization.

The assessment data collected, analyzed, and synthesized in an evaluation report provide a guide to understanding the needs and values that are meaningful from the client's perspective. For a group or population, the aggregation of site-specific data and the presentation of patterns should be provided in a manner that is credible and trustworthy. The report takes the reader logically through identifying the population's strengths and potential barriers to occupational performance and participation and the implications for the health of the population members. It also identifies areas to target in group interventions or population-based services and the occupational outcomes that are relevant, meaningful, and valued by the clients. If group interventions are recommended, one or more group protocols may be included in the report.

SUMMARY

As occupational therapists, we must be clear on identifying emerging practices as they arise. As we identify such areas of practice, we will need to identify how we evaluate our clients' skills and function. There are multitudes of possibilities for our future practices; a few have been outlined here

CASE EXAMPLE 14.10. COMMUNITY MENTAL HEALTH CLINIC: OCCUPATIONAL PERFORMANCE ANALYSIS

The occupational therapist who serves female clients who are mothers of young children in a **community mental health clinic** researches how the symptoms of mental illness inhibit clients' parent–child interaction and overall functioning as parents. She reviews the epidemiological data and finds information about the prevalence of single motherhood and the additional challenges to successful parenthood facing clients like those she serves. She decides to collaborate with some of her colleagues to organize some family group activities at the center, so that she can better understand how her clients actually interact with their children. In this way, she has the opportunity to observe some of the mothers interacting with their children. She uses the Social Profile (Donohue, 2013) and guidelines for observing parent–child interaction provided in the frame of reference for enhancing social participation (Olson, 2020).

CASE EXAMPLE 14.11. COMMUNITY-BASED PRACTICE AND OLDER ADULTS: OCCUPATIONAL PERFORMANCE ANALYSIS

For the **community-based practice** with older adults, the occupational therapy team uses the interdisciplinary processes for situational and ecological assessments to examine the needs of two different organizations providing educational and group activities for older adults. They synthesize the data already collected for each organization (through interviews and focus groups) with the relevant community health indicators and research literature to identify pilot occupation-based educational or group activities during which they can interact with a group in an activity. They also use the Social Profile (Donohue, 2013) to guide their observations of group member participation around the group activity.

CASE EXAMPLE 14.12. ELEMENTARY SCHOOL COMMUNITIES: OCCUPATIONAL PERFORMANCE ANALYSIS

The occupational therapist working on evaluating the programmatic needs of a **suburban school district's** kindergarten fine motor center program completes a literature review to increase her understanding of this population. In particular, she wants to identify the expected fine motor skill level of kindergarteners on the basis of research and the best practices for facilitating this development within a kindergarten curriculum.

She then works with the other school-based occupational therapists to develop a short screening tool for assessing the drawing, writing, and cutting skills of kindergarteners to meet the needs of this project. After creating this tool, she and the other occupational therapists pilot the tool in four kindergarten classes. With the help of graduate occupational therapy students, they organize the data into a database and then compare the results with what is reported in the literature about the expected skills of kindergarten students.

(primary care, telehealth, and evaluation of groups and populations). Occupational therapists show their value by using clear evaluation measures followed by tailored intervention approaches based on skilled assessment methods.

As our health care system evolves, we must be confident in our abilities to fill gaps in services for individuals across the continuum of care and for our emerging practice sites to allow us to do so.

QUESTIONS

1. From a primary care perspective, what is a holistic evaluation?
2. What is the importance of advocacy in the primary care setting?

3. What are three areas where telehealth might be especially useful, and three potential problems for the therapist in this type of setting? Identify ways that you might possibly deal with these potential problems.
4. What potential licensure issues pertain to occupational therapy practice in telehealth?
5. What are three potential problems for evaluating groups and populations from an occupational therapy perspective? How might you address with those problems?
6. What purpose would focus groups serve in evaluation of a group? Why would a literature review be helpful in evaluating groups?

REFERENCES

Accreditation Council for Occupational Therapy Education. (2018). 2018 Accreditation Council for Occupational Therapy Education (ACOTE®) standards and interpretative guide. *American Journal of Occupational Therapy, 72*(Suppl. 2), 7912410005. https://doi.org/10.5014/ajot.2018.72S217

Allen, J., Noser, A., Littlefield, A., Seegan, P., Clements, M., & Patton, S. (2018). Measuring self-efficacy in the context of pediatric diabetes management: Psychometric properties of the Self-Efficacy for Diabetes Scale. *Journal of Pediatric Psychology, 43*(2), 143–151. https://doi.org/10.1093/jpepsy/jsx094

American Occupational Therapy Association. (2014a). Occupational therapy practice framework: Domain and process (3rd ed.) *American Journal of Occupational Therapy, 68*(Suppl. 1), S1–S48. https://doi.org/10.5014/ajot.2014.682006

American Occupational Therapy Association. (2014b). The role of occupational therapy in primary care. *American Journal of Occupational Therapy, 68*(Suppl. 3), S25–S33. https://doi.org/10.5014/ajot.2014.686S06

American Occupational Therapy Association. (2015a). Occupational therapy code of ethics (2015). *American Journal of Occupational Therapy, 69*(Suppl. 3), 6913410030. https://doi.org/10.5014/ajot.2015.696S03

American Occupational Therapy Association. (2015b). Standards of practice for occupational therapy. *American Journal of Occupational Therapy, 69*, 6913410057. https://doi.org/10.5014/ajot.2015.696S06

American Occupational Therapy Association. (2017). AOTA occupational profile template. *American Journal of Occupational Therapy, 71*(Suppl. 2), 7112420030. https://doi.org/10.5014/ajot.2017.716S12

American Occupational Therapy Association. (2018). Telehealth in occupational therapy. *American Journal of Occupational Therapy, 72*, 7212410059. https://doi.org/10.5014/ajot.2018.72S219

Ayres, A. J. (1989). *Sensory Integration and Praxis Tests.* Los Angeles, CA: Western Psychological Services.

Bierman, R. T., Kwong, M. W., & Calouro, C. (2018). State occupational and physical therapy telehealth laws and regulations: A 50-state survey. *International Journal of Telerehabilitation, 10*(2), 3–54. https://doi.org/10.5195/ijt.2018.6269

Bischoff, H. A., Stähelin, H. B., Monsch, A. U., Iversen, M. D., Weyh, A., von Dechend, M. . . . Theiler, R. (2003). Identifying a cut-off point for normal mobility: A comparison of the timed "up and go" test in community-dwelling and institutionalized elderly women. *Age and Aging, 32*, 315–320. https://doi.org/10.1093/ageing/32.3.315

Brannan, A. M., Heflinger, C. A., & Bickman, L. (1997). The Caregiver Strain Questionnaire: Measuring the impact on the family of living with a child with serious emotional disturbance.

Journal of Emotional and Behavioral Disorders, 5, 212–222. https://doi.org/10.1177/106342669700500404

Braveman, P. (2006). Health disparities and health equity: Concepts and measurement. *Annual Review of Public Health, 27,* 167–194. https://doi.org/10.1146/annurev.publhealth.27.021405.102103

Braveman, B. (2016). Health Policy Perspectives—Population health and occupational therapy. *American Journal of Occupational Therapy, 70,* 7001090010. https://doi.org/10.5014/ajot.2016.701002

Brown, C. (2017). *The evidence-based practitioner: Applying research to meet client needs.* Philadelphia: Davis.

Brown, C. (2019). Ecological models in occupational therapy. In B. A. Boyt Schell & G. Gillen (Eds.), *Willard and Spackman's occupational therapy* (13th ed., pp. 623–632). Philadelphia: Wolters Kluwer.

Bruininks, R. H., & Bruininks, B. D. (2005). *Bruininks–Oseretsky Test of Motor Proficiency: Examiner's manual.* San Antonio, TX: Pearson.

Buysse, D. J., Reynolds, C. F., III, Monk, T. H., Berman, S. R., & Kupfer, D. J. (1989). The Pittsburgh Sleep Quality Index: A new instrument for psychiatric practice and research. *Psychiatry Research, 28*(2), 193–213. https://doi.org/10.1016/0165-1781(89)90047-4

Centers for Disease Control and Prevention. (2019). *Chronic diseases in America.* Retrieved from https://www.cdc.gov/chronicdisease/resources/infographic/chronic-diseases.htm

Chisholm, D., & Schell, B. A. B. (2019). Overview of the occupational therapy process and outcomes. In B. A. Boyt Schell & G. Gillen (Eds), *Willard and Spackman's occupational therapy* (13th ed., pp. 353–368). Philadelphia: Wolters Kluwer.

Clark, F., Blanchard, J., Sleight, A., Cogan, A., Florindez, L., Gleason, S., ... Vigen, C. (2015). *Lifestyle Redesign®: The intervention tested in the USC Well Elderly Studies* (2nd ed.). Bethesda, MD: AOTA Press.

Cole, M. B. (2018). *Group dynamics in occupational therapy: The theoretical basis and practice application of group intervention* (5th ed.). Thorofare, NJ: Slack.

Dahl-Popilizio, S., Rogers, O., Muir, S., Carroll, J., & Manson, L. (2017). Interprofessional primary care: The value of occupational therapy. *Open Journal of Occupational Therapy, 5*(3). https://doi.org/10.15453/2168-6408.1363

Dickerson, A. E., Meuel, D. B., Ridenour, C. D., & Cooper, K. (2014). Assessment tools predicting fitness to drive in older adults: A systematic review. *American Journal of Occupational Therapy, 68,* 670–680. https://doi.org/10.5014/ajot.2014.011833

Dillman, D. A., Smyth, J. D., & Christian, L. M. (2014). *Internet, phone, mail, and mixed-mode surveys: The tailored design method.* Hoboken, NJ: Wiley.

Donnelly, C., Brenchley, C., Crawford, C., & Letts, L. (2014). The emerging role of occupational therapy in primary care. *Canadian Journal of Occupational Therapy, 81,* 51–61. https://doi.org/10.1177/0008417414520683

Donohue, M. V. (2013). *Social Profile: Assessment of social participation in children, adolescents, and adults.* Bethesda, MD: AOTA Press.

Dreyer, N., Dreyer, K. A., Shaw, D. K., & Wittman, P. P. (2001). Efficacy of telemedicine in occupational therapy: A pilot study. *Journal of Allied Health, 30*(1), 39–42.

Dunn, W. (2014). *Sensory Profile–2.* San Antonio: Pearson.

Fazio, L. S. (2017). *Developing occupation-centered programs with the community* (3rd ed.). Thorofare, NJ: Slack.

Finlayson, M. (2017). Needs assessment research. In R. R. Taylor (Ed.), *Kielhofner's research in occupational therapy: Methods of inquiry for enhancing practice* (2nd ed., pp. 395–409). Philadelphia: Davis.

Folio, M., & Fewell, R. (2000). *Peabody Developmental Motor Scales* (2nd ed.). Austin, TX: Pro-Ed.

Forsyth, K., & Kviz, F. J. (2017). Survey research. In R. R. Taylor (Ed.), *Kielhofner's research in occupational therapy: Methods of inquiry for enhancing practice* (2nd ed., pp. 375–394). Philadelphia: Davis.

Gewurtz, R., & Kirsh, B. (2016). Organizational culture frameworks related to mental health: Implications and applications for occupational therapy. In T. Krupa, B. Kirsh, D. Pitts, & E. Fossey (Eds.), *Bruce & Borg's psychosocial frames of reference: Theories, models, and approaches for occupation-based practice* (4th ed., pp. 265–284). Thorofare, NJ: Slack.

Graf, C. (2008). The Lawton Instrumental Activities of Daily Living Scale. *American Journal of Nursing, 108*(4), 52–62. https://doi.org/10.1097/01.NAJ.0000314810.46029.74

Gummesson, C., Atroshi, I., & Ekdahl, C. (2003). The Disabilities of the Arm, Shoulder and Hand (DASH) Outcome Questionnaire: Longitudinal construct validity and measuring self-rated health change after surgery. *BMC Musculoskeletal Disorders, 4,* 11. https://doi.org/10.1186/1471-2474-4-11

Halle, A., Mroz, T., Fogelberg, D., & Leland, N. (2018). Occupational therapy and primary care: Updates and trends. *American Journal of Occupational Therapy, 72,* 7203090010. https://doi.org/10.5014/ajot.2018.723001

Harrison, P. L., & Oakland, T. (2015). *ABAS-3: Adaptive Behavior Assessment System.* Los Angeles: Western Psychological Services.

Health Insurance Portability and Accountability Act of 1996 (HIPAA), Pub. L. 104-191, 42 U.S.C. § 300gg, 29 U.S.C §§ 1181–1183, and 42 U.S.C. §§ 1320d–1320d9.

Hoffmann, T., Russell, T., Thompson, L., Vincent, A., & Nelson, M. (2008). Using the Internet to assess activities of daily living and hand function in people with Parkinson's disease. *NeuroRehabilitation, 23,* 253–261. https://doi.org/10.3233/NRE-2008-23307

Hollander, J. E., Davis, T. M., Doarn, C., Goldwater, J. C., Klasko, S., Lowery, C., . . . Carr, B. G. (2018). Recommendations from the first National Academic Consortium of Telehealth. *Population Health Management, 21,* 271–277. https://doi.org/10.1089/pop.2017.0080

Hwang, R., Mandrusiak, A., Morris, N. R., Peters, R., Korczyk, D., & Russell, T. (2017). Assessing functional exercise capacity using telehealth: Is it valid and reliable in patients with chronic heart failure? *Journal of Telemedicine and Telecare, 23,* 225–232. https://doi.org/10.1177/1357633X16634258

Institute of Medicine. (1994). *Defining primary care: An interim report.* Washington, DC: Author.

Jordan, K. (2019). Editorial—Occupational therapy in primary care: Positioned and prepared to be a vital part of the team. *American Journal of Occupational Therapy, 73,*10. https://doi.org/10.5014/ajot.2019.735002

Kairy, D., Tousignant, M., Leclerc, N., Côté, A., & Levasseur, M. (2013). The patient's perspective of in-home telerehabilitation physiotherapy services following total knee arthroplasty. *International Journal of Environmental Research and Public Health, 10,* 3998–4011. https://doi.org/10.3390/ijerph10093998

Koverman, B., Royeen, L., & Stoykov, M. (2017). Occupational therapy in primary care: Structures and processes that support integration. *Open Journal of Occupational Therapy, 5*(3). https://doi.org/10.15453/2168-6408.1376

Krueger, R. A., & Casey, M. A. (2015). *Focus groups* (5th ed.). Thousand Oaks, CA: Sage.

Krupa, T., Kirsch, B., Pitts, D., & Fossey, E. (2016). *Bruce & Borg's psychosocial frames of reference: Theories, models and approaches for occupation-based practice* (4th ed.) Thorofare, NJ: Slack.

Lamb, A. J. (2017). Unlocking the potential of everyday opportunities. *American Journal of Occupational Therapy, 71,* 71066140010. https://doi.org/10.5014/ajot.2017.716001

Law, M., Baptiste, S., Carswell, A., McColl, M. A., Polatajko, H. J., & Pollock, N. (2019). *Canadian Occupational Performance Measure* (5th ed., rev.). Altona, MB: COPM, Inc.

Little, L. M., & Wallisch, A. (2018). Let's Eat: Development and reliability of an eating behavior assessment for children with autism spectrum disorders. *Annals of International Occupational Therapy, 1*(1), 24–30. https://doi.org/10.3928/24761222-20180212-03

Little, L. M., Wallisch, A., Pope, E., & Dunn, W. (2018). Acceptability and cost comparison of a telehealth intervention for families of children with autism. *Infants and Young Children, 31,* 275–286. https://doi.org/10.1097/IYC.0000000000000126

Liu, X., Sawada, Y., Takizawa, T., Sato, H., Sato, M., Sakamoto, H., . . . Okamura, S. (2007). Doctor–patient communication: A comparison between telemedicine consultation and face-to-face consultation. *Internal Medicine, 46,* 227–232. https://doi.org/10.2169/internalmedicine.46.1813

Loring, K., Ritter, P., Villa, F., & Armas, J. (2009). Community-based peer-led diabetes self-management: A randomized trial. *Diabetes Education, 35,* 641–651. https://doi.org/10.1177/0145721709335006

Mallinson, T., Fischer, H., Rogers, J. C., Ehrlich-Jones, L., & Chang, R. (2009). Human occupation for public health promotion: New directions for occupational therapy practice with persons with arthritis. *American Journal of Occupational Therapy, 63,* 220–226. https://doi.org/10.5014/ajot.63.2.220

Mitchell, P., Wynia, M., Golden, R., McNellis, B., Okun, S., Webb, C. E., . . . Von Kohorn, I. (2012). *Core principles & values of effective team-based health care.* Washington, DC: Institute of Medicine.

Morgan-Brown, M., & Chard, G. (2014). Comparing communal environments using the Assessment Tool for Occupation and Social Engagement: Using interactive occupation and social engagement as outcome measure. *British Journal of Occupational Therapy, 77*(2), 50–58. https://doi.org/10.4276/030802214X13916969446994

Nasreddine, Z., Phillips, N., Bedirian, V., Charbonneau, S., Whitehead, V., Collin, I., . . . Chertkow, H. (2005). The Montreal Cognitive Assessment: A brief screening tool for mild cognitive impairment. *Journal of the American Geriatric Society, 53,* 695–699. https://doi.org/10.1111/j.1532-5415.2005.53221.x

Nicholas, M. K. (2007). The pain self-efficacy questionnaire: Taking pain into account. *European Journal of Pain, 11,* 153–163. https://doi.org/10.1016/j.ejpain.2005.12.008

Ninnis, K., Van Den Berg, M., Lannin, N. A., George, S., & Laver, K. (2019). Information and communication technology use within occupational therapy home assessments: A scoping review. *British Journal of Occupational Therapy, 82,* 141–152. https://doi.org/10.1177/0308022618786928

Nobakht, Z., Rassafiani, M., Hosseini, S. A., & Ahmadi, M. (2017). Telehealth in occupational therapy: A scoping review. *International Journal of Therapy and Rehabilitation, 24,* 534–538. https://doi.org/10.12968/ijtr.2017.24.12.534

Olson, L. J. (2020). Enhancing social participation frame of reference. In P. Kramer, J. Hinojosa, & T. Howe (Eds.), *Frames of reference for pediatric occupational therapy* (4th ed., pp. 461–496). Baltimore: Lippincott Williams & Wilkins.

Podsiadlo, D., & Richardson, S. (1991). The Timed "Up & Go": A test of basic functional mobility for frail elderly persons. *Journal of the American Geriatric Society, 39,* 142–148. https://doi.org/10.1111/j.1532-5415.1991.tb01616.x

Public Health Ontario. (2015). *At a glance: The six steps for planning a health promotion program.* Toronto: Author.

Ratzon, N. Z., Lunievsky, E. K., Ashkenasi, A., Laks, J., & Cohen, H. A. (2017). Simulated driving skills evaluation of teenagers with attention deficit hyperactivity disorder before driving lessons. *American Journal of Occupational Therapy, 71,* 7103220010. https://doi.org/10.5014/ajot.2017.020164

Reese, R. M., Jamison, R., Wendland, M., Fleming, K., Braun, M. J., Schuttler, J. O., & Turek, J. (2013). Evaluating interactive videoconferencing for assessing symptoms of autism. *Telemedicine and E-Health, 19,* 671–677. https://doi.org/10.1089/tmj.2012.0312

Reitz, S. M., & Graham, K. (2019). Health promotion theories. In B. A. Boyt Schell & G. Gillen (Eds.), *Willard and Spackman's occupational therapy* (13th ed., pp. 675–692). Philadelphia: Wolters Kluwer.

Roberts, P., Farmer, M., Lamb, A. J., Muir, S., & Siebert, C. (2014). The role of occupational therapy in primary care. *American Journal of Occupational Therapy, 68,* S25–S33. https://doi.org/10.5014/ajot.2014.686S06

Robinson, B. C. (1983). Validation of a caregiver strain index. *Journal of Gerontology, 38,* 34–348. https://doi.org/10.1093/geronj/38.3.344

Rollnick S., & Miller, W. (1995). What is motivational interviewing? *Behavioural and Cognitive Psychotherapy, 23,* 325–334. https://doi.org/10.1017/S135246580001643X

Royeen, L. (2020). *Occupational therapy as part of a team-based approach in primary care settings.* Unpublished doctoral dissertation, Western Michigan University, Kalamazoo, MI.

Russell-Babin, K., & Wurmser, T. (2016). Transforming care through top-of-license practice. *Nursing Management, 47*(5), 24–28. https://doi.org/10.1097/01.NUMA.0000482527.15743.12

Scaffa, M. E. (2019). Occupational therapy interventions for groups, communities and populations. In B. A. Boyt Schell & G. Gillen (Eds.), *Willard and Spackman's occupational therapy* (13th ed., pp. 436–447). Philadelphia: Wolters Kluwer.

Scaffa, M. E., & Brownson, C. A. (2014). Program planning and needs assessment. In M. Scaffa & S. M. Rietz (Eds.), *Occupational therapy in community-based practice settings* (2nd ed., pp. 61–79). Philadelphia: Davis.

Serwe, K. M., & Bowman, C. (2018). Telehealth experiential learning: A pilot study of the client's experience. *Journal of Occupational Therapy Education, 2*(2), 5. https://doi.org/10.26681/jote.2018.020205

Serwe, K. M., Hersch, G. I., Pickens, N. D., & Pancheri, K. (2017). Caregiver perceptions of a telehealth wellness program. *American Journal of Occupational Therapy, 71,* 7104350010. https://doi.org/10.5014/ajot.2017.025619

Spitzer, R., Kroenke, K., Williams, J., & Lowe, B. (2006). A brief measure for assessing generalized anxiety disorder. *Archives of Internal Medicine, 166,* 1092–1097. https://doi.org/10.1001/archinte.166.10.1092

Stake, R. (2014). *Qualitative research: Studying how things work.* New York: Guilford Press.

Stephenson, S., Anderson-Tome, A., Fischer, S., Guzman, A., Meredith, W, & Somers, C. (2019). Pilot study: Using the Bioness Integrated Therapy System (BITS) to examine the correlation between skills and success with on-the-road driving evaluations. *American Journal of Occupational Therapy, 73,* 7311515280. https://doi.org/10.5014/ajot.2019.73S1-PO4054

Stillerova, T., Liddle, J., Gustafsson, L., Lamont, R., & Silburn, P. (2016). Could everyday technology improve access to assessments? A pilot study on the feasibility of screening cognition in people with Parkinson's disease using the Montreal Cognitive Assessment via Internet videoconferencing. *Australian Occupational Therapy Journal, 63,* 373–380. https://doi.org/10.1111/1440-1630.12288

Taylor, R. R. (2017). *Kielhofner's research in occupational therapy: Methods of inquiry for enhancing practice* (2nd ed.). Philadelphia: Davis.

Thomson, L., & Robnett, R. (2016). *Kohlman Evaluation of Living Skills.* (4th ed.). Bethesda, MD: AOTA Press.

Uniform Data System for Medical Rehabilitation. (2012). The FIM® instrument: Its background, structure, and usefulness. Buffalo, NY: Author.

Wallisch, A., Little, L., Pope, E., & Dunn, W. (2019). Parent perspectives of an occupational therapy telehealth intervention. *International Journal of Telerehabilitation, 11*(1), 15–22. https://doi.org/10.5195/ijt.2019.6274

Ethical Issues in Evaluation

Wayne L. Winistorfer, MPA, OTR, FAOTA

CHAPTER HIGHLIGHTS

- What are ethics?
- Six ethical principles of beneficence, nonmaleficence, autonomy, justice, veracity, and fidelity, and their role in occupational therapy evaluation
- Difference between ethics and laws

KEY TERMS AND CONCEPTS

- Autonomy
- Beneficence
- Code of conduct
- Core values
- Due care
- Ethics
- Evidence-based practice
- Fidelity
- Harm
- Justice
- Laws
- Moral code
- Moral norms
- Nonmaleficence
- *Occupational Therapy Code of Ethics*
- Professional judgment
- Related Standards of Conduct
- Satisficing
- Veracity

INTRODUCTION

Throughout this text, there are mentions of ethical principles, ethical issues, and the application of mindful and ethical considerations to the topic of evaluation. Occupational therapy evaluation and ethics do not appear to have a natural connection, but occupational therapists recognize its importance. When patients or clients are seen for an occupational therapy evaluation, the process is likely well established within the setting, and occupational therapists proceed on the basis of their knowledge, experience, and habits. Therapists are expected to follow the practice standards of the profession and the setting as they apply to the person, group, or population. They must also adhere to the applicable regulations and any specific requirements relative to the source of reimbursement for services. This is considered good practice.

However, whenever an occupational therapy evaluation process is undertaken, it reflects decisions and patterns established by and consistent with values and ethics. Applying ethical principles may not occur at the level of conscious awareness or as the result of deliberate, objective discernment. Using the term *discernment* is common in the realm of ethics; the equivalent term in occupational therapy is **professional judgment.** The application of ethical principles is an essential foundational element for how assessments are actually selected, presented to the client, and interpreted and how an occupational therapy evaluation process is delivered in practice. In addition, the results of an evaluation, how and with whom they are shared, and how they lead to appropriate intervention plans are certainly affected by general ethical principles and specific professional ethics codes and standards.

All health care professions define, adopt, and attempt to enforce profession-specific codes of ethical conduct. These codes are meant to ensure that, when entering into relationships with health care professionals, members of the public can expect to be treated safely, fairly, and competently. Professional codes of ethics typically address the profession's higher calling and virtues in the form of principles. Honoring these principles is the ethical ideal of the profession and is considered to be aspirational in nature. Problems of professional ethics usually arise from conflicts of values (Beauchamp & Childress, 2013).

This chapter reviews ethics and ethical principles and analyzes how the principles relate to broad areas of occupational therapy evaluation. Applicable standards and ethical dilemmas that may arise with occupational therapy assessment and the occupational therapy evaluation process are discussed. Case examples and guidance for critical analysis, recommended behaviors, and application to evaluation as a component of ethical occupational therapy practice are presented.

WHAT ARE ETHICS?

When people says they are being ethical, they are referring to beliefs, behaviors, or actions that they have judged as the right thing to do. The Preamble to the American Occupational Therapy Association (AOTA) *Occupational Therapy Code of Ethics* includes the admonition,

> Ethical action goes beyond rote compliance with these Principles and is a manifestation of moral character and mindful reflection. It is a commitment to benefit others, to virtuous practice of artistry and science, to genuinely good behaviors, and to noble acts of courage. (AOTA, 2015a, p. 2)

Although people may have no conscious awareness of why an action is correct, they arrive at a proper personal conclusion as a product of the influences and experiences that have occurred throughout their lifetime. Learning and life experience results in the development of personal values: people's own *moral code.* The influences and values developed from personal experiences, as well as from shared cultural, societal, and organizational expectations, result in shared *moral norms* (Beauchamp & Childress, 2013).

Defining *Ethics*

In the case of occupational therapy or other health care practitioners, biomedical ethics and professional ethics also influence the underlying foundational values and moral norms that guide ethical behavior in professional practice. Beauchamp and Childress (2013), in their classic book *Principles of Biomedical Ethics,* defined **ethics** as a generic term covering several "different ways of understanding and examining the moral life" (Beauchamp & Childress, 2013, p. 7). These well-respected authors have devoted efforts over many years to advancing the features of and challenges unique to biomedical ethics. AOTA has consistently relied on the work of ethicists, as well as the ethical codes of other professions, when regularly updating the *Occupational Therapy Code of Ethics* (hereinafter referred to as the *Code of Ethics;* AOTA, 2015a) and the numerous resources and advisory opinions published in the *Reference Guide to the Occupational Therapy Code of Ethics* (Scott & Reitz, 2017; Slater, 2016). Revisions, accomplished at approximately 5-year intervals, have focused on emerging cultural issues, technological advances, and evolving areas of practice that generate contemporary ethical dilemmas (AOTA, 2015a).

Codes of Conduct

A profession's embrace of ethical principles does not represent professional obligations, nor do the principles form the basis for disciplinary action of members of the profession who violate them (American Psychological Association, 2016). A *code of conduct* has detailed descriptions of requirements and prohibitions intended to minimize vagueness and define clear boundaries for professional behavior. Although a profession's foundational values likely remain constant, the specific expected behaviors and prohibitions may be revised over time. Revisions are typically made in response to emerging issues, cultural or societal evolution, and emerging practice areas and challenges.

At times, specific abhorrent or egregious behavior of a member of a profession reaches a critical level of public awareness. When public notoriety rises to the level of scandal, the unethical behavior may reveal a gap in the breadth or scope of a professional code of conduct. Although the scandal may be blatantly incongruous with the core values of the profession, the violation may not be adequately addressed within the expected or prohibited behavioral standards of the ethics code or code of conduct. The "this has never happened before" response may prompt a professional association to examine its ethics code or code of conduct and adopt new prohibitions designed to address the specific concern, objectionable behavior, or notorious event. The motivation for the association is to ensure that similar offenses do not occur and to preserve the profession's integrity (Beauchamp & Childress, 2013).

Occupational Therapy Code of Ethics

Professional ethics for the occupational therapy profession did not just begin in 1975 when the AOTA Representative Assembly passed Resolution 461-75 to establish the Commission on Ethics (Slater, 2016). The genesis of concern for the ethical practice of occupational therapy certainly began

CORE VALUE	APPLICATION TO OCCUPATIONAL THERAPY
Altruism	Demonstrate concern for the welfare of others
Equality	Treat all people impartially and free of bias
Freedom	Honor personal choice Values and desires of the client guide practice
Justice	A state in which diverse communities are inclusive Organize and structure communities such that all members can function, flourish, and live a satisfactory life
Dignity	Promote and preserve individuality by treating the client with respect in all interactions
Truth	Provide accurate information in all forms of oral, written, and electronic communication
Prudence	Use clinical and ethical reasoning skills, use sound judgment and reflection to make decisions in professional roles

TABLE 15.1. *Occupational Therapy Code of Ethics* Core Values

Note. Adapted from "Occupational Therapy Code of Ethics (2015)," by the American Occupational Therapy Association, 2015, *American Journal of Occupational Therapy, 69*(Suppl. 3), 6913410030. Adapted with permission.

before the adoption of the first *Code of Ethics* in 1977 (Slater, 2016). Yet, not until that time could occupational therapy professionals point to a guiding document that addressed ethical behavior and delineated the mechanisms intended "to serve Association members and the public through development, review, interpretation, and education . . . the process whereby they are enforced" (Article 7, Section 7; Slater, 2016, p. 3). The purpose of the *Code of Ethics* has remained constant since its adoption: "to promote quality care and professional conduct" (Slater, 2016, p. 3).

The intention of professional principles is to guide practitioners' interactions and behavior. As the occupational therapy professional *Code of Ethics* was established, a set of **core values** was codified as the foundation that led to the ethical principles on which the current *Code of Ethics* is structured (Table 15.1).

The core values of the occupational therapy profession lay the foundation for how practitioners come to know that an action is ethical or unethical. They do not provide an authoritative framework or description of specific behaviors that dictate the professional, ethical practice of occupational therapy. The *Code of Ethics* (AOTA, 2015a) is the document that brings the profession's core values into the realm of application. The *Code of Ethics* uses six ethical principles that, along with the associated **Related Standards of Conduct** (RSCs; AOTA, 2015a), bring clarity to an array of activities and situations that present ethical dimensions and ethical dilemmas. RSCs prescribe expected, virtuous behaviors and an assortment of prohibitions that are relevant to the contemporary, ethical practice of occupational therapy (AOTA, 2015a).

Standards of Practice

AOTA's (2015b) *Standards of Practice* include an ethics requirement by which occupational therapy practitioners are expected to abide: "An occupational therapy practitioner abides by the *Occupational Therapy Code of Ethics 2015*" (Standard I, No. 4; p. 3). It is important to know that the AOTA *Standards of Practice* and the *Code of Ethics* do not directly have legal consequences for any occupational therapy practitioner. An AOTA member's membership status can be adversely affected when unethical behavior leads to the application of the *Enforcement Procedures of the Occupational Therapy Code of Ethics* (AOTA, 2019; Slater, 2016). AOTA membership status, pursuant to a substantiated ethics violation, is within the jurisdiction of the AOTA Ethics Commission.

Occupational therapy practitioners who are not AOTA members are guided by AOTA standards, yet violations of the standards are not enforceable within the realm of the national professional association. The National Board for Certification in Occupational Therapy uses its own code of conduct separate from AOTA (see Exhibit 15.1). A number of state and territorial professional regulatory authorities (state licensure laws or codes), however, identify adherence to the professional standards of practice as a legal, enforceable requirement for their license holders. In these states, when a licensee violates the state-specific scope of practice, the state may choose to exercise its authority to apply the AOTA (2015b) *Standards of Practice* or the AOTA (2015a) *Code of Ethics* to sanction or otherwise enforce disciplinary action regarding the practitioner's license within that jurisdiction (AOTA, State Affairs Group, 2019).

Occupational Therapy Code of Ethics and Evaluation

The *Code of Ethics* (AOTA, 2015a) directly relates to occupational therapy evaluation. While performing assessments and evaluations, occupational therapy practitioners who violate or do not conform to accepted, recognized standards could be subject to complaints and adverse action by their state or territorial jurisdiction, in addition to sanctions that could be imposed by the national professional association, AOTA. Ethical practice requires that the occupational therapy evaluation process honor general ethical principles enumerated within the *Code of Ethics*. More specifically, several RSCs provide authoritative statements of professional expectations and behavioral directives, as well as some prohibitions, that apply to assessments and the process of occupational therapy evaluation. The *Code of Ethics* (AOTA, 2015a) serves as a framework with which to explore issues in occupational therapy assessment and evaluation. Each ethical principle offers specific opportunities to practice ethically and also introduces potential challenges and ethical dilemmas related to practice. Table 15.2 describes how the six ethical principles relate to evaluation.

Throughout the remainder of this chapter, the *Code of Ethics* (AOTA, 2015a) and relevant RSCs are used as the structure for definitions, illustrations, case examples, and analysis.

BENEFICENCE

The principle of **beneficence** includes all forms of action intended to benefit other persons. The term *beneficence* connotes acts of mercy, kindness, and charity (Beauchamp & Childress, 2013). Beneficence requires taking action to help others, promote good, prevent harm, and remove the

---

EXHIBIT 15.1.	Code of Conduct of the National Board for Certification in Occupational Therapy

It is noteworthy that the National Board for Certification in Occupational Therapy® (NBCOT®) uses its own code of conduct and does not apply the AOTA *Code of Ethics*. The NBCOT Candidate/Certificant Code of Conduct (NBCOT, 2015), which is based on the same foundational core values embraced by AOTA, is used to review complaints about incompetent or impaired practitioners. NBCOT also applies its own procedures for disciplinary action. However, just as only AOTA members are directly the subject of, and under the jurisdiction of, the AOTA *Code of Ethics* and the enforcement procedures, the NBCOT Code of Conduct applies only to those holding current certification. Initial NBCOT certification is the accepted qualification to be eligible for an initial state license. However, continuing NBCOT certification is a requirement for licensure in only one state, South Carolina. NBCOT is concerned about ethical practice, but disciplinary action for unethical practice is not applicable to those occupational therapy practitioners who do not hold a current NBCOT certification (Registered Occupational Therapist or Certified Occupational Therapy Assistant).

TABLE 15.2.   Ethical Principles for Occupational Therapy Evaluation

ETHICAL PRINCIPLE	CODE OF BEHAVIOR	RELEVANCE TO EVALUATION
Beneficence	All forms of action intended for the well-being and safety of clients	Appropriate evaluation, intervention, reassessment, and reevaluation are provided in a client-centered and evidence-based manner within the scope of occupational therapy practice.
Nonmaleficence	Abstain from causing harm to others	Undue internal and external influences on evaluation that may compromise the occupational therapy process should be avoided.
Autonomy	Respect clients' rights to self-determination, privacy, confidentiality, and consent	Always seek consent before evaluation, and maintain privacy and confidentiality of the reports and results.
Justice	Promote fairness and objectivity	Timely response to referral as determined by law, regulation, or policy and nondiscriminatory behavior
Veracity	Truthfulness when representing occupational therapy	Refrain from making false claims on the basis of the evaluation.
Fidelity	Commitment to treat clients and others with respect, fairness, discretion, and integrity	Treat clients and others with respect, and establish collaborative communication.

potential for harm. Examples of beneficence include protecting and defending the rights of others, preventing harm from occurring to others, removing conditions that will cause harm to others, helping persons with disabilities, and rescuing persons in danger (Beauchamp & Childress, 2013).

Beneficence and Related Standards of Conduct

The *Code of Ethics* RSCs that are consistent with the principle of beneficence, highlighting only those areas that pertain to evaluation, are as follows:

- Provide appropriate evaluation and a plan of intervention for recipients of occupational therapy services specific to their needs.
- Reevaluate and reassess recipients of service in a timely manner to determine whether goals are being achieved and whether intervention plans should be revised.
- Use, to the extent possible, evaluation, planning, intervention techniques, assessments, and therapeutic equipment that are evidence based, current, and within the recognized scope of occupational therapy practice. (AOTA, 2015a, pp. 2–3)

The first RSC applicable to the ethical principle of beneficence directs occupational therapy personnel to "provide appropriate evaluation . . . for recipients . . . specific to their needs" (AOTA, 2015a, p. 2), which leads to the question, "What is an appropriate evaluation? The second RSC relates to the timely reevaluation and reassessment. The third RSC describes the use of evaluations that are "evidence based, current, and within the recognized scope of occupational therapy practice" (AOTA, 2015a, p. 2). Law and MacDermid (2008) described ***evidence-based practice*** as "integrating clinical experience with the best available external clinical evidence from systematic research" (p. 5). Their focus on the balance between clinical experience and

systematic research relates to the clinical decision-making process to choose appropriate evaluation tools that will lead to evidence-based interventions. Decisions "should be made on the basis of judicious clinical reasoning, sound judgment, insight, experience, and available research" (Slater, 2016, p. 181).

Beneficence: Practical Application to Evaluation

When selecting ethically beneficent occupational therapy assessments and evaluation processes, therapists must consider several questions.

Is this assessment current?

When examining the age and current applicability of an assessment, therapists should consider
- The original development date of the assessment,
- When the assessment was last updated, and
- Whether the most current edition of the assessment is available and in their possession.

Using the most current version of an assessment is always indicated as the best and most ethical approach. Many assessments are updated on a regular basis. Keeping current requires research and awareness of developments in the profession and specific areas of practice. The expense of purchasing updated versions is a concern, but best practice requires having the most recent assessments, recording forms, and tools. Practitioners are responsible for using the most recent version of any assessment.

Determine whether an assessment developed during an earlier time period is still relevant to the current situation. For example, the first edition of the Bay Area Functional Performance Evaluation (Bloomer & Williams, 1979) used a paper bank deposit slip, which was later revised because of concerns related to cultural experience and relevance. With the emergence of digital financial transactions, paper bank deposit slips may be foreign to any number of patients referred to occupational therapy. Likewise, a patient who is indigent, has no bank account, and exclusively uses cash for purchases may have little or no exposure to banking in either paper or electronic formats (Houston et al., 1989).

In another example, the original Kohlman Evaluation of Living Skills (KELS; McGourty, 1978) used a bound, paper telephone directory and a desk phone to assess cognition and functional performance. Today, these tools may be unknown to a generation with touch-screen personal cellphones that have Contacts features and search functions to access websites and links to contact local businesses. The most current KELS added online banking and bill-pay simulations (Thomson & Robnett, 2016).

Is this assessment evidence based?

To determine whether an assessment is evidence based, therapists should ask,

- What is the assessment's validity and reliability?
- Am I accessing and referencing the most recent data on research applications of the tool?
- Has research been published within the past 5 years that validates the use of this tool?

Many widely used assessments are the subject of research. Occupational therapists have an ethical duty to access research findings and determine their applicability to practice. Research data that verify test validity and performance norms can affect the contemporary interpretation of results and skew a comparison of a person's performance to the results expected of a cohort population.

Affirmative findings pertaining to these questions may bring therapists peace of mind. However, when the currency, applicability, and evidence of an assessment's currency are compromised, practitioners need to consider using other tools or procuring the most recent edition of a tool. Less-than-perfect assessment tools require therapists to be judicious when reporting evaluation results, which are likely to be compromised in some way. Clinical experience and expertise can supplement the validity of evaluation results, but therapists must also be aware and recognize the shortcomings of the situation and acknowledge them in any reports. Most importantly, the therapist has an ethical responsibility to choose the best assessment based on the needs of the client, which is the essence of beneficence.

Is this evaluation within the scope of the profession or appropriately used by occupational therapists?

It is incumbent on therapists to know whether the assessments they are using, or want to begin using, are appropriately used within the domain of occupational therapy. An easy indicator is that the evaluation tool was designed, developed, and researched by occupational therapy practitioners for populations frequently seen by occupational therapy practitioners. Some tools are available for purchase or use only by members of specific professions or by occupational therapists with specialized skills or certification.

For example, only certified speech-language pathologists may use the American Speech–Language–Hearing Association's (2020) Functional Communication Measures to submit data to the National Outcomes Measurement System. Similarly, an occupational therapist with a

bachelor's-level education must hold certification and have additional training in assessment to purchase and use the Sensory Integration and Praxis Tests (Ayres, 1989).

Are You Honoring the Principle of Beneficence?

What are occupational therapists to do when they are presented with a patient in need of occupational therapy evaluation and the available assessments are not current or not quite appropriate?

A decision-making strategy from the field of administration and management can serve as a method for resolving the challenges of the less-than-perfect solution. *Satisficing* entails exploring the available alternatives until an acceptable threshold is met. This mash-up of the words *satisfy* and *suffice,* first introduced by Herbert A. Simon (1956), was popularized by John Rawls (1971) in *A Theory of Justice.* Satisficing explains decision making for circumstances in which an optimal resolution cannot be determined or achieved.

For example, an immediate request to evaluate a patient when optimal tools are not available does not release the occupational therapist from completing the assigned task, but the therapist must choose the most appropriate assessment to meet the needs of the client. Satisficing allows the therapist to do what is requested in ways that are satisfactory for the situation and within the constraints of the environment and available resources. Using a previous version of a standardized assessment may be necessary when there is no other option. Eliminating one component of an assessment tool when the tools or equipment are outdated or broken can fulfill the basics of the questions to be answered by the evaluation process. These variations must be clearly noted when reporting or documenting assessment results. In addition, any limitations or compromises must be considered while identifying priorities for the development of an intervention plan.

However, satisficing is not an acceptable response when an evaluation request is outside the scope of the occupational therapy domain of practice. In the face of this practice dilemma, ethical responses could include offering alternative assessment tools or strategies, suggesting that other professionals or professions perform the evaluation, or simply declining the referral and declining to provide the service (Fleming & Rucas, 2015; Case Example 15.1).

NONMALEFICENCE

The principle of *nonmaleficence* "obligates us to abstain from causing harm to others" (Beauchamp & Childress, 2013, p. 150). It also includes an obligation to not impose risk of harm even if the potential risk is without malicious or harmful intent. The standard of *due care* "requires that the goals pursued justify the risks that must be imposed to achieve those goals" (Beauchamp & Childress, 2013, p. 154). The concept of *harm* in health care often means that a health care practitioner injured or wronged a patient. However, a patient could be harmed by "thwarting, defeating or setting back of some party's interests" (Beauchamp & Childress, 2013, p. 153).

Health care practitioners perform services that may cause pain to a client, but their direct intention is not to harm. Actions that cause harm may sometimes be inadvertent. At

CASE EXAMPLE 15.1. KANDI: BENEFICENCE AND EVALUATION

Kandi, a new graduate, just started her first job as an occupational therapist providing services to inpatients in an acute care hospital. Kandi is assigned to Marquis, a seasoned occupational therapist and long-term employee, for orientation to the setting and to the varied caseload. In the Rehabilitation Services department, Marquis is known as a clinical expert who always connects with patients and their families. A physical therapist in the department told Kandi that Marquis is the best person in the department for bringing focus to the critical issues for safe transition to home, home health, or other care settings. While orienting Kandi to her new job, Marquis stated strongly that "there is no evaluation tool that captures the functional deficits and rehab needs of our caseload. I've been doing this for years. I can tell when someone is or isn't going to be safe at home." Kandi found this odd because during her occupational therapy education program, she learned of several assessments that she understood could be appropriately used in this setting. Kandi knew she had an understanding of assessment tools to effectively identify occupational deficits and characterize the contexts applicable to the person being served, yet Kandi was unsure how to respond to Marquis's comments.

Into the second week of working alongside one another, Marquis regularly checked in with Kandi regarding her day. Kandi's assigned schedule included a medical staff–ordered occupational therapy evaluation of and treatment for an elderly man admitted to the hospital on observation status from the Emergency Department the prior evening. The man had a serious fall at home, resulting in multiple contusions to his face and suspected concussion and rib fractures. Kandi completed a records review and learned that the man lives alone. It was unclear from the available documentation whether the man's recent fall was a first or repeat occurrence. The documentation from the staff in the Emergency Department reflected that the man was unsure whether, or when, he had fallen in the past, but he reported that he "gets tipsy" at home. The early morning case management notes say, "Because no fractures were found on X-ray, plan to transition home in early afternoon, as soon as cleared by therapies."

Kandi told Marquis about the case and that she brought with her the equipment to administer the Allen Cognitive Level Screen (ACLS–5; Allen et al., 2007), which she intended to use with this elderly man. Marquis questioned why Kandi was using the ACLS–5. Kandi shared what she knew about repeat falls and the level of risk for those with cognitive impairments and that men are less likely to report fall occurrences than women (AOTA, 2017; Bergen et al., 2016).

Marquis scoffed, "I know about that Allen thing. I went to a workshop back in the 1990s, and I know it works for psych patients. I haven't been to any workshops in a long time, but I've been an OT for decades. How is leather lacing going to prevent this old guy from falling again? Just recommend a home health visit. He's going home today, and he'll be just fine!"

Foundational ethics question:

- How does the ethical principle of beneficence apply to this scenario?

Considerations:

- How might Kandi approach this conflict with Marquis?
- What standards are applicable, and what resources might Kandi use to advance ethical practice?
- How can cognitive assessment contribute to an ethical occupational therapy evaluation when there are only one or two occupational therapy encounters before discharge from an acute care setting?
- How does using appropriate assessment tools address individual needs and the development of an ethical intervention plan?
- Why is it important to use, to the extent possible, evaluations that are evidence based, current, and within the recognized scope of occupational therapy practice?
- Is it reasonable to believe that an assessment by occupational therapy could influence the development of a comprehensive and safe transition plan?
- Are there any ethical concerns about Marquis's participation in continuing professional development activities?
- How might Kandi address these ethical concerns?

other times, it may be difficult to identify the specific harm that resulted from a health care practitioner's action or lack of action. When harm is the direct intent of an action, the principle of nonmaleficence is certainly violated. However, clear malevolent intent and proven harm by a health care professional could also result in disciplinary action or even criminal liability.

Nonmaleficence and Related Standards of Conduct

The *Code of Ethics* RSCs illustrate several scenarios in which an occupational therapist might violate the principle of nonmaleficence while engaging in the evaluation process. The *Code of Ethics* RSCs that are consistent with the principle of nonmaleficence are as follows:

- Recognize and take appropriate action to remedy personal problems and limitations that might cause harm to recipients of service, colleagues, students, research participants, or others.
- Avoid compromising the rights or well-being of others on the basis of arbitrary directives (e.g., unrealistic productivity expectations, falsification of documentation, inaccurate coding) by exercising professional judgment and critical analysis.

- Avoid exploiting any relationship established as an occupational therapy clinician, educator, or researcher to further one's own physical, emotional, financial, political, or business interests at the expense of recipients of services, students, research participants, employees, or colleagues. (AOTA, 2015a, pp. 3–4)

Are You Honoring the Principle of Nonmaleficence?

In honoring the principle of nonmaleficence, occupational therapists have a duty to take action when their personal limitations have the potential to result in insufficient service, as illustrated in Case Example 15.2. Applying the principle of nonmaleficence requires practitioners to address any harm that may result from engaging in relationships and delivery of service that could be considered exploitative or result in lack of due care. For example, devoting an atypical and unnecessary amount of time and charging extended service time for the evaluation of a patient reflects a violation of nonmaleficence if the therapist's motivation is to ensure a desired number of work hours and the size of the next paycheck. When this occurs, the patient and the therapist's employer are both victims of maleficent intent and unethical behavior.

Conversely, occupational therapists who devote too little time to the completion of a thorough evaluation of a patient, as a result of an organization's unachievable productivity demands, are also acting in a manner contrary to the patient's best interests. Therapists have a duty to focus on the benefit to the patient and not harm the patient by engaging in behaviors and actions that violate the principle of nonmaleficence.

AUTONOMY

Autonomy is often referred to as the "self-determination" principle. Occupational therapy's core value of freedom

---

CASE EXAMPLE 15.2. SHEILA: NONMALEFICENCE AND EVALUATION

Sheila works as an outpatient occupational therapist specializing in neurological conditions. She is also a sexual assault survivor, but she has not made this known to her coworkers. Sheila is fully aware of situations that might trigger her anxiety and the overwhelming symptoms of posttraumatic stress disorder that she sometimes experiences.

Today, Sheila had a new, middle-aged male patient on her schedule for an initial evaluation after a mild cerebrovascular accident with residual upper-extremity (UE) impairments and related limitations in activities of daily living. Sheila was surprised to discover that the patient was accompanied by a staff member from a local Community Corrections Transitional Living Center. Sheila introduced herself to the patient and opened the patient's electronic medical record. She immediately discovered personal red flags indicating that the patient was listed on the state's Sex Offender Registry. After a deep breath, Sheila excused herself from the patient and his attendant. She quickly checked with her Outpatient Department's registration and scheduling staff to see whether another therapist might be available to complete this initial evaluation. Discovering that no one else had an opening in their schedule, Sheila returned to the patient, feeling her heart racing and her breathing become shallow and labored. Sheila asked the patient to describe some of his functional limitations and to demonstrate UE functional movements. The patient reported having difficulty controlling the movement of his right hand and, without prompting, stood up in front of Sheila and demonstrated his challenges with unzipping his pants and tightening his belt. Sheila startled and moved away from the patient as she recognized her skyrocketing anxiety.

After having spent less than 6 minutes with this patient, Sheila informed him and the attendant that the evaluation was completed. Sheila informed the patient, "There is nothing I can do for you" and directed him and his attendant to leave the building. At the same time, she left the treatment area. Sheila immediately documented a brief evaluation report and included a discharge notation: "No therapy indicated at this time." As Sheila left the building, she abruptly announced to the registration staff that she was ill and asked them to cancel her patients for the rest of the day.

Foundational ethics question:

- How does the ethical principle of nonmaleficence apply to this scenario?

Considerations and discussion:

The patient has a diagnosis of stroke and functional impairments resulting from that stroke. His condition would typically be considered eligible for occupational therapy evaluation and intervention.

- Does a personal challenge experienced by a therapist justify early termination of an evaluation session?
- Does the reason a therapist experiences distress make a difference in supporting the early termination of an evaluation session?
- Is a therapist acting ethically when discharging a patient for personal reasons when the patient could reasonably have benefited from occupational therapy services?

Did the occupational therapist harm this patient?

What other options might Sheila have explored or used? Abandoning a patient or providing a service that does not

(Continued)

CASE EXAMPLE 15.2. SHEILA: NONMALEFICENCE AND EVALUATION *(Cont.)*

meet the expected standard is a violation of the principle of nonmaleficence. Intention is always a factor in evaluating nonmaleficence, and justification of the harmful action is obligatory. Sheila terminated the evaluation session without gathering sufficient information about the patient's status. Compelling personal challenges prevented her from fulfilling her professional role at the level of the expected standard of performance. A severe emotional crisis could serve as a rational justification for prematurely terminating an evaluation session. Alternatively, the recommendations for no intervention and immediately discharging the patient appear to be violations of the principle of nonmaleficence. Although no other therapist was immediately available to perform the evaluation, Sheila could have ended the session and directed the patient to reschedule with another therapist at a future date.

Some factors can be considered legitimate when there is a serious barrier to the establishment of a therapeutic relationship. An occupational therapist can take steps to prevent being assigned a new patient for evaluation when there is a risk that the patient's personal characteristics or history will generate a serious adverse emotional reaction and moral distress. Self-disclosure of one's life story is optional, but refusing to serve a patient in need of occupational therapy requires an explanation and request for accommodations. A more egregious violation of the principle of nonmaleficence is a therapist refusing to serve a patient for reasons that most would label as bigoted or racist in some way.

Other violations of the principle of nonmaleficence include exploitation of the therapist–patient relationship. Nonmaleficence can also be violated with the blurring of professional boundaries when personal relationships between the therapist and the patient encroach on professional objectivity.

---

honors personal choice and acknowledges that the wishes and values of the client guide the ethical practice of the profession. The right to self-determination also recognizes the patient's right "to hold views, to make choices, and to take actions based on [his or her] values and beliefs" (Beauchamp & Childress, 2013, p. 106). This principle means that the client should have the occupational therapy evaluation fully explained to them, an opportunity to express their views about the evaluation process, and the choice of whether to engage in it.

Autonomy and Related Standards of Conduct

The *Code of Ethics* RSCs that are consistent with the principle of autonomy are as follows:

- Respect and honor the expressed wishes of recipients of service.
- Fully disclose the benefits, risks, and potential outcomes of any intervention; the personnel who will be providing the intervention; and any reasonable alternatives to the proposed intervention.
- Obtain consent after disclosing appropriate information and answering any questions posed by the recipient of service or research participant to ensure voluntariness.
- Establish a collaborative relationship with recipients of service and relevant stakeholders to promote shared decision making.
- Respect the client's right to refuse occupational therapy services temporarily or permanently, even when that refusal has potential to result in poor outcomes.
- Maintain the confidentiality of all verbal, written, electronic, augmentative, and nonverbal communications, in compliance with applicable laws, including

all aspects of privacy laws, and exceptions thereto (e.g., Health Insurance Portability and Accountability Act of 1996 [P. L. 104-191], Family Educational Rights and Privacy Act of 1974 [P. L. 93-380]).

- Facilitate comprehension and address barriers to communication (e.g., aphasia; differences in language, literacy, culture) with the recipient of service (or responsible party), student, or research participant. (AOTA, 2015a, pp. 4–5)

Are You Honoring the Principle of Autonomy?

Patients have the right to be fully informed of the process of occupational therapy evaluation and to consent or refuse to participate in all or any portion of an assessment (see Case Example 15.3). When a patient has been legally declared incompetent or two physicians have examined the patient and determined a temporary or permanent lack of capacity to make decisions about medical care or treatment, an authorized agent must be relied on to engage in decision making. A patient who is in a coma or too ill to make their own decisions may have someone who holds a health proxy make decisions for them. Additionally, parents have a right to make health decisions for their children who are under the age of majority (general age 18 years).

JUSTICE

The ethical principle of *justice* refers to the fair, equitable, and impartial treatment of persons (Beauchamp & Childress, 2013). When occupational therapy practitioners use the principle of justice, they consistently follow established rules and demonstrate a concern for fairness. It is important to emphasize that fair and equitable is not the

CASE EXAMPLE 15.3. SETH: AUTONOMY AND EVALUATION

An 18-year-old high school senior, **Seth,** has been treated for severe symptoms of attention deficit hyperactivity disorder since he was a young child. Seth's wealthy grandfather decided it was time for Seth to be more independent and gifted Seth with a new sport utility vehicle as an 18th birthday present. Seth's parents have refused to allow Seth to test for or obtain his driver's license because they are concerned that Seth will not be sufficiently attentive to drive safely.

Seth's father heard about the Safe Driver Program at the local rehabilitation center, which serves drivers of all ages. Seth's father scheduled an appointment for Seth to have a comprehensive occupational therapy evaluation focused on driving skills. Seth complained to his father about having to take a special test when his friends already have their license. Seth decided to go to the session because his father told him, "You're going to take this test since I'm paying for it. And if you don't I'm selling your car!"

On arrival for his appointment, Seth was asked to sign a Consent to Evaluation and Treatment form. Seth read it carefully, signed the form, and informed his father that he would refuse to take the driving evaluation if his father did not leave the building. Seth's father decided to "let Seth win one" and informed Seth he would return in about 90 minutes. Peggy, the occupational therapist, engaged Seth in the standard protocol of assessments of the driving skills evaluation. Peggy identified several deficits, including Seth's environmental scanning, impulse control, and inappropriate attention to distracting stimuli presented within the assessment tool. On completion of the evaluation, Peggy summarized the identified deficits and formulated an intervention plan intended to help Seth be successful in his pursuit of the IADL of driving. Peggy finished sharing her findings and recommendations with Seth just as Seth's father returned. As Peggy began to share the evaluation findings with Seth's father, Seth yelled, "I know my rights! You can't tell him how I did unless I say so!" Seth's father admonished Seth, saying, "I paid for this so I have a right to know what Peggy thinks." Seth stormed out of the building. Seth's father told Peggy, "I'll call you!" as he quickly followed Seth out the door.

Foundational ethics question:

- How does the ethical principle of autonomy apply to this scenario?

Considerations and discussion:

Seth exercised his newly acquired right to consent to an occupational therapy evaluation and also to have his right to privacy honored. Adults who have the capacity to make their own medical decisions have the right to choose whether and with whom their personal information can be shared. Seth's father is demonstrating his recent former role of parent of a child by exercising his paternalistic impulses. Seth's father is struggling with the fact that the parent of an adult child who has reached the age of consent and who has capacity to make his or her own decisions has no right to that child's health care information (Berg et al., 2001). The fact that Seth's father paid for the evaluation may be relevant but is legally inconsequential to his request to learn about what is now Seth's protected health information.

When Seth's father contacts Peggy to learn about the occupational therapy evaluation and her recommendations, Peggy is bound by federal law, as well as the ethical principle of autonomy, to observe Seth's wishes and refuse to provide any information to Seth's father. If and when Seth consents to having his evaluation results shared with his father, Peggy can reveal the outcome and recommendations. Seth could also decide to personally share the evaluation results with anyone of his choice. If Seth never consents to a release of information, he alone is the client with whom Peggy can confer regarding next steps.

---

equivalent of equal. *Equal* denotes the same, whereas equitable refers to even-handed treatment or fair distribution of benefits or resources according to individual or group need (Beauchamp & Childress, 2013).

The process of occupational therapy evaluation emphasizes the unique nature of each person's occupations, contexts, and preferences. When two distinct individuals are treated equally, the perception, the outcome, and the impacts may have disparate results. Providing an equal amount of time or fair amount of services is a matter of subjective judgment. For example, two male patients, both with newly diagnosed rheumatoid arthritis, may be scheduled for the same length of time for their initial occupational therapy evaluation, yet their unique client factors, performance deficits, occupational choices, and priorities could result in one evaluation requiring a second session for completion, and the findings of both evaluations will result in two substantially different occupational therapy intervention plans.

Justice and Related Standards of Conduct

The *Code of Ethics* RSCs that are consistent with the principle of justice are as follows:

- Respond to requests for occupational therapy services (e.g., a referral) in a timely manner as determined by law, regulation, or policy.
- Maintain awareness of current laws and AOTA policies and official documents that apply to the profession of occupational therapy.
- Hold requisite credentials for the occupational therapy services they provide in academic, research, physical, or virtual work settings.

- Bill and collect fees legally and justly in a manner that is fair, reasonable, and commensurate with services delivered.
- Ensure that documentation for reimbursement purposes is done in accordance with applicable laws, guidelines, and regulations. (AOTA, 2015a, pp. 5–7)

Are You Honoring the Principle of Justice?

It is the responsibility of all occupational therapists to honor the principle of justice in evaluation. They must follow state laws, hold the requisite state license, and bill according to their work site and the services that have been provided to the patient. Most importantly, therapists must provide evaluations equitably to all patients on the basis of patients' individual needs (see Case Example 15.2). This does not mean providing the same amount of time or the same assessment tool to each patient; rather, therapists must determine what each individual needs and provide the evaluation that is appropriate for that person.

VERACITY

The principle of *veracity* refers to comprehensive, accurate, and objective transmission of information and includes fostering an understanding of that information

---

CASE EXAMPLE 15.4. VERONICA: JUSTICE AND EVALUATION

Veronica, an occupational therapist working in a community mental health center, received a referral for occupational therapy evaluation of Mildred, a 49-year-old woman with a long history of depression and bipolar affective disorder. Mildred is experiencing some troubling symptoms that are resulting in significant difficulties with organizing and performing IADLs, so much so that she has recently been tardy to or absent from her job cleaning offices.

At the time of registration for the occupational therapy evaluation, Mildred presented her insurance card from her employer-sponsored health insurance. On first meeting Veronica, Mildred informed her that her insurance requires a $25 per-visit copay, which she had paid in cash. Mildred went on to share that she also had a separate deductible of $2,000. Mildred told Veronica that coming up with $25 was difficult, but she knew it is worth it because an occupational therapist was a big help to her a few years ago. Mildred also explained that she did not know where she will get the money to pay her sizable insurance deductible.

Veronica reassured Mildred that the financial advocate at the center could help with her financial concerns. Veronica knew that in her setting, when patients are not able to pay for services, grant funding and government programs allow for "writing off" their bill. However, when patients have insurance, their insurance benefits are accessed, and patients are responsible for their portion of the fees. Veronica takes her job in community mental health seriously. She is proud of her role and passionate about promoting social justice by providing her services to people who are economically and socially disadvantaged (Braveman & Bass-Haugen, 2009).

As Veronica engaged Mildred in gathering an occupational profile and analyzed Mildred's occupational performance skills and patterns, she identified several comorbid upper-extremity neuromuscular dysfunctions that likely impede Mildred's independent performance of activities of daily living. The evaluation took much more time than Veronica had estimated, and she had to consider more assessment components than anticipated. When Veronica documented the evaluation results, she realized that she had completed an occupational therapy evaluation of high complexity and *CPT® (Current Procedural Terminology)* code 97167 should be charged (American Medical Association, 2019). Veronica was well informed about the charge categories and that her employer had established a higher charge for each progressive level of complexity of occupational therapy evaluation. Veronica felt that she really connected with Mildred, and she empathized with Mildred's financial concerns. Veronica entered the charge for Mildred's occupational therapy evaluation as the low-complexity CPT 97165, knowing that Mildred's total bill for occupational therapy services would be a challenge for Mildred, regardless of the final cost.

Foundational ethics question:

- How does the ethical principle of justice apply to this scenario?

Considerations and discussion:

Veronica is demonstrating concern for her client and is making accommodations that Mildred might appreciate. However, Veronica is not acting justly for Mildred's best interests or for the best interests of her employer. Reporting that Mildred's occupational therapy evaluation was less complex than it really was may result in Mildred being ineligible for the intensity of occupational therapy services that may be warranted by her current limitations. The insurance reviewer, whose job it is to authorize occupational therapy services, may raise questions about the service provided when comparing the clinical documentation with the billed charge. On the basis of a charge for a low-complexity evaluation, the insurance reviewer could legitimately limit Mildred's number of authorized occupational therapy visits. Limited authorization for a low frequency and duration of approved services could well result in insufficient progress for Mildred's independence.

Veronica's intentional undercharging violates the principle of justice in terms of being untruthful and

(Continued)

CASE EXAMPLE 15.4. VERONICA: JUSTICE AND EVALUATION *(Cont.)*

undervaluing her services. Veronica is also not being just to her employer because the organization will be reimbursed for less time and service than Veronica devoted to Mildred's occupational therapy evaluation. Veronica's social justice mindset is clearly violating the broader application of the principle of justice.

The occupational therapy profession identifies justice as one of the profession's core values; it is also one of the six ethical principles that frame the *Code of Ethics.* The

core value of justice highlights inclusion and the development of communities where people can "function, flourish and live a satisfactory life" (AOTA, 2015a, p. 2; see Table 15.1). The *Code of Ethics* directs occupational therapy practitioners to relate in a respectful, fair, and impartial manner, and respect laws and standards. Honoring the core value of justice and abiding by the ethical principle of justice are imperatives for all occupational therapy practitioners.

(Beauchamp & Childress, 2013). Truthfulness and honesty are the hallmarks of the principle of veracity. When occupational therapists evaluate a patient, that patient has the right to a full and accurate accounting of the findings and recommendations. Sharing the documentation produced at the end of an evaluation, with abbreviations, medical terminology, and documentation formats that are foreign or beyond the patient's reading comprehension level, is contrary to honoring the principle of veracity. (See Chapter 11, "Interpretation and Documentation of the Evaluation Process.") Occupational therapy practitioners have the duty to inform patients and make every effort to ensure that patients understand what is being shared and receive the assistance they need to comprehend the importance of that information to the development of their individualized intervention plan.

Veracity and Related Standards of Conduct

The *Code of Ethics* RSCs that are consistent with the principle of veracity are as follows:

- Represent credentials, qualifications, education, experience, training, roles, duties, competence, contributions, and findings accurately in all forms of communication.
- Refrain from using or participating in the use of any form of communication that contains false, fraudulent, deceptive, misleading, or unfair statements or claims.
- Record and report in an accurate and timely manner, and in accordance with applicable regulations, all information related to professional or academic documentation and activities. (AOTA, 2015a, pp. 7–8)

Are You Honoring the Principle of Veracity?

Occupational therapy practitioners must accurately and truthfully represent their professional competence, experience, and conformance to professional standards. An occupational therapist who claims expertise in the evaluation of populations or skill with specific assessments without proper training and experience is clearly violating the principle of veracity.

If an occupational therapist is called on to perform an evaluation for a patient diagnosed with a rare condition

with which the therapist has no experience, the principle of veracity requires that the therapist make the patient aware of the limits of their competence or refer the patient to a more experienced therapist. That does not mean the patient must be turned away. In some settings and in underserved geographic regions, the less experienced occupational therapist may be the only practitioner available to provide any level of service. In these situations, the therapist must honor the principle of veracity by informing the patient of the resources and skills offered and rely on the patient to exercise autonomy and accept or refuse the less-than-ideal occupational therapy service. This could mean the patient makes the choice to go without services.

Occupational therapy assistants work under the supervision of occupational therapists. They may perform specific evaluations independently with supervision but require supervision to use evaluative data for setting goals and intervention planning. Once the occupation therapy assistant performs an evaluation, they are required to review the evaluation data with the supervising occupational therapist (see Case Example 15.5). Together they can decide on the areas of strength and limitations for the patient. Following this the occupational therapist and the occupational therapy assistant can, as a team, develop the goals for the client and the course of intervention.

FIDELITY

The ethical principle of *fidelity* is derived from the Latin root *fidelis,* meaning loyal. *Fidelity* refers to the duty one has to keep a commitment once it is made (Veatch et al., 2010). Health professions make a commitment to fidelity when vowing to be loyal to their clients and to be, consistent, attentive, and acting in the best interests of the person being served. Occupational therapy practitioners would rarely inform patients that they will be loyal to them, but in the interest of establishing a therapeutic relationship, therapists often tell their patients, "I'm here to help you accomplish your goals" and "We're in this together!" The therapist who most embodies the ethical principle of fidelity is the one who is always willing to take on the difficult patient.

Fidelity and Related Standards of Conduct

The *Code of Ethics* RSCs that are consistent with the principle of fidelity are as follows:

CASE EXAMPLE 15.5. ELLEN: VERACITY AND EVALUATION

Great Life Senior Care, Inc. (GLSC) is a continuing care community funded by resident funds, local government block grant funding, or, when residents' personal funds are depleted, by state and federal Medicaid. The GLSC brochures and website describe a wide array of services, including professional occupational therapy services. Amelia, the daughter of Enid, a soon-to-be new resident, is eager to have a comprehensive evaluation of her mother's functional status. The GLSC transition specialist promptly scheduled Enid for time with **Ellen,** their "very skilled OT" for a comprehensive independent living and community skills evaluation. The transition specialist stated that "the goal of time with the OT is to learn about Enid's challenges and to develop a 'living well plan'" for Enid's residence at GLSC.

When Amelia brought her mother to the scheduled appointment, they were welcomed by Ellen, who is an occupational therapy assistant (OTA). Amelia, an educated health care consumer, questioned Ellen: "You're an OTA; where is the occupational therapist?" Ellen chuckled and replied, "Oh, don't worry. I know what I'm doing. Since we're a community program, I take care of all occupational therapy evaluations. I've been doing these evaluations for over 15 years! There isn't an OTR at GLSC and we really don't need one."

Foundational ethics question:

- How does the ethical principle of veracity apply to this scenario?

Considerations and discussion:

Clearly, the OTA in this scenario is not conforming to the AOTA *Standards of Practice* (AOTA, 2015b) or the AOTA *Guidelines for Supervision, Roles, and Responsibilities During the Delivery of Occupational Therapy Services* (AOTA, 2014). This OTA is almost certainly violating the state's licensure statute or administrative code by both claiming to provide and providing what she is representing as an occupational therapy evaluation. Speaking with authority and denigrating the organization's need for a properly trained and credentialed occupational therapist violates the principle of veracity. The organization is not providing what it purports to offer, and consumers are not getting what they expect. The client is bound to suffer from receiving an inadequate evaluation and appropriate intervention plan. The OTA is demeaning the profession and likely damaging the otherwise good reputation of this assisted living facility.

Questions to consider:

- What might Amelia, Enid's daughter, do to address this situation?
- What other options might these consumers pursue?

- Promote collaborative actions and communication as a member of interprofessional teams to facilitate quality care and safety for clients.
- Respect the practices, competencies, roles, and responsibilities of their own and other professions to promote a collaborative environment reflective of interprofessional teams.
- Use conflict resolution and internal and alternative dispute resolution resources as needed to resolve organizational and interpersonal conflicts, as well as perceived institutional ethics violations.
- Self-identify when personal, cultural, or religious values preclude, or are anticipated to negatively affect, the professional relationship or provision of services, while adhering to organizational policies when requesting an exemption from service to an individual or group on the basis of conflict of conscience. (AOTA, 2015a, pp. 8–9)

Are You Honoring the Principle of Fidelity?

Fidelity also applies to developing respect for and acting respectfully toward other occupational therapy practitioners and all other professionals encountered in the practice environment. Behaviors that demonstrate disrespect or that discount the value or contributions of others violate fidelity both within an interdisciplinary team and within organizations and systems (Purtilo & Doherty, 2011).

Adherence to the principle of fidelity also requires occupational therapists to share information in ways that promote the patient's understanding of the information and, with the patient's consent, engagement of those invited to participate in the occupational therapy evaluation. Fidelity is violated when therapists opt out of sharing objective assessment findings with patients in the interest of not upsetting or demoralizing them and their hopes and goals for improvement (Veatch et al., 2010). See Case Example 15.6.

ETHICS AND LAWS

The case studies in this chapter focus on ethical dilemmas and application of ethical principles to dilemmas that an occupational therapy practitioner may encounter while administering assessments and engaging in the totality of the evaluation process. The majority of these case scenarios also referenced a legal standard, cited an applicable law, or described an action that clearly violated an organizational policy or even included fraudulent documentation or billing. It is important to understand that ethics and laws are not the same, yet most laws have, at their core, a value or ethical principle. **Laws** are enacted for the good of the public and describe what is prohibited and the consequences of violating a specific law (Kornblau, 2019). Unethical behavior may also be illegal. However, strict adherence to laws that are deemed by some to be unjust may in fact be the best and most justifiable path to upholding ethical principles.

CASE EXAMPLE 15.6. HECTOR: FIDELITY AND EVALUATION

Hector Garcia, a middle-aged man, is referred to a comprehensive outpatient postconcussion rehabilitation program to aid his recovery from a serious concussion that occurred during a scaffold collapse at his construction job. Mr. Garcia emigrated from Central America as a teenager, and his primary language is Spanish. Although Mr. Garcia is known to be fluent in English, since the accident he has almost exclusively spoken Spanish and reportedly has had difficulty comprehending spoken English.

The protocol for the postconcussion rehabilitation program includes comprehensive evaluations, which are completed on Day 1. The first team member to evaluate Mr. Garcia was Carmen, an occupational therapist trained in Puerto Rico. Carmen is new to the postconcussion program. Mr. Garcia was then evaluated by other members of the team, including Jim, a physical therapist, and Erin, a speech–language pathologist.

On Day 2 of the program, the interdisciplinary treatment team typically meets with the patient, so Mr. Garcia and his Workers' Compensation case manager were invited to attend a team meeting to hear the evaluation findings, review recommendations, and arrive at an interdisciplinary intervention plan specific to Mr. Garcia's needs. Because of illness, Carmen is absent from work on Mr. Garcia's Day 2 meeting. Juana, another occupational therapist at the rehabilitation center, volunteered to review the occupational therapy evaluation report before the team meeting and participate in the interdisciplinary team conference in Carmen's place.

As the team conference began, Erin expressed concern about Mr. Garcia's comprehension of the information to be discussed. Erin shared that she had asked Leona, a physical therapy assistant at the clinic who is fluent in Spanish, to join the meeting to provide English-to-Spanish translation for Mr. Garcia. On hearing this, Juana scoffed and blurted out, "He's been in this country for over 30 years. He understands English! My ex-husband was from Mexico, and when I'd ask him to do something he didn't want to do, he'd act like he didn't understand English. What a waste of Leona's time!" Despite Juana's objection, Leona joined the meeting and greeted Mr. Garcia, who nodded and smiled in response to Leona's greeting, "Buenos dias."

As Erin shared results of the speech therapy cognitive assessments she had performed with Mr. Garcia, Juana interrupted and questioned why Erin used one of the assessments and why she thought it was appropriate for a postconcussion assessment. Erin calmly explained her rationale and proceeded to deliver the remainder of her report.

When Juana's turn came to report the occupational therapy evaluation results, she stated, "I hate to say this, but Carmen didn't know what she was doing! She really doesn't have the skill or experience to evaluate anyone with this level of head injury. I'm not going to share the garbage that she documented! I need to see this *cholo* after our meeting today to start over and use the right occupational therapy evals!" Jim, Erin, and the case manager were so stunned by Juana's statements that they did not speak for a full 20 seconds. Leona observed that Mr. Garcia appeared confused, and she interpreted this to mean that Mr. Garcia did not understand what was going on. Leona invited Mr. Garcia to join her in leaving the meeting, and they both exited the room. The Workers' Compensation case manager followed behind. Juana also left the room, exclaiming to Erin and Jim, "I've had it! Carmen is on her way out of this department!"

Foundational ethics question:

- How does the ethical principle of fidelity apply to this scenario?

Considerations and discussion:

The emotional responses likely elicited by the event described in this case example must be addressed before moving on to the foundational ethical concerns this encounter presents. Any reader of this case example would no doubt initially focus on the uncivil behaviors exhibited by Juana, the occupational therapist. "Disrespectful and rude" is certainly an accurate characterization of Juana's treatment of her colleagues. Juana's referring to Mr. Garcia as *cholo* (a slang term of disrespect) and the skepticism she voiced about the need for language translation were insensitive, bigoted, and clinically inappropriate.

Let's start with by focusing on what's going on with Juana and why. Is this behavior out of character for Juana? Has she ever acted in this way before? Why would she make statements about her ex-husband in the presence of a patient she did not know? Why would Juana refer to Mr. Garcia in a derogatory manner? What might the answers to these questions have to do with Juana's behavior? Anyone who values the ethical principles of fidelity and beneficence would consider Juana's behavior to be absolutely unacceptable.

Some additional background may help shine a light on Juana's behavior:

- Juana has been a clinical specialist in the treatment of head injury for more than a decade. Erin has less than 1 year of experience as a speech-language pathologist. Jim is a contract therapist on a 3-month, contracted assignment, but he has expertise in the treatment of persons with head injuries.
- Juana knows that Carmen transferred to the postconcussion rehab program just before she was to be terminated from her job at another rehabilitation center in the same organization.
- Juana has been assigned as Carmen's mentor since Carmen transferred to this program site more than 2 months ago. Juana has helped the department

(Continued)

CASE EXAMPLE 15.6: HECTOR: FIDELITY AND EVALUATION *(Cont.)*

manager structure a formal learning plan for Carmen. In Juana's assessment, Carmen is seriously lagging in achieving the objectives of her learning plan.

- Although other team members are unaware of it, Juana's very recent divorce left her struggling with her personal finances and the care of her three teenage children. Her ex-husband, who was a college exchange student when they married, recently returned to his home country of Mexico. Juana's ex-husband has not contributed any financial support for their children since his departure.

Do any of these intervening circumstances justify Juana's behavior? Likely not.

Let's agree that Juana behaved badly but consider some potentially rational justifications, consistent with the principle of fidelity, that underlie Juana's issues.

- Could Juana be correct that Carmen did not use relevant assessments tools or processes for the occupational therapy evaluation of Mr. Garcia?
  - Juana is a clinical specialist in this area of practice. We can be confident that Juana's clinical judgment regarding appropriate assessments is sound.
- Do we know whether Carmen has demonstrated the clinical competence to evaluate a person in need of postconcussion rehabilitation?
  - Juana is serving in a role that requires her to assess and rate Carmen's clinical performance.
- By what authority did Juana make such bold statements about Carmen's performance?
  - Juana has been assigned as mentor. Juana has a professional duty to critique the assessment tools selected and the documentation Carmen produced.

Juana's primary violations of the ethical principle of fidelity were her disrespectful statements about the patient, her lack of explanation for how Mr. Garcia could have been more appropriately evaluated by an occupational therapist, and her intrusive and disruptive behaviors during an interdisciplinary team meeting. Juana also violated the principle of fidelity by unfairly and publicly questioning the credibility of a colleague, Erin, in this interdisciplinary setting. Juana violated the principle of fidelity by attacking Carmen's performance without discussing the issues with Carmen and also by vociferously denouncing Carmen's work.

A request by Juana to be exempted from care on the basis of a personal bias or personal challenge is one way to honor the principle of fidelity. Because of what appears to be a negative bias, which one can assume was prompted by Juana's spillover feelings about her ex-husband, Juana could have requested to be excused from serving as Carmen's mentor, and she should not have volunteered to participate in this interdisciplinary team meeting. Without question, Juana should not take on the task of reevaluating Mr. Garcia from an

occupational therapy perspective. Juana's actions clearly violate any sense of loyalty or freedom from bias, and she should not be allowed to provide evaluation or treatment services for this patient whom she clearly does not respect.

There is more to this scenario that specifically honors the principle of fidelity.

- Carmen, an appropriately credentialed occupational therapist, meets the legal requirements for performing evaluations in an outpatient rehabilitation program. We must assume that Carmen was loyal in fulfilling her assigned job to evaluate Mr. Garcia by selecting and using assessments, and her skills, to do her best.
- Erin, the speech-language pathologist, identified that Mr. Garcia's current comprehension of English could be hampered by the effects of the head injury. Erin acknowledged Mr. Garcia's right to understand the meaningful information being shared by members of the interdisciplinary team.
- Erin also took affirmative action to invite Leona, the physical therapy assistant fluent in Spanish, to act as a translator. Erin and Leona honored Mr. Garcia's challenges in comprehending the information so he could adequately participate in formulating his own intervention plan.
- Team members attending this meeting could have addressed Juana's behavior when it first occurred early in the meeting. Erin could have ignored or objected to Juana's questioning and certainly could have been insulted. Yet Erin did not appear to take Juana's questioning personally, and she diplomatically and respectfully responded to Juana's objections in a professional manner.
- Jim missed the opportunity to support his colleague, Erin. Jim could have defended Erin's choice or otherwise interrupted and advised Juana to wait to ask her questions until after the meeting. Professional respect and collaboration are expectations consistent with the principle of fidelity.
- We must grant Juana due respect for her role as a clinical specialist. Juana devoted her energy and has made a moral commitment to providing high-quality occupational therapy evaluation and treatment to a vulnerable population. Although it may be difficult to discern, fidelity is likely at the core of Juana's concerns.

Additional questions to consider:

- How could Juana have supported her statements (and delivered her opinion of Carmen's work) in ways that better honor the ethical principle of fidelity?
- How could Juana have supported her coworkers and respected the interdisciplinary team process in ways that honor the ethical principle of fidelity?

QUESTIONS

1. Why should occupational therapy practitioners be concerned with the ethical application of assessment and evaluation processes?
2. Which of the core values of the occupational therapy profession would you consider to be the most important influence on assessment and evaluation processes?
3. Which of the six ethical principles included in the AOTA (2015a) *Occupational Therapy Code of Ethics* would you consider to be the most valuable in ensuring your ethical practice related to occupational therapy assessment and evaluation?
4. Review the case examples. Although each case example focuses on a single ethical principle, each case has at least one additional, secondary ethical principle that is applicable to the resolution of the dilemma. Focus on the principle or principles that have the most impact on occupational therapy assessment and the occupational therapy evaluation process. What do you notice?
5. For each case example, which additional ethical principle is most applicable in the context of occupational therapy evaluation and assessment?

REFERENCES

Allen, C. K., Austin, S. L., David, S. K., Earhart, C. A., McCraith, D. B., & Riska-Williams, L. (2007). *Manual for the Allen Cognitive Level Screen–5 (ACLS–5) and Large Allen Cognitive Level Screen–5 (LACLS–5)*. Camarillo, CA: ACLS and LACLS Committee.

American Medical Association. (2019). *Current Procedural Terminology: CPT® 2019 professional edition*. Chicago: Author.

American Occupational Therapy Association. (2014). Guidelines for supervision, roles, and responsibilities during the delivery of occupational therapy services. *American Journal of Occupational Therapy, 68*(Suppl. 3), S16–S22. https://doi.org/10.5014/ajot.2014.686S03

American Occupational Therapy Association. (2015a). Occupational therapy code of ethics (2015). *American Journal of Occupational Therapy, 69*(Suppl. 3), 6913410030. https://doi.org/10.5014/ajot.2015.696S03

American Occupational Therapy Association. (2015b). Standards of practice for occupational therapy. *American Journal of Occupational Therapy, 69*(Suppl. 3), 6913410057. https://doi.org/10.5014/ajot.2015.696S06

American Occupational Therapy Association. (2017). *Fact sheet: Occupational therapy and prevention of falls*. Retrieved from https://www.aota.org/About-Occupational-Therapy/Professionals/PA/Facts/Fall-Prevention.aspx

American Occupational Therapy Association. (2019). Enforcement procedures for the *AOTA Occupational Therapy Code of Ethics*. *American Journal of Occupational Therapy, 73*(Suppl. 2), 7312410003. https://doi.org/10.5014/ajot.2019.73S210

American Occupational Therapy Association, State Affairs Group. (2019, June). *Occupational therapy profession—Scope of practice definitions*. Retrieved from https://www.aota.org/~/media/Corporate/Files/Advocacy/Licensure/StateRegs/Scope-of-Practice-Chart-2019.pdf

American Psychological Association. (2016). *Ethical principles of psychologists and code of conduct (including 2010 and 2016 amendments)*. Washington, DC: Author. Retrieved from https://www.apa.org/ethics/code/

American Speech-Language-Hearing Association. (2020). *National Outcomes Measurement System (NOMS)*. Retrieved from https://www.asha.org/noms/national-outcomes-measurement-system/

Ayres, A. J. (1989). *Sensory Integration and Praxis Tests*. Los Angeles: Western Psychological Services.

Beauchamp, T. L., & Childress, J. F. (2013). *Principles of biomedical ethics* (7th ed.). New York: Oxford University Press.

Berg, J. W., Appelbaum, P. S., Lidz, C. W., & Parker, L. S. (2001). *Informed consent: Legal theory and clinical practice* (2nd ed.). New York: Oxford University Press.

Bergen, G., Stevens, M. R., & Burns, E. R. (2016). Falls and fall injuries among adults aged ≥65 years—United States, 2014. *Morbidity and Mortality Weekly Report, 65*, 993–998. https://doi.org/10.15585/mmwr.mm6537a2

Bloomer, J. S., & Williams, S. K. (1979). *Bay Area Functional Performance Evaluation* (research ed.). Palo Alto, CA: Consulting Psychologists Press.

Braveman, B., & Bass-Haugen, J. D. (2009). Social justice and health disparities: An evolving discourse in occupational therapy research and intervention. *American Journal of Occupational Therapy, 63*, 7–12. https://doi.org/10.5014/ajot.63.1.7

Family Educational Rights and Privacy Act of 1974, Pub. L. 93–380, 20 U.S.C. § 1232g; 34 CFR Part 99.

Fleming, A., & Rucas, K. (2015). Welcoming a paradigm shift in occupational therapy: Symptom validity measures and cognitive assessment. *Applied Neuropsychology: Adult, 22*, 23–31. https://doi.org/10.1080/23279095.2013.822873

Health Insurance Portability and Accountability Act of 1996 (HIPAA), Pub. L. 104–191, 42 U.S.C. § 300gg, 29 U.S.C. §§ 1181–1183, and 42 U.S.C. §§ 1320d–1320d9. Retrieved from https://www.govinfo.gov/app/details/PLAW-104publ191

Houston, D., Lang Williams, S., Bloomer, J., & Mann, W. C. (1989). The Bay Area Functional Performance Evaluation: Development and standardization. *American Journal of Occupational Therapy, 43*, 170–183. https://doi.org/10.5014/ajot.43.3.170

Kornblau, B. L. (2019). Understanding the law. In K. Jacobs & G. L. McCormack (Eds.), *The occupational therapy manager* (6th ed., pp. 565–570). Bethesda, MD: AOTA Press.

Law, M. C., & MacDermid, J. (2008). *Introduction to evidenced-based practice*. In M.C. Law & J. MacDermid's Evidenced-Based Rehabilitation: A Guide to Practice (2nd ed). Thorofare, NJ: Slack

McGourty, L. K. (1978). *Kohlman Evaluation of Living Skills*. Seattle: KELS Research.

National Board for Certification in Occupational Therapy®. (2015). *NBCOT® candidate/certificant code of conduct*. Retrieved from https://www.nbcot.org/-/media/NBCOT/PDFs/Code_of_Conduct.ashx?la=en

Purtilo, R., & Doherty, R. (2011). *Ethical dimensions in the health professions* (5th ed.). Philadelphia: Saunders/Elsevier.

Rawls, J. (1971). *A theory of justice.* Cambridge, MA: Belknap Press.

Simon, H. A. (1956). Rational choice and the structure of the environment. *Psychological Review, 63*(2), 129–138. https://doi.org/10.1037/h0042769

Scott, J. B., & Reitz, S. M. (2017). *Practical applications for the Occupational Therapy Code of Ethics (2015).* Bethesda. MD: AOTA Press

Slater, D. Y. (2016). *Reference guide to the Occupational Therapy Code of Ethics.* Bethesda, MD: AOTA Press.

Thomson, L. K., & Robnett, R. (2016). *KELS: Kohlman Evaluation of Living Skills* (4th ed.). Bethesda, MD: AOTA Press.

Veatch, R. M., Haddad, A. M., & English, D. C. (2010). *Case studies in biomedical ethics.* New York: Oxford University Press.

Occupational Therapy Evaluation and Evidence-Based Practice

16

Jennifer S. Pitonyak, PhD, OTR/L, SCFES

CHAPTER HIGHLIGHTS

- Defining *evidence-based practice*
- How to evaluate quantitative and qualitative evidence
- Contemporary evidence-based practice model for occupational therapy
- Generating, gathering, and disseminating data
- Additional uses of evaluation data for knowledge translation

KEY TERMS AND CONCEPTS

- Baseline data
- Bias
- Case studies
- Correlation coefficient
- Correlation research
- Database
- Descriptive or observational studies
- Evidence-based practice
- Evidence-informed practice
- External validity
- Impact factor
- Internal validity
- Meta-analysis
- Nonexperimental studies
- Peer-reviewed journals
- Professional reasoning
- Publication
- Qualitative research
- Quantitative research
- Quasi-experimental research
- Randomized controlled trials
- Research Pyramid
- Respected opinions
- Single-hierarchy models
- Single-subject design

INTRODUCTION

This chapter discusses how evidence-based practice (EBP) in occupational therapy influences the evaluation of clients. It begins with a history and description of traditional EBP and also presents current thinking in the profession on aligning EBP with theory-directed practice and the epistemology of the profession (Fleming-Castaldy & Gillen, 2013; Hinojosa, 2013; Tomlin & Borgetto, 2011).

From that base, the chapter presents ways to use data from evaluation and reevaluation to inform decision making in practice and offers examples of evidence-based literature that informs the occupational therapy process. Using evaluation data, occupational therapy practitioners can develop evidence needed to support their practice. The collection, organization, and examination of aggregate evaluation data builds evidence for assessment methods and suggests specific interventions. The chapter concludes with a discussion on how to disseminate the evidence to promote evidence-based decision making in practice as well as additional uses of evaluation data beyond day-to-day practice.

Occupational therapy students, practitioners, educators, researchers, and policy makers must understand the importance of EBP for the profession. The objectives of this chapter are:

- To describe the process of EBP and its relationship to occupational therapy evaluation,
- To examine traditional and emerging EBP models for usefulness in occupational therapy evaluation, and
- To apply EBP principles to occupational therapy evaluation through examples from the literature.

WHAT IS EVIDENCE-BASED PRACTICE?

EBP in health care is a process that combines current published evidence with practitioner expertise and client preferences to guide practitioner decision making throughout the occupational therapy process (Ilott, 2003; Law & Baum, 1998; Sackett et al., 1996; Straus et al., 2019). There are various definitions of *EBP* in the literature, and most reflect this interaction among evidence; expertise; and client values, beliefs, and preferences. Sackett et al. (1996) advised that the best evidence comes from combining clinical expertise and knowledge gained through practice with pertinent published research.

More recently in occupational therapy and other health professions, scholars have called for *evidence-informed practice* to be more clearly differentiated from EBP (Miles & Loughlin, 2011; Nevo & Slonim-Nevo, 2011; Tomlin &

Dougherty, 2014). For example, in occupational therapy, Tomlin and Dougherty (2014) pointed out that there is a fundamental duality in the concept of *EBP* and proposed that "evidence-supported practice would provide a solid body of published research demonstrating the effectiveness of health profession services in bringing about desirable outcomes for health and quality of life," whereas *evidence-informed practice* "describes the approach of the practitioner who makes use of all sources of evidence, internal and external, in making decisions about client care" (p. 15).

Whether termed *evidence-informed practice* or *EBP*, the underlying process evolved from the concept of *evidence-based medicine*, a phrase first coined during the 1980s at McMaster Medical School in Canada (Rosenberg & Donald, 1995). Supporters of EBP recognize that the ability to provide best care requires the integration of current best evidence, practitioner expertise, and client preferences (Law & MacDermid, 2013; Lee & Miller, 2003; Sackett et al., 1996; Tomlin & Dougherty, 2014).

EBP requires **professional reasoning** and constant reflection, similar to the occupational therapy evaluation process. Before one can consider this relationship between EBP and evaluation, it is first necessary to understand the process of EBP and how occupational therapy practitioners use this thinking in practice. The occupational therapy process is client centered; as such, the process is dynamic and varied both within and across client situations and requires complex thinking about how to evaluate and measure evidence-based, client-centered outcomes (Mroz et al., 2015).

EBP requires occupational therapy practitioners to be inquisitive; engage in self-directed, lifelong learning; be willing to consider evidence that conflicts with their current knowledge and beliefs; and be able to communicate research findings with clients and their families. Practitioners need to select and examine the best available evidence in the form of published reviews or expert opinions. Furthermore, consumers of evidence need to be able to critically analyze existing research to determine whether findings translate to practice (Thomas & Law, 2013).

Occupational therapy practitioners begin engaging in EBP at the first step of the occupational therapy process, when they receive a referral to evaluate a client. Practitioners use procedural professional reasoning to select the assessment methods most commonly used for screening individuals with the referral problem. The screening further informs the practitioner about which evidence-based and theory-directed assessments to use. As the evaluation continues, the practitioner develops a clear and searchable question related to client needs or the planned method of assessment. Once the practitioner identifies the question, they should search the literature for the most current and relevant evidence (Ilott, 2003; Rosenberg & Donald, 1995; Taylor, 1997).

EBP requires that occupational therapy practitioners be able to locate evidence quickly and easily (Dysart & Tomlin, 2002; Ilott, 2003; Lloyd-Smith, 1997). Searching databases for literature is a skill that improves with experience. Practitioners are encouraged to use resources such as reference librarians at public or university libraries and online tutorials.

After locating relevant literature, the occupational therapy practitioner carefully reviews the information and notes previous findings about the planned assessments and their use. The practitioner combines the located evidence with their own practice experience. Areas of focus for decision making about the assessment methods may also include information provided about the particular client issues and the client's (and family's) particular values, beliefs, and preferences (Ilott, 2003; Taylor, 1997). This merging of information, both external to the practitioner–client relationship and internal to the relationship, reinforces the point that evidence derived solely from research may be insufficient for decision making in practice (Tomlin & Dougherty, 2014). Evidence-based evaluation includes the use of assessment and administration methods that best match with the client's needs and practitioner-identified theoretical perspective, rather than just the use of clinically available assessments reported in the research literature.

Throughout the occupational therapy intervention process, occupational therapy practitioners continually evaluate the outcomes of intervention (Ilott, 2003). These occupational therapy intervention outcomes may be in such areas as client performance, quality of life, or intervention effectiveness. When assessing outcomes, practitioners must consider the validity of assessment methods for operationalizing the outcome of interest and the accuracy in measuring change.

Using an evidence-based perspective is important for informing occupational therapy practitioner decision making in practice and requires that practitioners upgrade their knowledge for this decision making (Taylor, 1997; Tomlin & Dougherty, 2014). EBP helps practitioners justify and demonstrate the effectiveness of their interventions to clients, families, and payers of health care services (Lloyd-Smith, 1997). EBP allows for effective use of resources by enabling the practitioner and the client to focus efforts on interventions that have a greater likelihood of success (Taylor, 1997). Differentiating between EBP and evidence-informed practice is also important for practitioner decision making in situations where assessment methods and intervention approaches may be part of standard practice but have not yet been recognized as best practice (Law & MacDermid, 2013). In this situation, practitioners can build evidence by systematically documenting client outcomes in their daily practice, compiling these findings, and disseminating this practice-based evidence in various forms (Tomlin & Dougherty, 2014).

Tickle-Degnen (2002) identified several ways occupational therapists can use EBP during the early rapport-building stages of a practitioner–client interaction. Early rapport building is ongoing in the initial evaluation of a client. As described earlier, it is important that occupational therapy practitioners explore the literature to identify the most appropriate, valid, and reliable assessments and administration methods to gather pertinent client information.

During this exploration, occupational therapy practitioners focus on the specific assessments used. A practitioner may also explore more descriptive or qualitative literature that provides information about the occupational desires, needs, and lifestyles of people with similar diagnoses or characteristics as their clients. Practitioners may find this information useful when using qualitative or nonstandardized methods of collecting data for the client's occupational profile. Information obtained in the descriptive or qualitative literature may be helpful as a point of discussion with the client to identify similarities and differences with the client's situation and allow the practitioner an opportunity to show interest, knowledge, and awareness of others in similar situations. The practitioner may choose to share current understanding regarding the efficacy of therapeutic interventions as part of the client's education in the occupational therapy process.

HOW TO ENGAGE IN EVIDENCE-BASED PRACTICE

In the traditional use of EBP, occupational therapy practitioners base decisions for evaluations, interventions, and outcomes on the best available published evidence, their professional reasoning, and the client's response to the occupational therapy process. This section first presents traditional EBP models from medicine applied in occupational therapy, then examines a more contemporary EBP model that more closely aligns with the occupational therapy process.

Peer-Reviewed Journals

Traditionally, the best evidence for practice is information obtained from *peer-reviewed journals.* Peer-reviewed publications provide expert evaluation of the material before dissemination; therefore, readers know that experts have evaluated the manuscript to determine that it has sufficient trustworthiness for publication. These research publications can use either quantitative or qualitative methods. In the realm of peer-reviewed publications, the best evidence for practice comes from journals with a high impact factor, which establishes the journal's reputation. The *impact factor* refers to an index calculated by the the average number of citations received by the articles published in a given journal; it is generally accepted that the more reputed journals have higher number of citations for their published articles.

Occupational therapy practitioners need evidence to support decision making about the occupational therapy process. The relevance of research findings to practice depends on the direct applicability of the study, the design of the study, the method of intervention used in the study, and the number of study participants. Common sense indicates that the closer a study is to the practice situation under question, the more applicable it will be. Studies that have the same population as the client or group in question will be more generalizable than those with populations with different conditions. Often the best available evidence may be in the literature of a related population or field, so practitioners need to interpolate the evidence from related studies that best fits the situation under consideration.

The more rigorous the design of the study, the more likely it is that occupational therapy practitioners can use the findings to support their practice decisions. Experimental studies with appropriate controls, interventions, and measures may increase confidence in the study findings. Practitioners, however, need to consider the artificiality of controlled experiments against the reality of practice; therefore, they need to understand the strengths and weaknesses of various research methods.

Empirical Observations

Occupatioal therapy practitioners can also obtain evidence from empirical observations. These can range from clinical observations made in practice settings to tightly controlled observations in experimental research. Each type of observation has its own limitations. Generally, clinical observations are limited by small sample sizes and, more important, by the observer's biases. Similarly, there are limitations to observations in experimental research because of the strictly controlled environment of the study.

Research Hierarchies

In the literature, experts have presented many hierarchies that rank the rigor of various research methods and their applicability to practice (Lloyd-Smith, 1997; Sackett, 1989; Tomlin & Borgetto, 2011). The experts who have developed most of these hierarchies regard sophisticated quantitative research methods as providing more valid results. *Quantitative research* refers to the systematic investigation with analysis based on statistical or mathematical techniques. Figure 16.1 portrays a commonly used hierarchy.

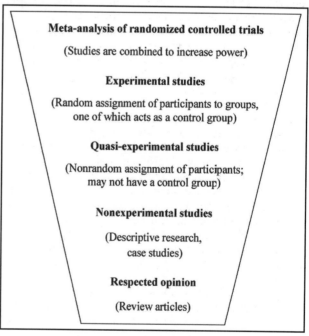

FIGURE 16.1.   Hierarchy of support for evidence-based practice.

Meta-analysis of randomized controlled trials

(Studies are combined to increase power)

Experimental studies

(Random assignment of participants to groups, one of which acts as a control group)

Quasi-experimental studies

(Nonrandom assignment of participants; may not have a control group)

Nonexperimental studies

(Descriptive research, case studies)

Respected opinion

(Review articles)

Source. From "Evidence-Based Practice and Occupational Therapy," by W. Lloyd-Smith, 1997, *British Journal of Occupational Therapy, 60,* 474–479. Copyright © 1997 by Sage Publications. Adapted with permission.

One characteristic that all hierarchies share is the basic structure of evidence systematically vetted by experts in the field as the most valid research evidence, giving it a top tier, while less stringent or less applicable evidence goes in lower tiers. Some experts in medicine base their hierarchies on scientists' studies in highly controlled laboratory settings. These studies take place in artificial environments and often use tissue samples or animals as subjects. Although these studies have the most rigor in terms of experimental validity, laboratory studies are usually difficult to apply to occupational therapy.

The hierarchy presented in Figure 16.1 was developed on the basis of in vivo studies involving human beings. It was adapted from Lloyd-Smith (1997), who put meta-analyses at the top and respected opinion at the base. The following sections describe in more detail the levels of evidence included in this hierarchy and strategies for evaluation of quantitative data.

How to Evaluate Quantitative Evidence

The first level on the quantitative research hierarchy of evidence presented in Figure 16.1 is respected opinion. *Respected opinions* from knowledgeable people in a field can be a good start for guiding decision making in practice when they are supported with appropriate scientific evidence to provide trustworthiness. An example in occupational therapy related to assessment is the discussion between scholars Gillen and Hinojosa (2015), published in the *Open Journal of Occupational Therapy,* in which they suggest opportunities for better use of assessments in practice.

Respected opinion is useful in applied fields such as occupational therapy, where publication of research commonly lags behind the publication of theory, opinion, and other reviews. For example, practitioners may use information on psychometrics published in assessment manuals to guide decision making about best methods of assessment for clients. Furthermore, practitioners need to read reviews of assessments that are published in journals and periodicals, because these reviews may be more critical than the manuals.

When research studies about evaluation or assessment methods are not available, the best available evidence is that of published opinion, including published reviews. For example, a recent review article by Hemphill (2015) presented spiritual assessment tools for use in practice, guidelines for selecting a spiritual assessment tool, and a case study illustrating use of assessment tools. In addition to review articles published in journals, common places for finding reviews of assessments are the *Mental Measurement Yearbook* website (https://buros.org/mental-measurements-yearbook), the Rehabilitation Measures Database (https://www.sralab.org/rehabilitation-measures), and the Stroke Engine website (https://www.strokengine.ca/assess). Chapter 3, "Assessment Identification and Selection," presents further discussion regarding resources for selection of instruments.

Nonexperimental studies

Moving up the hierarchy, the next level of evidence comprises *nonexperimental studies,* which are research studies that either have no manipulation or have an intervention that the researcher does not control. Such studies describe observation of an already occurring or ongoing event. There are generally three types of studies classified as nonexperimental: (1) descriptive studies, (2) case studies, and (3) correlation research.

Descriptive or observational studies describe an event or characteristic of a group. When examining these studies relative to evaluation, occupational therapy practitioners need to consider the specific assessments used to determine outcomes. An example of descriptive evidence that informs assessment selection in occupational therapy is Kramer et al.'s (2010) study of the validity of the Child Occupational Self-Assessment (Keller et al., 2005).

Case studies, another type of nonexperimental research, are used to develop clinical knowledge. They are in-depth studies of one client and their disease course and response to intervention. Case studies are directly applicable to client care. However, because case studies use only one or a few participants, their generalizability to other clients or other environments is limited. When reading a case study, occupational therapy practitioners need to review the occupational therapy process, including the assessments used and how outcomes were measured. Because of the nature of case studies, practitioners should be attentive to the methodology and interpretations of the author and to the reliability and validity of the assessments and process used. For example, a case study published in the *American Journal of Occupational Therapy* examined the process of applying a cognitive approach for improving participation after stroke (Henshaw et al., 2011).

Correlation research examines relationships between variables, or, in the situation of test development, correlation is used to establish interrater, test–retest, or other types of reliability. The strength of the relationship between variables is measured with a statistic called a ***correlation coefficient,*** which is a statistical measure that ranges between –1.0 and 1.0. An example of the use of correlation to establish test reliability in the *American Journal of Occupational Therapy* is the study of a new assessment for near-task home lighting for older adults with low vision (Perlmutter et al., 2013). It is important to understand that correlation research does not demonstrate a causal relationship between independent variables but rather indicates that the variables are somehow linked, as is the case with test reliability.

Quasi-experimental research

The third level from the base of the hierarchy is ***quasi-experimental research,*** which involves manipulation of an independent variable and measurement of a dependent variable. Quasi-experimental studies do not randomly assign participants to groups; these studies may have only one group under study, or they may involve multiple groups. If more than one group is used, the groups are non-equivalent, because participants within the groups are not randomly assigned.

With respect to evaluation, again, occupational therapy practitioners need to attend to the specific assessments used and the measurement of the dependent variable. The results of quasi-experimental studies generally have less internal validity than true experiments, but, because they study preexisting groups, the results may have greater external validity or generalizability compared with true experiments (Portney & Watkins, 2009). These types of studies may have great applicability to practice. For example, in a recent quasi-experimental study, Chippendale (2019) used multiple assessment methods as outcome measures to evaluate feasibility of the Stroll Safe outdoor fall prevention program.

Experimental studies

The fourth level from the base of the hierarchy of evidence contains studies that use true experimental designs, commonly referred to as *randomized controlled trials.* These studies are designed within experimental parameters; participants are randomly assigned to intervention or no-intervention groups, and independent and dependent variables are defined by the researcher. Just as when reviewing quasi-experimental studies, practitioners need to focus on the assessments used. For example, Pyatak et al. (2019) conducted a pilot randomized controlled trial to examine effectiveness-implementation of a Lifestyle Redesign® occupational therapy intervention in a primary care setting. The researchers used a variety of clinical and health behavior outcome measures to assess implementation of the intervention.

Meta-analysis of randomized controlled trials

The top level in the quantitative research hierarchy consists of studies that use *meta-analysis,* a statistical procedure for combining data from multiple studies to determine the effect of the intervention. Unlike a review article, the meta-analysis does not merely summarize the results from individual studies. Combining individual randomized controlled trials increases the power of meta-analysis over that of a single study, improving the estimate of the effect size the intervention provides and the ability to generalize the results (Portney & Watkins, 2009).

Meta-analyses usually involve studies with the same target population and intervention, providing greater certainty of the effect of an intervention. Because meta-analyses pool data from many randomized controlled trials, they also increase the external validity of the results. The results are generalized more readily to multiple settings. Unfortunately, there are relatively few meta-analyses in the occupational therapy and health profession literature. In meta-analysis, because the concern lies with the variables of interest, the authors do not identify or discuss assessments in great depth. Although meta-analytic studies are important pieces of evidence, they usually do not have much relevance to EBP in evaluation.

How to Evaluate Qualitative Evidence

Occupational therapy practitioners may not find published quantitative evidence that directly supports their question about the occupational therapy process, or quantitative information may not be the best form of evidence for decision making in a particular practice situation. Therefore, another area from which to find evidence is the field of qualitative research. This section covers evaluation of qualitative studies for EBP.

Similar to other study designs, when appraising qualitative literature for evidence to inform the occupational therapy process, practitioners should review any assessments used by the study authors to determine the assessments' appropriateness for the client's needs, the reliability and validity of the data collected, and the manner in which the assessments were used. *Qualitative research* refers to systematic investigation of gathering and analyzing non-numerical data and provides practitioners with evidence that may help inform their understanding of how clients live their lives and what they value. This understanding can guide practitioners in how to evaluate a client to obtain the most pertinent information to guide client-centered practice (Hammell, 2004; Mroz et al., 2015).

Occupational therapy practitioners need to evaluate the various types of qualitative research, just like with quantitative research, for trustworthiness and credibility. However, unlike quantitative research, qualitative research does not have a hierarchy that ranks the rigor of the research. Nevertheless, many publications suggest how to evaluate qualitative research for EBP (Cohen & Crabtree, 2008; Devers, 1999; Dixon-Woods et al., 2004; Giacomini & Cook, 2000; Greenhalgh & Taylor, 1997; Henderson & Rheault, 2004; Popay & Williams, 1998). Practitioners need to determine whether the research article addresses their question about evaluation in some meaningful way. Often, qualitative research studies address a broad query without extensive detail on evaluation. In the process of addressing the query, however, the authors may present ideas on how they gained access to the participants and built trust and rapport, which may be important when practitioners are initiating or carrying out an evaluation. Practitioners can use information from these examples to refine methods of evaluating a client.

A major issue with qualitative research is the potential for *bias.* Qualitative researchers are the data-collection tool for their studies (Toma, 2006). When examining phenomena, the researcher decides which data are relevant and which to collect. Inductive reasoning drives data analysis. Qualitative researchers reflect on their own personal perspectives, values, and interests and the way these influence the research process (Patton, 2015; Toma, 2006). The researcher addresses personal bias in the Method section with a discussion on reflexivity that demonstrates how potential researcher bias was handled in data collection and data analyses.

Occupational therapy practitioners should carefully read the qualitative research article findings and conclusions. The researcher should clearly describe the themes that emerged and present evidence from the findings and the literature to support their conclusions. Furthermore, when reading such articles through the lens of an evaluator, practitioners should examine carefully the assessments used and their appropriateness given the study. Although qualitative studies may not use formal assessments, they provide rich data for the therapist to determine how to evaluate clients.

For example, a recent mixed-methods study examined how the Canadian Occupational Performance Measure (COPM; Law et al., 2019) can be used as an assessment in primary care settings (Donnelly et al., 2017). The researchers used focus groups to understand the practitioners' experience of using the COPM in this emerging practice setting. Practitioners with questions about the feasibility of using the COPM in new practice settings may benefit from translating the qualitive findings of this study to their practice situation. The researchers found that the COPM was a useful tool because of its focus on function; however, they also concluded that the nature of the primary care practice setting made it difficult to consistently readminister the COPM (Donnelly et al., 2017).

In general, practitioners may find that qualitative research is more accessible and perhaps more directly related to practice. However, practitioners need to consider the individual nature of the reality addressed through qualitative research and carefully consider how the assessments were used in the studies.

CONTEMPORARY EBP MODEL FOR OCCUPATIONAL THERAPY

Vision 2025 of the American Occupational Therapy Association (AOTA, 2017b) calls for occupational therapy to be *effective,* defined as evidence based, client centered, and cost-effective, and scholars of the profession agree that translating evidence to practice is important for demonstrating effectiveness of occupational therapy services (Fleming-Castaldy & Gillen, 2013; Hinojosa, 2013; Lin et al., 2010; Thomas & Law, 2013). However, scholars, both within occupational therapy and from other health professions, have also voiced concern about definitive acceptance of research evidence over practitioner expertise and client response in single-hierarchy EBP models (Hinojosa, 2013; Murad et al., 2016; Tomlin & Borgetto, 2011; Tomlin & Dougherty, 2014).

For example, important qualitative constructs of the occupational therapy profession, such as client-centeredness, conflict with single-hierarchy models that rank true experimental designs over all other types of evidence. Client-centered occupational therapy evaluation requires practitioners to select appropriate assessment methods supported not only by science but also by theory and characteristics of the client and contexts influencing their occupational performance (Pitonyak et al., 2015). Single-hierarchy EBP models are often inconsistent with the professional reasoning of practitioners (Hinojosa, 2013; Tickle-Degnen & Bedell, 2003; Tomlin & Borgetto, 2011; Tomlin & Dougherty, 2014) and lack the ability to evaluate qualitative evidence. However, Hinojosa (2013) proposed several directions for action to bridge EBP and theory-directed practice, most important, the need for an evidence-based model in occupational therapy that comprehensively evaluates evidence relevant to occupation.

Tomlin and Borgetto (2011) introduced a more comprehensive model of the research hierarchy to occupational therapy, the Research Pyramid, portrayed in Figure 16.2. The Research Pyramid more closely aligns with the philosophical underpinnings of the profession and addresses some of the limitations of single-hierarchy EBP models, one being the oversimplification and confounding of criteria of rigor (i.e., internal validity) and applicability (i.e., external validity). The ranking of evidence in single-hierarchy EBP

models suggests that research designs with stronger internal validity also have stronger external validity. *Internal validity* is the rigor and trustworthiness of the procedures of a study to avoid confounding. *External validity* is the generalizability or transferability of the outcomes of a study to the real world or other settings.

Single-hierarchy models rank research designs such as randomized controlled trials with high internal validity as best evidence, yet statistically significant results in a controlled trial may not translate to meaningful or usable evidence in real-world situations. This assumption of single-hierarchy models fails to consider the limitations in generalizing findings of tightly controlled trials carried out with systematic procedures to diverse practice settings and real-world situations. Occupational therapy evaluation carried out in practice and real-world settings requires both quantitative and qualitative evidence to inform fully occupational therapy decision making.

As shown in Figure 16.2, the *Research Pyramid* addresses this concern with two orthogonal axes: (1) quantitative–qualitative and (2) internal–external validity. The Research Pyramid is constructed of three faces: (1) experimental research, (2) qualitative research, and (3) outcome research, providing a model that evaluates comprehensive forms of evidence and better aligns with professional reasoning used during occupational therapy evaluation.

The Research Pyramid also addresses the limited consideration given to large-scale, population-based outcome studies in single-hierarchy models. Population-based outcome studies use observational methods and therefore lack the ability to randomly assign participants to various conditions. However, the inherently low internal validity of population-based outcome studies is tempered by the increased generalizability of this research design to real-life situations.

FIGURE 16.2. Research Pyramid.

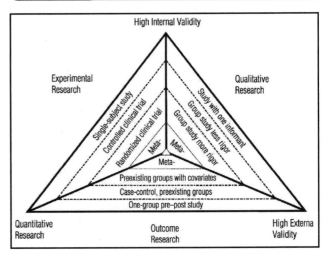

Source. From "Research Pyramid: A New Evidence-Based Practice Model for Occupational Therapy," by G. Tomlin & B. Borgetto, 2011, *American Journal of Occupational Therapy,* Vol. 65, p. 191. Copyright © 2011 by the American Occupational Therapy Association. Used with permission.

Note. Meta = meta-analyses.

Ciro (2011) called for the profession to increase use of observational or epidemiological methods. Epidemiological research designs inform the understanding of various health conditions, which for occupational therapy practitioners means understanding occupational performance disabilities and related factors. Intervention effectiveness, the focus of single-hierarchy models that rank controlled trials as best evidence, is certainly important to occupational therapy; however, observational and qualitative research designs may offer better evidence for informing decision making in the overall occupational therapy process. Figure 16.2 illustrates the Research Pyramid's consideration of observational or outcome research.

WHAT ARE THE DATA FROM THE OCCUPATIONAL THERAPY PROCESS?

When neither quantitative nor qualitative evidence is available to support occupational therapy practitioner decision making, the best support for practice decisions is practice itself. To use individual practice data as support for subsequent decisions, the practitioner needs to know what data are available that support practice, how to evaluate the source of the data, how to compile the data, and how to disseminate findings so others can benefit from them.

An evidence-based perspective on occupational therapy practice as it relates to evaluation can lead occupational therapy practitioners to think about the data they generate through practice. The practitioner must decide how to document outcomes and the efficacy of occupational therapy interventions. The practitioner may begin to seek evidence that a particular intervention strategy, whether an old favorite or a new approach, is most effective in helping clients regain occupational performance. When designing new programs, the practitioner may conscientiously include evaluative outcome measures that will assist in the creation of practice-based evidence. Administrators and third-party payers may have practitioners justify the effectiveness of their interventions. Justifying the effectiveness of interventions and providing evidence to support practice requires practitioners to identify the data that support practice and consider carefully what other data they should collect and analyze.

The occupational therapy process is rich with potential areas of data collection to support occupational therapy intervention, explore the therapeutic process, and understand better the lived experience of clients receiving occupational therapy services. For example, consistent use of the AOTA Occupational Profile Template (AOTA, 2017a) may guide occupational therapy practitioner decision making about best assessment methods for gathering information about the client, their environment, and their goals. Furthermore, data from the occupational therapy process can be relevant when practitioners are analyzing the impact of occupational therapy intervention, to help determine whether changes resulted specifically from occupational therapy intervention or from a combination of factors.

These sources of data are important in determining the impact of intervention and applicability of outcomes data. One example of a secondary analysis informing the lived experience of clients with multiple sclerosis is a study by Finlayson et al. (2012) examining the degree to which age, gender, work status, and impairment moderated fatigue-management program outcomes. Thoughtful consideration of evaluation and reevaluation data can help practitioners produce outcomes data either in a prospective analysis of practice or in a retrospective chart review (see Exhibit 16.1).

Determining the efficacy of intervention requires that occupational therapy practitioners look at the outcome measurement for intervention strategies. Depending on the goal of outcomes assessment, practitioners may choose to collect data on the basis of a specific guideline for intervention. For example, if the therapist uses the person–environment–occupation approach (Law et al., 1996), they may set out to collect specific data on the person's skills, abilities, experiences, or roles; environmental set-up, cues, barriers, or supports; the occupations the client engages in or wishes to engage in; and the relationship of all these components to occupational performance and occupational therapy intervention. Practitioners then can relate the results of their research back to the theoretical approach, further validating that approach as an appropriate guide to practice (Ottenbacher & Hinderer, 2001).

Generating Data

It is often difficult to apply the findings of studies to practice settings. It may be impossible to find any published literature that provides direct evidence for decision making about the occupational therapy process. However, practice itself offers a rich opportunity to accumulate the data necessary to make informed decisions. Although it is difficult to conduct randomized controlled trials within the confines of practice, two types of studies are feasible in practice settings and offer occupational therapy practitioners the ability to gather data through practice: (1) case studies and (2) single-subject designs. Case studies are a form of nonexperimental research, and single-subject designs qualify as quasi-experimental research.

Case studies often start with an interesting problem in practice. Unlike a single-subject study, case studies typically do not involve systematic collection of baseline data before the implementation of intervention. Rather, case studies are often retrospective; the practitioner recognizes later that a case is interesting or unique or that a unique intervention produced optimal outcomes. Case studies arise out of the

---

EXHIBIT 16.1.	Questions for Evidence-Based Practice

Some questions that occupational therapy practitioners can use to guide selection of assessments and develop strategies for documenting evidence-based evaluation findings include:

- What data are intervention decisions based on?
- Are data derived from standardized assessments that have been determined to be valid and reliable?
- Can data collected from nonstandardized assessments be generalized to other client situations or to other practice settings?
- Do evaluation and reevaluation results demonstrate that occupational therapy intervention was effective for a particular client or population?

general course of practice. Unlike research that is undertaken for the sake of gaining new knowledge, case studies are the documentation of new knowledge gained serendipitously through practice. For example, in a case report, Marx et al. (2019) described changes in activity engagement for a person with dementia using the Tailoring Activities for Persons With Dementia and Their Caregivers protocol along with other outcome measures.

Case studies offer occupational therapy practitioners a unique opportunity to generate evidence for decision making in practice. A well-documented case study can provide evidence to inform practice and contribute to the generation of hypotheses for more formal research endeavors. By documenting cases in a systematic manner, practitioners can begin to amass the data necessary for other types of research design.

A typical *single-subject design* starts with the measurement of *baseline data,* which represents the state of the outcome variable or target behavior before any intervention. Occupational therapy practitioners can obtain baseline data as part of the initial evaluation process. Then they compare the baseline state of the target behavior with new data after phases in the study during which they apply or withdraw interventions. Practitioners collect data during all phases of the study and can incorporate this data collection into reassessment practices. Data collection usually results from objective, quantitative measures. Data often address the frequency of occurrence of the target behavior in the presence or absence of the interventions.

Qualitative evidence from evaluation and reevaluation also can provide data for a single-subject study. These qualitative data can describe the roles a person has, how they are valued, and whether this changes over the course of intervention. One strategy to collect this type of data may be through use of the COPM (Law et al., 2019) during evaluation and reevaluation. Qualitative data also can describe the process of an intervention and whether the client values it, thereby providing information on the likelihood of carryover of recommendations. In addition, qualitative data can provide important information about cultural values and beliefs that can affect occupational therapy outcomes, including those related to illness, disability, and role performance.

Gathering Data

Practice generates large volumes of data from day-to-day evaluation, intervention, reassessment, and reevaluation of clients, as well as through case studies and single-subject studies. To use these data to demonstrate outcomes and provide evidence for practice, occupational therapy practitioners need to organize the data and ensure that the information obtained about individual clients is available for later use. An easy and efficient method of compiling data is to develop a *database.* Practitioners can easily create a database using readily available word processing programs.

The first step in setting up a database is determining what data are important to compile. In general, a database should start with the variables that describe clients. The first descriptor should be a unique identification number for each individual in the database. It is important to adhere to Health Insurance Portability and Accountability Act of 1996 (P. L. 104-191) regulations and protect the anonymity of individuals when assigning identifiers. The use of patient numbers and Social Security numbers is inappropriate because these numbers can be connected easily to a client's private information. Therefore, the numbers used for a database should be unique and not connected to the client other than for the purpose of the database. Occupational therapy practitioners must keep Social Security numbers, patient numbers, and other unique identifiers secure and separate from the overall database.

Once identifiers are determined, the next category of descriptive information is demographic data, such as age, race, gender, diagnosis, and medical history. Occupational therapy practitioners need to collect demographic data to describe the characteristics of the individuals in a given group. Demographic data are also important sources of potential confounding variables when practitioners attempt to determine the effectiveness of an intervention. Access to these data allows for analysis of the impact of these variables on the outcome of interest.

The second source of data available to occupational therapy practitioners is information generated from assessments used in the evaluation and reevaluation of individual clients. It is important that practitioners collect all the pertinent outcome information during evaluations and reevaluations. These data also need to be coded and recorded in the database. Use of standardized assessments ensures that the data collected are both valid and reliable. This strengthens the conclusions drawn from the data and aids in replication of the interventions.

When setting up a database, it is best to collect as much data as possible. It is better to have data available and not needed than to need the data and not have them. Therefore, practitioners should include all information possible pertaining to the occupational therapy process—not just interventions provided by the occupational therapy practitioners but concomitant treatments as well, including all medication. This information will be helpful in future analyses to explain other possible causes for the outcomes. For example, Dunn et al. (2009) used personal information profiles from a previous qualitative research study to examine how clients with spinal cord injury responded after developing a low-grade pressure ulcer.

Databases provide valuable archival information. It is important to take sufficient time to set up a comprehensive and well-documented database; otherwise, practitioners may find they have data that are not clearly defined, not adequately documented, or too difficult to compile after the fact. Taking the time to plan and set up a well-thought-out database ensures that when it comes time to analyze and disseminate the data, they will be in a usable form. Furthermore, there will be a clear record of exactly what information the practitioner collected for each variable without having to rely on human memory or information from other sources.

Disseminating Data

The knowledge base in any field is highly dependent on the dissemination of information in a public forum. In general, scientific knowledge progresses through the sharing of results, the critical evaluation of the results over time, and the replication of results in other settings. Without this cycle, occupational therapy practitioners and researchers rely on outdated or erroneous information. EBP is dependent on the public sharing of the newest and best available information for practice.

There are many levels in the dissemination of information. The first level consists of colleagues in the occupational therapy practitioner's own institution or immediate community. This informal sharing of information can provide an initial level of critique that helps a practitioner refine ideas and processes. Journal clubs, brown bag lunches, and online discussion forums are ideal and low-pressure methods for bringing ideas into a public forum. However, practitioners should not stop at this level, because peer reviews of articles often focus on the content rather than an analysis of the credibility of the study.

Once assured by colleagues that the results are interesting, the occupational therapy practitioner has a professional and moral obligation to disseminate them to a wider forum. Publications and conference presentations are the two major avenues for disseminating new information. Publications provide the broadest dissemination and the greatest level of critical review. Conference presentations may be particularly effective if the proceedings of the conference are published. Although conference presentations move information to the public more quickly, they are not optimal, because the level of critical review is not the same as for a juried publication. Additionally, with a presentation, the audience is usually still limited and often biased toward a particular topic. However, conference presentations often provide interesting opportunities to discuss with colleagues outcomes, ways to improve the study, and the experiences of other professionals with specific assessments.

Publication is the primary way of disseminating information throughout the public domain and ensuring that the information will be retrievable in the future. Publication can take the form of journal articles, books and book chapters, magazines and newsletters, or other electronic forms. In general, journals serve the purpose of presenting new and interesting information, books and book chapters present reviews, and magazines and newsletters present new ideas. Journals are of two types: (1) peer-reviewed and (2) non–peer-reviewed. Peer-reviewed journals require that manuscripts undergo a process of evaluation by experts in the discipline who evaluate the manuscript on the basis of the current level of knowledge in the field. Peer review ensures that the presented information has sufficient rigor, interest, and uniqueness to warrant dissemination. Non–peer-reviewed journals generally do not have the same rigor, because manuscripts are reviewed only by an editor, who may not have expertise in the specific area.

Additional Uses of Evaluation Data for Knowledge Translation

Beyond informing occupational therapy practitioner decision making in day-to-day practice, evidence generated from the occupational therapy process can be used for broader areas of knowledge translation, such as developing new programs and measuring a wide variety of outcomes. Knowledge translation is a process with the aim of using evidence to improve health and enhance service delivery (Center on Knowledge Translation for Disability and Rehabilitation Research [KTDRR], 2019). An important component of the knowledge translation process is the identification of key stakeholders who work to adapt knowledge to the local situation; determine barriers and facilitators of knowledge use; create and implement new interventions or programs; and evaluate outcomes, including the continued use of knowledge (KTDRR, 2019).

Occupational therapy practitioners can use data gathered from the occupational therapy process, in combination with evidence from the literature, to develop new interventions and programs and evaluate the outcomes. For example, practitioners in school-based practice can synthesize data about goal achievement or the most frequently provided methods of specially designed instruction to help identify priority needs or gaps in programming to develop new intervention programs. This approach was used by Bazyk et al. (2015) to develop Every Moment Counts (EMC), a mental health promotion initiative informed by information from the occupational therapy process in school-based settings and research evidence on best methods for fostering mental health among children and youths. Bazyk et al. (2015) conducted a knowledge translation process focused on increasing practitioner knowledge and use of EMC and measuring outcomes of a community of practice as the mechanism for knowledge translation.

SUMMARY

It is critical that occupational therapy practitioners engage in EBP that supports the philosophical underpinnings of the profession and informs decision making using both external and internal information throughout the occupational therapy process. Comprehensive EBP models, such as the Research Pyramid, evaluate and inform the quantitative and qualitative evidence necessary for occupational therapy evaluation. As the practitioner gathers data about the client and chooses appropriate assessment methods, their decision making is guided by both external evidence from relevant, published literature and internal evidence from the practitioner–client relationship. Information gathered during effective practice can become future data for EBP and knowledge translation. When the practitioner uses these data from practice to provide evidence for practice, they not only aid practice but also, when disseminating findings, provide evidence to support the field of occupational therapy in general, develop new programs, and measure a wide variety of outcomes.

ACKNOWLEDGMENTS

The author acknowledges Michelle Cohen, PhD, and Pamalyn Kearney, EdD, OTR/L, who authored a previous version of this chapter on EBP; their early conceptualization of the relationship between EBP and occupational therapy evaluation is still evident in the structure of this chapter. Also, Virginia Stoffel, PhD, OT, BCMH, FAOTA, and Nikhil Tomar, MS, previously authored the chapter titled "Additional Uses of Evaluation Data." Ideas from their previous work have been incorporated into this current chapter.

QUESTIONS

1. Describe the relationship between EBP and evaluation. How can a therapist use evaluation data to support EBP?
2. Choose one assessment. How can you support your decision to use this tool through available evidence?
3. Choose one practice area. Identify the assessments commonly used in this practice area. In your opinion, does evidence support the use of these assessments?
4. Think about a practice site where you have been. What data have you seen there that a therapist could collect to use for future evidence for practice?
5. Search an online database for EBP. What information in that database might be useful to you in evaluation or assessment?

REFERENCES

American Occupational Therapy Association. (2017a). AOTA occupational profile template. Retrieved from https://www.aota.org/~/media/Corporate/Files/Practice/Manage/Documentation/AOTA-Occupational-Profile-Template.pdf

American Occupational Therapy Association. (2017b). Vision 2025. *American Journal of Occupational Therapy, 71*, 7130420010. https://doi.org/10.5014/ajot.2017.713002

Bazyk, S., Demirjian, L., LaGuardia, T., Thompson-Repas, K., Conway, C., & Michaud, P. (2015). Building capacity of occupational therapy practitioners to address the mental health needs of children and youth: A mixed-methods study of knowledge translation. *American Journal of Occupational Therapy, 69*, 6906180060. https://doi.org/10.5014/ajot.2015.019182

Center on Knowledge Translation for Disability and Rehabilitation Research. (2019). Knowledge translation. Retrieved from https://ktdrr.org/knowledge-translation/

Chippendale, T. (2019). Feasibility of the Stroll Safe outdoor fall prevention program. *American Journal of Occupational Therapy, 73*, 7304205060. https://doi.org/10.5014/ajot.2019.031294

Ciro, C. (2011). Enhancing our collective research acumen by using an epidemiological perspective. *American Journal of Occupational Therapy, 65*, 594–598. https://doi.org/10.5014/ajot.2011.000703

Cohen, D. J., & Crabtree, B. F. (2008). Evaluative criteria for qualitative research in health care: Controversies and recommendations. *Annals of Family Medicine, 6*, 331–339. https://doi.org/10.1370/afm.818

Devers, K. J. (1999). How will we know "good" qualitative research when we see it? Beginning the dialogue in health services research. *Health Services Research, 34*, 1153–1188.

Dixon-Woods, M., Shaw, R. L., Agarwal, S., & Smith, S. (2004). The problem of appraising qualitative research. *Quality and Safety in Health Care, 13*, 223–225. https://doi.org/10.1136/qhc.13.3.223

Donnelly, C., O'Neill, C., Bauer, M., & Letts, L. (2017). Canadian Occupational Performance Measure (COPM) in primary care: A profile of practice. *American Journal of Occupational Therapy, 71*, 7106265010. https://doi.org/10.5014/ajot.2017.020008

Dunn, C. A., Carlson, M., Jackson, J. M., & Clark, F. A. (2009). Response factors surrounding progression of pressure ulcers in community-residing adults with spinal cord injury. *American Journal of Occupational Therapy, 63*, 301–309. https://doi.org/10.5014/ajot.63.3.301

Dysart, A. M., & Tomlin, G. S. (2002). Factors related to evidence-based practice among U.S. occupational therapy clinicians. *American Journal of Occupational Therapy, 56*, 275–284. https://doi.org/10.5014/ajot.56.3.275

Finlayson, M., Preissner, K., & Cho, C. (2012). Outcome moderators of a fatigue management program for people with multiple sclerosis. *American Journal of Occupational Therapy, 66*, 187–197. https://doi.org/10.5014/ajot.2012.003160

Fleming-Castaldy, R., & Gillen, G. (2013). Ensuring that education, certification, and practice are evidence based. *American Journal of Occupational Therapy, 67*, 364–369. https://doi.org/10.5014/ajot.2013.006973

Giacomini, M. K., & Cook, D. J. (2000). Users' guides to the medical literature: XXIII. Qualitative research in health care B. What are the results and how do they help me care for my patients? *Journal of the American Medical Association, 284*, 357–362. https://doi.org/10.1001/jama.284.4.478

Gillen, G., & Hinojosa, J. (2015). He said—he said: A scholarly conversation about assessment. *Open Journal of Occupational Therapy, 3*(3). https://doi.org/10.15453/2168-6408.1198

Greenhalgh, T., & Taylor, R. (1997). How to read a paper: Papers that go beyond numbers (qualitative research). *British Medical Journal, 315*, 740–743. https://doi.org/10.1136/bmj.315.7110.740

Hammell, K. W. (2004). Dimensions of meaning in the occupations of daily life. *Canadian Journal of Occupational Therapy, 71*, 296–305. https://doi.org/10.1177/000841740407100509

Health Insurance Portability and Accountability Act of 1996, Pub. L. 104–191, 42 U.S.C. § 300gg, 29 U.S.C §§ 1181–1183, and 42 U.S.C. §§ 1320d–1320d9.

Hemphill, B. (2015). Spiritual assessments in occupational therapy. *Open Journal of Occupational Therapy, 3*(3). https://doi.org/10.15453/2168-6408.1159

Henderson, R., & Rheault, W. (2004). Appraising and incorporating qualitative research in evidence-based practice. *Journal of Physical Therapy Education, 18*, 35–40. https://doi.org/10.1097/00001416-200410000-00005

Henshaw, E., Polatajko, H., McEwen, S., Ryan, J. D., & Baum, C. M. (2011). Cognitive approach to improving participation after stroke: Two case studies. *American Journal of Occupational Therapy, 65*, 55–63. https://doi.org/10.5014/ajot.2011.09010

Hinojosa, J. (2013). The evidence-based paradox. *American Journal of Occupational Therapy, 67*, e18–e23. https://doi.org/10.5014/ajot.2013.005587

Ilott, I. (2003). Challenging the rhetoric and reality: Only an individual and systemic approach will work for evidence-based occupational therapy. *American Journal of Occupational Therapy, 57*, 351–354. https://doi.org/10.5014/ajot.57.3.351

Keller, J., Kafkes, A., Basu, S., Federico, J., & Kielhofner, G. (2005). *The Child Occupational Self Assessment (COSA; Version 2.1).*

Chicago: University of Illinois, College of Applied Health Sciences, Department of Occupational Therapy, MOHO Clearinghouse.

Kramer, J. M., Kielhofner, G., & Smith, E. V. (2010). Validity evidence for the Child Occupational Self Assessment. *American Journal of Occupational Therapy, 64,* 621–632. https://doi.org/10.5014/ajot.2010.08142

Law, M., Baptiste, S., Carswell, A., McColl, M. A., Polatajko, H., & Pollock, N. (2019). *Canadian Occupational Performance Measure* (5th ed., rev.). Altona, MB: COPM, Inc.

Law, M., & Baum, C. (1998). Evidence-based occupational therapy. *Canadian Journal of Occupational Therapy, 65,* 131–135. https://doi.org/10.1177/000841749806500301

Law, M., Cooper, B., Strong, S., Stewart, D., Rigby, P., & Letts, L. (1996). The Person–Environment–Occupation Model: A transactive approach to occupational performance. *Canadian Journal of Occupational Therapy, 63,* 9–23. https://doi.org/10.1177/000841749606300103

Law, M., & MacDermid, J. (Eds.). (2013). *Evidence-based rehabilitation: A guide to practice* (3rd ed.). Thorofare, NJ: Slack.

Lee, C. J., & Miller, L. T. (2003). The process of evidence-based clinical decision making in occupational therapy. *American Journal of Occupational Therapy, 57,* 473–477. https://doi.org/10.5014/ajot.57.4.473

Lin, S. H., Murphy, S. L., & Robinson, J. C. (2010). Facilitating evidence-based practice: process, strategies, and resources. *American Journal of Occupational Therapy, 64,*164–171. https://doi.org/10.5014/ajot.64.1.164

Lloyd-Smith, W. (1997). Evidence-based practice and occupational therapy. *British Journal of Occupational Therapy, 60,* 474–479. https://doi.org/10.1177/030802269706001103

Marx, K. A., Scott, J. B., Verrier Piersol, C., & Gitlin, L. N. (2019). Tailored activities to reduce neuropsychiatric behaviors in persons with dementia: Case report. *American Journal of Occupational Therapy, 73,* 7302205160. https://doi.org/10.5014/ajot.2019.029546

Miles, A. & Loughlin, M. (2011). Models in the balance: Evidence-based medicine versus evidence-informed individualized care. *Journal of Evaluation in Clinical Practice, 17,* 531–536. https://doi.org/10.1111/j.1365-2753.2011.01713.x

Mroz, T. M., Pitonyak, J. S., Fogelberg, D., & Leland, N. E. (2015). Client centeredness and health reform: Key issues for occupational therapy. *American Journal of Occupational Therapy, 69,* 6905090010. https://doi.org/10.5014/ajot.2015.695001

Murad, M. H., Asi, N., Alsawas, M., & Alahdab, F. (2016). New evidence pyramid. *Evidence Based Medicine, 21*(4), 125–127. https://doi.org/10.1136/ebmed-2016-110401

Nevo, I., & Slonim-Nevo, V. (2011). The myth of evidence-based practice: Towards evidence-informed practice. *British Journal of Social Work, 41,* 1176–1197. https://doi.org/10.1093/bjsw/bcq149

Ottenbacher, K. J., & Hinderer, S. R. (2001). Evidence-based practice: Methods to evaluate individual patient improvement. *American Journal of Physical Medicine and Rehabilitation, 80,* 786–796. https://doi.org/10.1097/00002060-200110000-00014

Patton, M. Q. (2015). *Qualitative research and evaluation methods: Integrating theory and practice* (4th ed.). Los Angeles: Sage.

Perlmutter, M. S., Bhorade, A., Gordon, M., Hollingsworth, H., Engsberg, J. E., & Baum, M. C. (2013). Home lighting assessment for clients with low vision. *American Journal of Occupational Therapy, 67,* 674–682. https://doi.org/10.5014/ajot.2013.006692

Pitonyak, J. S., Mroz, T. M., & Fogelberg, D. (2015). Expanding client-centred thinking to include social determinants: A practical scenario based on the occupation of breastfeeding. *Scandinavian Journal of Occupational Therapy, 22,* 277–282. https://doi.org/10.3109/11038128.2015.1020865

Popay, J., & Williams, G. (1998). Qualitative research and evidence-based healthcare. *Journal of the Royal Society of Medicine, 91,* 32–37. https://doi.org/10.1177/014107689809135s08

Portney, L. G., & Watkins, M. P. (2009). *Foundations of clinical research: Applications to practice* (3rd ed.). Upper Saddle River, NJ: Prentice Hall Health.

Pyatak, E., King, M., Vigen, C. L. P., Salazar, E., Diaz, J., Schepens Niemiec, S. L., . . . Shukla, J. (2019). Addressing diabetes in primary care: Hybrid effectiveness–implementation study of Lifestyle Redesign® occupational therapy. *American Journal of Occupational Therapy, 73,* 7305185020. https://doi.org/10.5014/ajot.2019.037317

Rosenberg, W., & Donald, A. (1995). Evidence-based medicine: An approach to clinical problem-solving. *British Medical Journal, 310,* 1122–1126. https://doi.org/10.1136/bmj.310.6987.1122

Sackett, D. L. (1989). Rules of evidence and clinical recommendations on the use of antithrombotic agents. *Chest, 25,* 25–35. https://doi.org/10.1378/chest.95.2_Supplement.2S

Sackett, D. L., Rosenberg, W. M. C., Gray, J. A. M., Haynes, R. B., & Richardson, W. S. (1996). Evidence-based medicine: What it is and what it isn't. *British Journal of Medicine, 312,* 71–72. https://doi.org/10.1136/bmj.312.7023.71

Straus, S. E., Glasziou, P., Richardson, W. S., & Haynes, R. B. (2019). *Evidence-based medicine: How to practice and teach EBM* (5th ed.). Edinburgh, Scotland: Elsevier.

Taylor, M. C. (1997). What is evidence-based practice? *British Journal of Occupational Therapy, 60,* 470–474. https://doi.org/10.1177/030802269706001102

Thomas, A., & Law, M. (2013). Research utilization and evidence-based practice in occupational therapy: A scoping study. *American Journal of Occupational Therapy, 67,* e55–e65. https://doi.org/10.5014/ajot.2013.006395

Tickle-Degnen, L. (2002). Client-centered practice, therapeutic relationship, and the use of research evidence. *American Journal of Occupational Therapy, 56,* 470–474. https://doi.org/10.5014/ajot.56.4.470

Tickle-Degnen, L., & Bedell, G. (2003). Heterarchy and hierarchy: A critical appraisal of the "levels of evidence" as a tool for clinical decision making. *American Journal of Occupational Therapy, 57,* 234–237. https://doi.org/10.5014/ajot.57.2.234

Toma, J. D. (2006). Approaching rigor in applied qualitative research. In C. F. Conrad & R. C. Serlin (Eds.), *The Sage handbook for research in education* (pp. 405–423). Thousand Oaks, CA: Sage.

Tomlin, G., & Borgetto, B. (2011). Research Pyramid: A new evidence-based practice model for occupational therapy. *American Journal of Occupational Therapy, 65,*189–196. https://doi.org/10.5014/ajot.2011.000828

Tomlin, G. S., & Dougherty, D. (2014). Decision-making and sources of evidence in occupational therapy and other health professions: Evidence-informed practice. *International Journal of Health Professions, 1,* 13–19. https://doi.org/10.2478/ijhp-2014-0001

Appendix A. AOTA Occupational Profile Template

The American Occupational Therapy Association (AOTA) encourages occupational therapy practitioners to complete an occupational profile, "a summary of a client's occupational history and experiences, patterns of daily living, interests, values, and needs" (AOTA, 2014, p. S13), for each client. An occupational profile is a requirement of the *CPT*® occupational therapy evaluation codes as of January 1, 2017.

American Occupational Therapy Association. (2017). AOTA occupational profile template. *American Journal of Occupational Therapy, 71*(Suppl. 2), 7112420030. https://doi.org/10.5014/ajot.2017.716S12

According to the *Occupational Therapy Practie Framework: Domain and Process* (3rd ed.; American Occupational Therapy Association [AOTA], 2014), an *occupational profile* is "a summary of a client's occupational history and experiences, patterns of daily living, interests, values, and needs" (p. S13). The information is obtained from the client's perspective through both formal interview techniques and casual conversation and leads to an individualized, client-centered approach to intervention.

Each item in the template provided here should be addressed to complete the occupational profile. Page numbers on the form correspond to the description in the *Framework*. A fillable version of the form is available to AOTA members at https://www.aota.org/~/media/Corporate/Files/Practice/Manage/Documentation/AOTA-Occupational-Profile-Template.pdf. Note that the template is a suggested approach; any template that incorporates the elements indicated in the AOTA template is appropriate.

An occupational profile is a requirement of the *CPT*® occupational therapy evaluation codes as of January 1, 2017; see https://www.aota.org/profile for more information on using the Occupational Profile Template in documentation. For more information on coding, visit http://www.aota.org/coding. ▲

References

American Occupational Therapy Association. (2014). Occupational therapy practice framework: Domain and process (3rd ed.). *American Journal of Occupational Therapy, 68*(Suppl. 1), S1–S48. https://doi.org/10.5014/ajot.2014.682006

American Medical Association. (2016). *Current procedural terminology: CPT*® *2017 professional edition.* Chicago: Author.

AOTA OCCUPATIONAL PROFILE TEMPLATE

"The occupational profile is a summary of a client's occupational history and experiences, patterns of daily living, interests, values, and needs" (AOTA, 2014, p. S13). The information is obtained from the client's perspective through both formal interview techniques and casual conversation and leads to an individualized, client-centered approach to intervention.

Each item below should be addressed to complete the occupational profile. Page numbers are provided to reference a description in the Occupational Therapy Practice Framework: Domain and Process, 3rd Edition (AOTA, 2014).

Client Report	**Reason the client is seeking service and concerns related to engagement in occupations**	Why is the client seeking service, and what are the client's current concerns relative to engaging in occupations and in daily life activities? (This may include the client's general health status.)
	Occupations in which the client is successful (p. S5)	In what occupations does the client feel successful, and what barriers are affecting his or her success?
	Personal interests and values (p. S7)	What are the client's values and interests?
	Occupational history (i.e., life experiences)	What is the client's occupational history (i.e., life experiences)?
	Performance patterns (routines, roles, habits, & rituals) (p. S8)	What are the client's patterns of engagement in occupations, and how have they changed over time? What are the client's daily life roles? (Patterns can support or hinder occupational performance.)

What aspects of the client's environments or contexts does he or she see as:

	Supports to Occupational Engagement	**Barriers to Occupational Engagement**
Environment	**Physical (p. S28)** (e.g., buildings, furniture, pets)	
	Social (p. S28) (e.g., spouse, friends, caregivers)	
Context	**Cultural (p. S28)** (e.g., customs, beliefs)	
	Personal (p. S28) (e.g., age, gender, SES, education)	
	Temporal (p. S28) (e.g., stage of life, time, year)	
	Virtual (p. S28) (e.g., chat, email, remote monitoring)	
Client Goals	**Client's priorities and desired targeted outcomes: (p. S34)**	Consider: occupational performance—improvement and enhancement, prevention, participation, role competence, health and wellness, quality of life, well-being, and/or occupational justice.

ADDITIONAL RESOURCES

For a complete description of each component and examples of each, refer to the *Occupational Therapy Practice Framework: Domain and Process, 3rd Edition.*

American Occupational Therapy Association. (2014). Occupational therapy practice framework: Domain and process (3rd ed.). *American Journal of Occupational Therapy, 68* S1–S48. https://doi.org/10.5014/ajot.2014.682006

The occupational profile is a requirement of the *CPT®* occupational therapy evaluation codes as of January 1, 2017. For more information visit www.aota.org/coding.

Index

Note. Page numbers in *italic* indicate exhibits, figures, and tables.